Supportive Care
for the Person
with Dementia

Supportive Care Series

Volumes in the series

Surgical Palliative Care
G.P. Dunn and A.J. Johnson

Supportive Care in Respiratory Disease
S.H. Ahmedzai and M. Muers

Supportive Care for the Renal Patient
E. Joanna Chambers, M. Germain, and E. Brown

Supportive Care for the Urology Patient
R.W. Norman and D. Currow

Supportive Care in Heart Failure
J. Beattie and S. Goodlin

Supportive Care for the Person with Dementia
J.C. Hughes, M. Lloyd-Williams, and G.A. Sachs

Supportive Care for the Person with Dementia

Edited by

Julian C. Hughes

Consultant in Old Age Psychiatry
and Honorary Professor of Philosophy of Ageing
North Tyneside General Hospital
Northumbria Healthcare NHS Foundation Trust
and Institute for Ageing and Health
Newcastle University, UK

Mari Lloyd-Williams

Professor and Director of Academic Palliative and Supportive Care
Studies Group (APSCSG)
School of Population, Community and Behavioural Sciences
University of Liverpool
Liverpool, UK

Greg A. Sachs

Professor of Medicine and Chief
Division of General Internal Medicine and Geriatrics
Indiana University School of Medicine
Investigator, IU Center for Aging Research
Regenstrief Institute, Inc.
Indianapolis, USA

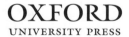

OXFORD
UNIVERSITY PRESS

OXFORD

UNIVERSITY PRESS

Great Clarendon Street, Oxford OX2 6DP

Oxford University Press is a department of the University of Oxford.
It furthers the University's objective of excellence in research, scholarship,
and education by publishing worldwide in

Oxford New York

Auckland Cape Town Dar es Salaam Hong Kong Karachi
Kuala Lumpur Madrid Melbourne Mexico City Nairobi
New Delhi Shanghai Taipei Toronto

With offices in

Argentina Austria Brazil Chile Czech Republic France Greece
Guatemala Hungary Italy Japan Poland Portugal Singapore
South Korea Switzerland Thailand Turkey Ukraine Vietnam

Oxford is a registered trade mark of Oxford University Press
in the UK and in certain other countries

Published in the United States
by Oxford University Press Inc., New York

© Oxford University Press, 2010

The moral rights of the author have been asserted
Database right Oxford University Press (maker)

First published 2010

British Library Cataloguing in Publication Data

Data available

Library of Congress Cataloging in Publication Data

Data available

Typeset in Minion by Glyph International, Bangalore, India
Printed in Great Britain
on acid-free paper by the MPG Books Group, Bodmin and King's Lynn

ISBN 978–0–19–955413–3

10 9 8 7 6 5 4 3 2 1

Oxford University Press makes no representation, express or implied, that the drug dosages in this book are
correct. Readers must therefore always check the product information and clinical procedures with the most
up-to-date published product information and data sheets provided by the manufacturers and the most recent
codes of conduct and safety regulations. The authors and the publishers do not accept responsibility or legal
liability for any errors in the text or for the misuse or misapplication of material in this work. Except where
otherwise stated, drug dosages and recommendations are for the non-pregnant adult who is not breastfeeding.

This book is dedicated to our patients and their families,
to all who work with us to provide them with care,
and to our own families for their continuing
love and support.

Preface to the supportive care series

Supportive care is the multi-disciplinary holistic care of patients with chronic and life-limiting illnesses and their families—from the time around diagnosis, through treatments aimed at cure or prolonging life, and into the phase currently acknowledged as palliative care. It involves recognizing and caring for the side effects of active therapies as well as patients' symptoms, comorbidities, psychological, social, and spiritual concerns. It also values the role of family carers and helps them in supporting the patient as well as attending to their own special needs. Supportive care is a domain of health and social care that utilizes a network of professionals and voluntary carers in a 'virtual team'. It is increasingly recognized by health care providers and governments as a modern response to complex disease management, but so far it can lay claim to little dedicated literature.

This is, therefore, one volume in a unique new series of textbooks on supportive care, published by Oxford University Press which has already established itself as a leading publisher for palliative care. Unlike 'traditional' palliative care, which grew from the terminal care of cancer patients, supportive care is restricted neither to dying patients nor to cancer. Thus, this series covers the support of patients with a variety of long-term conditions, who are currently largely managed by specialist and general teams in hospitals and by primary care teams in community settings. It will, therefore, provide a practical guide not only to supportive care of the patient at all stages of the illness, providing up-to-date knowledge of the scientific basis of palliation but practical guidance on delivering high quality multi-disciplinary care across health care sectors also. The volumes, edited by acknowledged leaders in the specific field of each volume, will bring together research, health care management, economics, and ethics through contributions from an international panel of experts of all disciplines. The underlying theme of the entire book is the application of the latest evidence-based knowledge, in a humane way, for patients with advancing stage of the disease.

As Series Editors, we hope to bring forth over four decades of research and clinical experience of acute medicine and palliative care. Our work has spanned St Christopher's Hospice and the Leicestershire Hospice in England—both of which have been inspirational leaders of traditional palliative care—together with the Academic Unit of Supportive Care at the University of Sheffield, England and the Harry Horvitz Center for Palliative Medicine in The Cleveland Clinic Foundation, USA. We have independently and jointly advocated the supportive care approach to cancer and other chronic disease management and are delighted to be collaborating in this series. Both of us are committed to delivering high quality of end-of-life care when it is necessary, but we are constantly seeking to influence our colleagues in all relevant health care disciplines to adopt the principles of modern supportive care to benefit a wider range of patients at earlier stages of illness. We aim, through this series, to inform and inspire other doctors, nurses, allied health professionals, pharmacists, social and spiritual care providers, and students, to improve the quality of living of all the patients and families in their care.

Sam Hjelmeland Ahmedzai
Professor of Palliative Medicine
Academic Unit of Supportive Care
The University of Sheffield
Royal Hallamshire Hospital
Sheffield, UK

Preface

We have no hesitation in recommending the model of supportive care for people with dementia and their carers for at least five reasons. First, its roots are strongly embedded in the fertile ground of palliative care, which we believe to be (as do many of the authors in this book) an appropriate grounding for the care of people with dementia. Secondly, supportive care is compatible with person-centred care, which has informed so much thinking about dementia and *people* with dementia over the past 20 years. Thirdly, supportive care is never nihilistic, and it also relieves some of the tensions that underlie other models of care: *of course* we need to encourage enthusiasm for better psychosocial approaches to people with dementia; *of course* we should pursue biomedical treatment with a good deal of vigour. For both approaches (as a package, not separately) are likely to make people's lives better. Fourthly, the supportive care model takes individuality seriously, recognizing that the care pathway for any particular person will be unique. Finally, supportive care does not sidestep the practical issue of implementation, but it allows that the logistics will be different in different places.

We could continue. Supportive care has much to commend it; but it is not a neat and tidy model waiting to be unpacked. And perhaps, this is another reason it seems so applicable to dementia care because dementia is not one thing, nor are the people who live with it. The contributors to this book amply demonstrate the length and breadth of dementia care, of what is required, and of the ways in which a supportive care model can help. For this reason, we are enormously grateful to them for their contributions and valuable work. They have put up with our cajoling with apparent good humour. Given their diverse backgrounds, we hope this book will be of interest to a range of professionals and others involved in the care of people with dementia. Readers may wish to focus on particular chapters, but we hope that the overall development of the theme of supportive care is conspicuous too.

It would certainly not be the book that it is without the initial encouragement of Sam Ahmedzai, co-editor for this OUP series. In addition, we have benefited enormously from the calm help of various OUP staff: Helen Hill, Eloise Moir-Ford, Georgia Pinteau, Nicola Ulyatt, and Jenny Wright. We are grateful to Priya Devaraj from CEPHA Imaging for her help with the production process, to Anne Hughes for contributing to proof reading, and to Agnes Muse and Lindsay Turner for secretarial support. To all of them we wish to express our sincere thanks, for this could not have been achieved without them. Beyond this book, however, our genuine concern is that the care of the person with dementia should improve, which is the intention of all who have written in these pages.

Julian C. Hughes
Mari Lloyd-Williams
Greg A. Sachs

Contents

List of contributors

Dag Aarsland is a professor of geriatric medicine at the University of Bergen and currently working as a professor of old age psychiatry at King's College London.

Kate Allan is a clinical psychologist, and previously worked at the Dementia Services Development Centre, University of Stirling, Scotland, exploring ways of enhancing communication between care staff and people with dementia.

Clive Baldwin is a senior lecturer in the Bradford Dementia Group, and holds a faculty position in the Department of Social Work, University of Bradford, UK.

Clive Ballard is professor of age-related diseases at King's College London, and the Institute of Psychiatry and director of research for the Alzheimer's Society, UK.

Bob Barber is consultant and honorary clinical senior lecturer in old age psychiatry in Northumberland, Tyne and Wear NHS Trust and the Institute for Ageing and Health, Newcastle University, UK. He leads for younger people with dementia.

Belinda Bilney is a senior physiotherapist and project manager at Ballarat Health Services in Victoria, Australia. Her research is in the management of people with Huntington's disease.

Mary Ann Cohen is clinical professor of psychiatry, Mount Sinai School of Medicine, USA, and performs psychodynamic psychotherapy privately. Her interests are psychosomatic medicine, AIDS, ethics, geriatrics, and addiction.

Helen Cooper, married, having three sons, worked as a GP in Newcastle upon Tyne until retirement, when she cared for her husband, who was a physician/geriatrician before he developed dementia.

Monica Crugel is specialist registrar in old age psychiatry. She completed her basic medical and speciality training in Bucharest (Romania) and has been working with Greenwich Older People's Services since 2005.

Wim Dekkers is an associate professor of philosophy of medicine and a senior researcher in the Radboud University Nijmegen Medical Centre in the Netherlands. He is trained in both medicine and philosophy.

Murna Downs is a professor of dementia studies and head of the Bradford Dementia Group, University of Bradford, UK, with interests in quality of life for people with dementia and their families.

Gillie Evans is a part-time principal in general practice at the Jenner Health Centre near Peterborough, UK. She is a founder member of a multidisciplinary Palliative Care in Dementia Group.

Jacquelyn Frank is assistant professor in Eastern Illinois University, USA, with an interest in the different needs of adult child and spouse caregivers of people with dementia.

Katherine Froggatt, based at the International Observatory on End of Life Care, Lancaster University, UK, co-leads research concerning older adults in supportive and palliative care.

Muriel Gillick is a geriatrician and palliative care specialist with Harvard Vanguard Medical Associates and a Clinical Professor in the Department of Ambulatory Care and Prevention, Harvard Medical School, USA.

Philip Hardman is professional and clinical lead for nursing within older adult services, Manchester Mental Health and Social Care Trust. He is also a part-time lecturer at Manchester University, UK.

Cees Hertogh is professor in geriatric ethics at the EMGO Institute for Health and Care Research of the VU University Medical Center Amsterdam, the Netherlands.

Julian Hughes is consultant in old age psychiatry and honorary professor of philosophy of ageing in Northumbria Healthcare NHS Trust and the Institute for Ageing and Health, Newcaslte University, UK.

David Jolley is a consultant in old age psychiatry in Tameside, and honorary reader at Manchester University in the Personal Social Services Research Unit, UK.

Alice Jordan is a specialist registrar in palliative medicine based in Newcastle upon Tyne. Her successful MD thesis through the Institute for Ageing and Health, Newcastle University, was entitled 'The assessment of good practice in pain management in severe dementia'.

John Keady is a professor of older people's mental health nursing, an appointment between the School of Nursing, Midwifery and Social Work, Manchester University, and GMW Mental Health NHS Foundation Trust, UK.

John Killick is a writer in residence for Alzheimer Scotland. A similar previous post involved working with persons with dementia. He was a research fellow at the University of Stirling.

Mari Lloyd-Williams is a professor of palliative and supportive care at the University of Liverpool, UK, and an honorary consultant in palliative medicine at the Royal Liverpool University Hospital and Marie Curie Hospice.

Jill Manthorpe, professor of social work at King's College London, UK, is director of the Social Care Workforce Research Unit with a background in the voluntary sector and higher education.

Meg Morris is professor and head of the School of Physiotherapy at The University of Melbourne, Australia. Her interests lie in Parkinson's disease, progressive neurological disorders, stroke, and gait disorders.

Deborah Parker is associate professor, acting director of the UQ/Blue Care Research and Practice Development Centre and acting director of the Australian Centre for Evidence Based Community Care in Australia.

Barbara Pointon lectured in music before taking early retirement to care for her husband, Malcolm, for 16 years and now campaigns internationally on behalf of people with dementia and their carers.

Louise Robinson, a GP and professor of primary care and ageing, Newcastle University, UK, is National Champion for Ageing and Older People in the Royal College of General Practitioners.

Steven Sabat, professor of psychology at Georgetown University, Washington, D.C., studies the intact cognitive and social abilities and subjective experiences of people with moderate to severe dementia.

Greg Sachs, professor of medicine at Indiana University, USA, and investigator in the IU Center for Aging Research of the Regenstrief Institute, is a geriatrician with interests in dementia, ethics, and palliative care.

Liz Sampson is an old age psychiatrist and senior lecturer in psychiatric and supportive care of the elderly at the Marie Curie Palliative Care Research Unit, University College London, UK.

Stephen Sapp is professor and chair of religious studies at the University of Miami, USA. His interests include ethical issues in dementia and the role of religion and spirituality in ageing.

Charles Schwartz is an internist and psychiatrist, educator, and associate professor at the Albert Einstein College of Medicine, USA. His interests are medicine, psychosomatic medicine, palliative medicine, bioethics, addiction and AIDS.

Sivaraman Shaji is chief psychiatrist at Bethsada Hospital, Perumbavoor, Kerala, India. He has been working as a research consultant to Alzheimer's and Related Disorders Society of India (ARDSI) since 1992.

Joseph Shega is a geriatrician and hospice and palliative care physician at the University of Chicago, USA. He specializes in the management of physical and psychological symptoms in persons with dementia.

Joyce Simard is a geriatric consultant based in Land O Lakes, Florida, USA, and in Prague in the Czech Republic. She specializes in developing activity programmes for people in all stages of Alzheimer's disease.

Philip Sloane is the Elizabeth and Oscar Goodwin Distinguished Professor of Family Medicine at the University of North Carolina at Chapel Hill, USA. He works in geriatric medicine and dementia care.

Graham Stokes is a consultant clinical psychologist and head of mental health at BUPA Care Services, UK. He specializes in person-centred care and the resolution of challenging behaviour in dementia.

Adrian Treloar is consultant and senior lecturer in old age psychiatry in London, UK. He developed a service specifically to help people with dementia to live at home until they die.

Ladislav Volicer is courtesy full professor in the University of South Florida, USA, and visiting professor at Charles University in Prague. He established one of the first Dementia Special Care Units.

Daphne Wallace is a retired psychiatrist (and psychotherapist) for older people. She chaired the Dementia Group of the Christian Council on Ageing and was a trustee of the Alzheimer's Society, UK.

Karen Watchman is a research fellow at the Centre for Research on Families and Relationships, University of Edinburgh, specializing in learning disability and dementia. She was the director of Down's Syndrome Scotland.

Heather Wilkinson is a co-director of the Centre for Research on Families and Relationships and the research director for the School of Health in Social Science, the University of Edinburgh, Scotland.

Sheryl Zimmerman is professor and director of aging research, School of Social Work, and co-director, program on aging, Sheps Center for Health Services Research, University of North Carolina, USA.

Chapter 1

Characterizing care

Julian C. Hughes, Mari Lloyd-Williams, and Greg A. Sachs

Introduction

This book is about practice: the practice of care for people with dementia. Initially, however, the most important thing is to get the concept right. In this chapter, therefore, we shall consider the conceptual problem. We shall try to reach a conceptual conclusion, but it might be that the real answer lies in the practical working out supplied by the rest of the book.

The conceptual problem: how do we characterize the care that is due to people with dementia in such a way as to capture all its possible, desirable, and necessary aspects? It is not immediately clear whether any characterization of care could be a sufficient response. To unpack the problem, we shall start by outlining some candidate answers and the difficulties associated with them, which will lead us to our favoured solution. To anticipate, we shall argue that the biomedical view is not psychosocial enough, and that the psychosocial approach is not biomedical enough. Palliative care, with its overtly biopsychosocial and spiritual approach, might seem to be a favourable candidate. As we shall see, however, even palliative care is not an unproblematic notion for dementia.

One thing that we do not intend to provide in this chapter is an analysis of the notion of 'care' itself. This would be a complex task, requiring attention to the ethics of care, the nature of the related virtue of compassion, the phenomenology of caring, the meaning of 'care', and so forth. It would also be an analysis which would be applicable to all conditions requiring care. No, our focus is on the way in which we characterize 'care' with respect to dementia.

Possible characterizations of care

Typical dementia care: a biomedical approach

To say that there is, in any strict sense, a biomedical approach to dementia care is probably a parody of most dementia care services. Talk of a biomedical model is often intended critically. Whilst there undoubtedly is a narrow biomedical model which encourages our understanding of dementia in terms of neuropathology (no bad thing in itself), it is very difficult to conceive how anyone offering *services* could avoid the plethora of psychosocial and ethical issues that arise, not only for people with dementia, but also for their carers.

Nevertheless, there is a narrow approach to dementia care that emphasizes illness, positions people with dementia *and their carers* as patients, and encourages 'a process of diagnostic overshadowing where all actions and expressions are attributed to the labelled condition' [1]. However one wishes to temper it, there is no denying that a biomedical model permeates dementia care. Although medical services providing dementia care will typically either refer or facilitate referral to social services, the emphasis is usually on *diagnosis* and the possibility of *treatment*, especially the prescribing of medications, with follow-up to allow monitoring of progress. In many such services (for reasons outlined later), once matters relating to diagnosis and treatment have been settled, patients can be discharged in the knowledge that they have an appropriate care package, which might involve home care, day care, and other social inputs that help to maintain the person in the community. In both the United States (US) and the United Kingdom (UK), it is broadly true that services for people with dementia either become available once patients and families have received a medical evaluation and diagnosis, or social services are uneasy at being involved unless there is or has been some sort of medical assessment. Our point is not that it is *bad* for people to receive both medical and social care. Rather, we note the primacy of the biomedical input, but the reality is that most of the care will be social. Healthcare services for people with dementia can be highly effective and hugely appreciated by stressed family carers. We shall, however, focus on two points of concern specific to the biomedical model.

First, in this model, undoubtedly for complicated sociocultural and economic reasons, despite lip-service to the importance of psychosocial approaches, it often seems that the only real alternative *is pharmacological*. This is most obvious in connection with behaviour that challenges. The consequence is frequently seen in terms of adverse reactions to the drugs used, growing evidence of higher mortality rates with the use of anti-psychotic drugs, and serious questions about their efficacy in this patient population. Secondly, inasmuch as care is centred on diagnosis and treatment, this model of care often involves patients *being discharged*. Hence, patients are often discharged for follow-up in the community by social work teams, which themselves (in the UK context) will often contract out the 'care' to private agencies. In the US, patients typically will be at risk of receiving services in a 'hit or miss' fashion since, unless they are enrolled in managed care or have the fortune to be referred to the Alzheimer's Association or similar agency, any source of comprehensive and coordinated access to services is unlikely. This tends to be the case even as patients receive ongoing care from an internist or other primary care physician.

Clinical services in the UK sometimes discharge people to long-term care, where the level of medical input will be variable. Patients on cholinesterase inhibitors (anti-dementia drugs) will be followed up, but current UK guidelines entail that at some stage the medication is stopped; subsequently, patients can be discharged. In the US, there is currently neither any parallel with respect to discharging patients with dementia from specialty care, nor are there guidelines for the discontinuation of anti-dementia drugs in more advanced stages of Alzheimer's disease (AD). However, it is still true that most cases of dementia are not even diagnosed, and when diagnosed, there is little coordination of care with other kinds of services – despite the ready access to any number of specialists. In the UK, meanwhile, people who suffer from vascular dementia, for whom the drugs are not indicated, need not be followed up by medical services at all, because once the diagnosis is made, given that there is no active treatment, there is 'nothing else medically to be done'.

In the US, in the absence of a National Health Service, there is a greater tendency for physicians to go ahead and prescribe medications for 'off label' purposes, such as anti-cholinesterase drugs in vascular and other types of dementia beyond AD. Nonetheless, despite perhaps an even greater employment of the biomedical model in dementia, there still appears to be a similar distancing of, or seemingly diminished interest from, physicians for patients in the later stages of dementia as the illness progresses with or without medications.

The effect of such discharge policies or distancing is that, when people with dementia die they are often *not* in touch with services that specialize in dementia care. Perhaps they do not need to be; but if this is true, it must be predicated on the view that the person's dementia no longer warrants specialist biomedical 'dementia' input. And this is a contentious viewpoint. If this view were true, it would indicate that the biomedical approach to dementia is relatively circumscribed, involving only the early part of the disease. But it is false and, hence, it is an indictment of specialist services if they are not involved at the end of a person's life.

Person-centred dementia care: taking the psychosocial view

The notion of person-centredness is the bedrock of the new culture of dementia care promoted by Kitwood [2] and discussed by Downs in Chapter 25 of the present volume. Brooker [3] recently summarized this, stressing the importance of valuing the individual and the need to take the psychological and social life of the person seriously. Rather than focussing on the neuropathology of the person, he or she is regarded as a locus of meaning [4], able to communicate a unique perspective [5], and any attempts to position the person, on account of his or her dementia, in an unfavourable light is regarded as malignant. Sabat [6] further pursues these ideas in Chapter 24.

The advocates of person-centred care are currently still in the business of offering a much needed corrective to the perceived over-medicalization of dementia. As such, they play down (to some extent) the biology of dementia. Whatever the uncertainties, however, there is a pathological basis to dementia that does respond to drug treatment. Moreover, there are effective drug treatments for the symptoms and signs that arise in the course of dementia (see Chapter 12), even if the counsel of perfection is to try psychosocial approaches first (as described in Chapter 17) [7]. Furthermore, in the severe stages of dementia, there is a variety of physical symptoms that need to be attended to, which result directly or indirectly from the advancing pathology [8]. Even if the correct psychosocial approach might alleviate or prevent unnecessary morbidity, the *changing biology of* the dementias needs to be taken into consideration.

Although each individual's dementia will be different, science offers potential ways to understand these differences, e.g. the individual genetically determined differences in terms of people's susceptibility to AD. Similarly, the dementias themselves are biologically different, and it might be that there will be a variety of ways in which to modify the progression of different dementias. There is, therefore, plenty for biomedicine to say about the dementias.

Moreover, at the heart of the person-centred approach is the notion of personhood itself. If this is characterized by saying that the person is a situated embodied agent [9], then it follows that, in addition to it being important that biomedicine does not overlook the imperative of the person's situated agency (with all that this entails from the psychosocial point of view), it is at least as important that person-centredness should not ignore the full implications suggested by the person's being embodied. Physical concerns should remain at the heart of good dementia care.

In this section, which is supposed to be about person-centred care, it may seem that we have been less than generous to those who advocate the undoubted benefits of psychosocial approaches. It can be argued with some justification that to ignore the broader issues that face people with dementia and their carers and to concentrate solely on the notion of a biomedical fix is detrimental to the person's care. It may have a tendency – by its emphasis on the *deficits* of the *patient* – to undercut the very personhood of people with dementia that it should be intended to maintain. Taking a balanced view, therefore, *fully* recognizing what being a person entails, is a way to avoid throwing out the baby with the bathwater. This applies whether one's bathwater is the biomedical or the psychosocial approach!

Palliative dementia care: a new approach!

Whilst the person-centred, psychosocial approach is a necessary corrective to the reductive tendencies of biomedicine, it may be that the immediate appeal of the palliative approach as a potential model of care lies precisely in its holism.

> Palliative care is an approach that improves the quality of life of patients and their families facing the problems associated with life-threatening illness, through the prevention and relief of suffering by means of early identification and impeccable assessment and treatment of pain and other problems, physical, psychosocial, and spiritual [10].

This definition of the palliative care approach immediately makes it plain that a broad view has to be taken. The recognition that dementia is a 'life-threatening illness' has led to a growing interest in the possibility of adopting this model for dementia care [11]. The benefits of the approach are that it can focus attention on aspects of care that are sometimes neglected, such as pain (see also Chapter 14) and breathlessness [12, 13]. As recorded in Chapter 31 of this volume, the need for better end-of-life care has been recognized and researched in the US for many years [14], though barriers to the provision of good quality terminal care for people with dementia continue to be exist there [15].

But the model also suggests the possibility that dementia care should be regarded as a palliative approach right from the moment of diagnosis. Attempts to put this into effect (see for example Chapter 5) are already providing some room for optimism [16]. A key ingredient in this approach is that there should be effective advance care planning, to which, in the present volume, we have devoted two chapters (Chapters 28 and 29 and see [17]). So there is much to commend the palliative care approach. Indeed, direct comparisons have been made between the palliative care approach and Kitwood's person-centred care [18, 19]. It could be considered an advantage that the palliative approach does not need to play down the importance of physical care: holism automatically involves the amelioration of symptoms by physical, psychosocial, and spiritual means; neither does this approach ignore the person's carers; nor does it seem irrelevant even in the last moments of the person's life. Does this provide, however, the answer to the question about how to characterize the care that is due to people with dementia?

An analysis of the problem

We have argued so far that the biomedical view is not psychosocial enough and that the psychosocial approach is not biomedical enough. The advantage of palliative care is precisely that it is an overtly biopsychosocial and spiritual approach. It is not, however, unproblematic. First, there is the lurking distinction between cure and palliation. Secondly, there is the need to add longitudinal depth and variety to palliative care's sense of holism. The characterization of care that we are seeking needs to face these problems.

Cure or care

In the early days of the hospice movement, the dichotomy between curative and non-curative care played a useful role. Many of us have witnessed what we have regarded as an inappropriate application of a model of care that aimed solely at cure when what was required was an acceptance of the reality that cure was no longer going to be possible. It becomes apparent for many patients at some stage that what they really need is good quality palliative care. A failure to see this or to understand how to provide such care was the impetus behind the hospice movement.

Even if the dichotomy between cure and non-cure was once appropriate, Ahmedzai has shown convincingly how changes in medical practice have made such a distinction less relevant [20]. For instance, he argues that 'in many areas of medicine the best palliation may well be achieved through measures which are in fact designed to cure or prolong life' [20]. An antipathy towards the dichotomy is also sensed in Hertogh writing about nursing homes and rehabilitation:

> This is not care medicine . . . nor is it cure medicine. In fact such dichotomies as *cure* versus *care* and *curative* versus *palliative* no longer hold true here. . . [21].

Ahmedzai also demonstrates the extent to which there is a tension between the rhetoric of palliative care that makes it plain that it derives from cancer care, where the reality was (and often is) that palliative care aims at end-of-life issues, and the rhetoric that proclaims palliative care should be extended to other non-cancer conditions, where the reality is that many (if not most) palliative issues arise a long time before the terminal phases of the condition.

The palliative care movement might reply that actually it has been careful to make distinctions between levels of palliative intervention: *specialist palliative care* might in many instances only be required at the end-of-life (however defined), but the *palliative care approach* is applicable to all long-term, progressive, and non-curable conditions. Whilst this acknowledges and deals with the conceptual problem at one level (ignoring the tendency to encourage the cure–care dichotomy), at another level, it calls into question the distinctive essence of palliative care: is not the palliative care approach in connection with dementia no more than good quality person-centred dementia care? What is it that is distinctive about palliative care over the whole course of a chronic disorder? Once it moves away from its roots in caring for the dying, 'palliative care' can start to seem like (albeit laudable) flag-waving.

There are several points to make against this line of reasoning. First, there will continue to be a need for expertise in dealing with the end of life – expertise that is difficult for the specialist in a particular condition to acquire. The second response is only partly true: perhaps there is something that does define palliative care across the course of a chronic illness. Perhaps it is the idea that palliative care is not 'aggressive'. This makes some intuitive sense in that palliative care is likely to stress 'being with' patients as much or more than 'doing to' them. But Reiter and Chambers have argued: first, that the notion of 'aggressive care' is better thought of as 'restorative care'; secondly, that both restorative and palliative care can be 'aggressive'; and thirdly, that notions of care can be subsumed by the broader view of 'supportive care' [22]. More broadly, the palliative care approach (when it works properly) is different with its attention to physical, psychological, social, and spiritual needs and, very importantly, the needs of the family too. It may be that there is something intangible here because – contrary to the suggestion we made above – clinical experience too frequently reveals that even 'good quality' dementia care falls short of the sort of holism that is the essence of palliative care.

It is worth commenting that, although it may seem premature even to suggest that there is such a thing as 'cure' in dementia, there are some types of dementia that can receive 'curative' treatment (e.g. normal pressure hydrocephalus) and it may, in any case, be that curative efforts (i.e. using means that aim at 'curing' some of the pathology) will be good forms of palliative care. Acetylcholinesterase inhibitors might be thought of in this light, and newer treatments might add to the effect.

A final, but not inconsequential, point in connection with the cure-care dichotomy is that it is associated with a model of care in which at some point curative effort is stopped and palliation starts. As Ahmedzai comments,

> This may be efficient and convenient for the services, but it leads to discontinuity from the point of view of the recipients [20].

A consequence might be, in the field of cancer care, that the person experiences a sense of abandonment and hopelessness. Inevitably, because of its associations with the end of life, the offer of palliative care might inspire mostly doom. Indeed, because of these associations it seems quite difficult to start talking in terms of palliative care at the time of diagnosis to people with dementia, who might be ten years away from death and still some years from any significant interruption to their present way of life, especially if pre-dementia diagnoses, such as 'mild cognitive impairment' [23] become routine.

Multidimensional holism and variety

These considerations lead to the second problematic area for palliative care, to do with the length and depth of dementia. First, palliative care needs to deal with the longitudinal nature of many non-curable, chronic conditions. Secondly, it needs to recognize the implications of dementia not being a single diagnostic entity. The first point means that at various times in the trajectory of an illness for a particular person, the main focus might well be on an area of expertise far removed from the knowledge and skills of those who offer palliative care. They might yet argue, as we have noted, that the holism of the palliative care approach should still apply. But notwithstanding the depth implied by the characterization of the person as a biopsychosocial and spiritual being, at any particular point it might be that the focus of concern for some time is purely biomedical, without any detriment to the person. Huntington's disease (discussed in Chapter 7) makes this point clear, as would Parkinson's disease. In both, the rehabilitative care and the medication management in these diseases, respectively, is not typically what a palliative care specialist will know well. Similarly, simple routine follow-up for someone on a cholinesterase inhibitor might suffice for a while. To call this palliative care is accurate, but perhaps unnecessary. Occam's razor might suggest that the concept 'palliative' adds nothing; certainly nothing more than might be added by the adjective 'clinical.'

Palliative care might be thought of as an appropriate approach at particular moments, but it does not seem to be a useful way to characterize the longer term commitment to the different types of care that might be needed. Bearing in mind the second point about the variety of conditions that can lead to dementia, if we are to characterize the care that is due to people with dementia in such a way as to capture all its possible, desirable and necessary aspects, we shall need to discuss investigations that might (rarely) lead to curative treatments (if, say, normal pressure hydrocephalus were picked up at an early stage; or if cognitive impairment turned out to result from a treatable brain tumour; or if primary prevention were able to eradicate HIV dementia (concerning which see Chapter 8)). The notion of palliative care would need to expand to accommodate prevention, direct treatment of pathophysiology, rehabilitation, and even cure or 'restorative care'. Expanding the concept of palliative care in this way cannot be prohibited, but it seems to be stretching a point. No doubt palliative care can have an impact throughout the course of dementia, but perhaps it should be seen as just one component – of tremendous importance – in an approach that, at best, should include a good deal of flexibility and, over time, might include attempts to prevent the underlying pathological processes (e.g. by treating cardiovascular risk factors), to cure the condition (e.g. by inserting shunts for hydrocephalus), to rehabilitate (e.g. following an in-patient stay for delirium), and so on. A broader characterization of the type of care required is, arguably, to call it supportive care.

Supportive care in dementia

The notion of supportive care provides a framework with the potential to include a biomedical approach, psychosocial and spiritual holism, along with the broader concerns (e.g. for the family and their bereavement) of palliative care. Having highlighted reasons for not wishing to call everything palliative care, it is important to stress that the insights of palliative care do indeed remain potent throughout the course of dementia, albeit alternative characterizations might seem apposite from time to time. Palliative care remains the thread that runs through the supportive care approach. Hence,

> . . . it has been argued that palliative care, as a component of comprehensive supportive care, can play a part at all stages of disease. In many cases, there is an overlap of curative and life-prolonging therapy, and then, a further overlap as life-maintaining priorities take over. At all stages there is a place for supportive care, defined as including palliative care but with a broader scope, including contributions from psychologists, rehabilitation, physiotherapy, occupational therapy, dietetics, complementary therapies as well as pain specialists, social workers, and chaplains [24].

Thus,

> If we use this approach, seeing palliative care as having a contribution – within a supportive care framework – even when curative or life-prolonging therapy is the first priority of clinicians, then

the contribution of palliative care to dementia care becomes more relevant throughout the illness [19].

The 'Sheffield model' of comprehensive supportive care [20, 24] makes a distinction between an explanatory model, which covers disease-directed, patient-directed, and family-directed therapies, and the logistical step, which considers how care is delivered to the patient and the family. The different directions of therapy outlined in the explanatory model are integrated within the logistical step of service provision. It may be that the exact components of the model need to be altered to match the circumstances of dementia care. But the overall aims of the model do seem to characterize the care that is due to people with dementia in such a way as – at least potentially – to capture all its possible, desirable, and necessary aspects.

For instance, as Ahmedzai recognizes:

> . . . supportive care needs may arise at any point in the disease trajectory: they certainly do not only surface when 'the disease is no longer curable.' Providing supportive care for patients' and families' needs at the earliest possible stage should be just as desirable as the current concentration on starting disease-directed therapies as early as possible [20].

The supportive care model allows that there will be a time for screening and investigations, some attempts (where possible) to cure the condition, efforts both to maintain and prolong life in accordance with the best interests of the person, but all the while a focus on the person, and on his or her family and close supporters, with attention to grief and bereavement. All of this activity should be supported, however, by multidisciplinary and interdisciplinary teams and continuity of care.

The aspiration here is no more than that there should be a complete mixture of biomedical dementia care, with good quality, person-centred, psychosocial, and spiritual care under the broad umbrella of holistic palliative care throughout the course of the person's experience of dementia. There remain numerous questions concerning how such care might be provided in practice, but the essential characterization of the care that is required is clear. There should be no dichotomies between which we should have to choose: no division between the need to cure and the need to care, no battle concerning whether the care is high or low tech, no tension between whether the care is biological or social, no concern over whether it is patient- or carer-centred, no debate about whether dementia care is mostly about 'being with' or 'doing to.' The supportive care model allows us to say that people with dementia deserve all of these approaches whenever and wherever they are applicable, from the time of diagnosis to the moment of death.

Conclusion

In this chapter, we have discussed the conceptual problems concerning how we can characterize the care that is due to people with dementia in such a way as to capture all its possible, desirable, and necessary aspects. We identified the problems lying behind the conceptual question as being to do with the dichotomies and divisions inherent in the different approaches to dementia care. Our conceptual conclusion has led us in the direction of supportive care. We believe this is a suitable way to characterize the nature of the care owing to people with dementia. Even at this preliminary stage, the supportive care model we envisage allows room for the full benefits of the palliative care approach and good quality end-of-life care to be harnessed, whilst still accommodating the biopsychosocial and spiritual dimensions of holistic care from the time of diagnosis.

We have not delved further into the logistics of how this care is to be provided. On our view, this will certainly involve a multidisciplinary and interdisciplinary team providing comprehensive and continuing (supportive) care. Nor have we examined in detail the content of such care. However, as we suggested at the start, it might be that the real answers lie in the practical working out of solutions to the difficulties that people with dementia and their carers are confronted with. In the chapters that follow we shall see how, in a great variety of ways, this might be achieved.

References

1. Downs M, Clare L, Mackenzie J (2006). Understandings of dementia: explanatory models and their implications for the person with dementia and therapeutic effort, in Hughes JC, Louw SJ, Sabat SR (eds) *Dementia: mind, meaning, and the person*, pp. 235–258. Oxford: Oxford University Press.
2. Kitwood T (1997). *Dementia reconsidered: the person comes first*. Buckingham and Philadelphia: Open University Press.
3. Brooker D (2004). What is person centred care? *Rev Clin Gerontol*, **13**, 215–222.
4. Sabat SR, Harré R (1994). The Alzheimer's disease sufferer as a semiotic subject. *Philos Psychiatry Psychol*, **1**, 145–160.
5. Sabat SR (2001). *The experience of Alzheimer's disease: life through a tangled veil*. Oxford: Blackwell.
6. Sabat SR (2006). Mind, meaning, and personhood in dementia: the effects of positioning, in Hughes JC, Louw SJ, Sabat SR (eds) *Dementia: mind, meaning, and the person*, pp. 287–302. Oxford: Oxford University Press.
7. Ballard C, O'Brien J, Swann A, James I (2001). *Treating behavioural and psychological symptoms of dementia*. Oxford: Oxford University Press.
8. Regnard C, Huntley ME (2006). Managing the physical symptoms of dying, in Hughes JC (ed) *Palliative care in severe dementia*, pp. 22–44. London: Quay Books.
9. Hughes JC (2001). Views of the person with dementia. *J Med Ethics*, **27**, 86–91.
10. World Health Organization (2002). *WHO definition of palliative care*. Available at: http://www.who.int/cancer/palliative/definition/en/. [accessed on 8th December 2006].
11. Hughes JC, Robinson L, Volicer L (2005). Specialist palliative care in dementia. *Br Med J*, **330**, 57–58.
12. Lloyd-Williams M (1996). An audit of palliative care in dementia. *Eur J Cancer Care*, **5**, 53–55.
13. Lloyd-Williams M, Payne S (2002). Can multidisciplinary guidelines improve the palliation of symptoms in the terminal phase of dementia? *Int J Palliat Nurs*, **8**, 370–375.
14. Volicer L, Hurley A (1998). *Hospice care for patients with advanced progressive dementia*. New York, NY: Springer Publishing Company.
15. Sachs GA, Shega JW, Cox-Hayley D (2004). Barriers to excellent end-of-life care for patients with dementia. *J Gen Int Med*, **19**, 1057–1063.
16. Shega JW, Levin A, Hougham GW *et al.* (2003). Palliative excellence in Alzheimer care efforts (PEACE): a program description. *J Palliat Med*, **6**, 315–320.
17. Hertogh CM (2006). Advance care planning and the relevance of a palliative care approach in dementia. *Age Ageing*, **35** (6), 553–555.
18. Hughes JC, Hedley K, Harris D (2006). The practice and philosophy of palliative care in dementia, in Hughes JC (ed) *Palliative care in severe dementia*, pp. 1–11. London: Quay Books.
19. Small N, Downs M, Froggatt K (2006). Improving end-of-life care for people with dementia – the benefits of combining UK approaches to palliative care and dementia care, in Miesen BML, Jones GMM (eds) *Care-giving in dementia – research and applications, volume 4*, pp. 365–392. London and New York: Routledge.
20. Ahmedzai SH (2005). The nature of palliation and its contribution to supportive care, in Ahmedzai SH, Muers MF (eds) *Supportive care in respiratory disease*, pp. 3–33. Oxford: Oxford University Press.
21. Hertogh CM (2006). Medical care for chronically ill elderly people: nursing home medicine as functional geriatrics, in Miesen BML, Jones GMM (eds) *Care-giving in dementia – research and applications, volume 4*, pp. 219–239. London and New York: Routledge.

22. Reiter GS, Chambers J (2004). The concept of supportive care for the renal patient, in Chambers EJ, Germain M, Brown E (eds) *Supportive care for the renal patient*, pp. 15–26. Oxford: Oxford University Press.

23. O'Brien J (2008). Mild cognitive impairment, in Jacoby R, Oppenheimer C, Dening T, Thomas A (eds) *Oxford textbook of old age psychiatry*, pp. 407–415. Oxford: Oxford University Press.

24. Ahmedzai S, Walsh D (2000). Palliative medicine and modern cancer care. *Semin Oncol*, **27**, 1–6.

Chapter 2

An introduction to the dementias: a clinical view

David Jolley

Introduction: fears and reality

'Dementia' as a word (Latin: *de* from, *mens* mind — out of one's mind) has not been welcomed within professional or lay vocabularies, but the condition it describes is currently brandished as a major public health threat, a world epidemic and personal, family, and economic plague which deserves recognition as a national priority [1]. Media interest has been attracted, always to the most gripping or heartrending of cases. Television soaps feature the condition as one way to fade out well-loved characters; celebrities share their personal or parental stories. Being recognized as old is not what most people desire. Being old and becoming witless, carrying a diagnosis of dementia and seen to be a burden to others is a nightmare. Popularizing the term 'dementia' comes from the best of intentions but carries risks.

It is understood that people change during their life course. Some aspects of intellect, memory and even personality become altered when people enter their seventh and subsequent decades free of brain pathology. Memory contains many experiences acquired over the years, and these remain important, often favoured reflections. Paul McCartney has mused on the feeling of a 'Memory Almost Full' [2]. Taking in new ideas becomes less easy and takes longer. Yet learning new tricks with reliance on fluid memory remains possible [3], if less proficient. Difficulty in remembering proper names embarrasses some of us through life, but comes to many others as an acquired but non-pathological feature of ageing.

Dementia is a clinical concept. It is characterized by loss of particular core abilities and is often complicated by the presence of additional abnormalities of mood, perception, and behaviour. The primary losses are still as described by Lishman: 'a syndrome characterized by acquired global impairment of intellect, memory, and personality without impairment of consciousness' [4]. These changes usually begin quietly and insidiously, becoming apparent only in retrospect after a period of months. They are noted most clearly by those closest to the individual, but usually not by the individuals, who often declare they are fine and are irritated by the reasonable concerns which others begin to express. In other instances onset may be sudden and symptoms fluctuating. There may be more awareness or insight, either of core cognitive difficulties or additional symptoms such as altered mood, sleep disturbance, intrusive illusions, or hallucinations.

Whilst dementia amongst individuals who are in their 80s or older can be wrongly attributed to age alone, it can occur in much younger people and may then be wrongly attributed to laziness, insolence, moodiness, or depression.

Symptoms of anxiety or depression may accompany loss of health, vigour, and abilities; or may arise in response to changes of circumstance: retirement from work, change of residence, or the impact of ill health or death amongst close relatives or friends. Such symptoms may lead to dulling of interest and reduced concentration and persistence in tasks. They may lead to ruminations that the brain, like the rest of the body, is failing.

Neither the normal changes of ageing nor the symptoms of depression constitute evidence of dementia. But they must be acknowledged and considered within the spectrum of differential diagnoses alongside symptomatic confusional states or delirium (where consciousness is clouded, symptoms appear more suddenly, and are more changeable), hearing impairment [5], learning disability, or other long-standing mental disorders.

The clinical syndrome of dementia may be symptomatic of an underlying body or brain disorder such as anaemia, vitamin deficiency, endocrine abnormality, or pressure from a tumour or other intracranial lesion. Sometimes it is due to chronic toxicity from a prescribed or self-administered medicine. Thus, assessment and investigation are essential once the possibility of dementia is being considered [6].

Pathological substrate

The common dementia illnesses are: Alzheimer's disease (AD), vascular dementia (VaD), dementia with Lewy bodies (DLB), and frontotemporal dementia (FTD) [7].

Alzheimer's disease

Many of the brain changes found in AD are similar to those seen at post-mortem in the brains of normal people who have survived into their eighties and beyond. In AD, these are more marked and more widespread [8]. The brain becomes shrunken; it weighs less and takes up less space. These changes were evident to Alois Alzheimer when investigating the brain of Auguste D more than a hundred years ago [9], as were characteristic intra-neuronal tangles and extra-neuronal plaques that stain with silver. Auguste D was a woman in her forties when she developed the degenerative disease which is now recognized as a world wide epidemic. Early Onset Alzheimer's was deemed an interesting but rare disorder, awful for the patient and their family, but of limited economic importance. It has become apparent, however, that these neuro-pathological characteristics are shared by the much more common degenerative disorder which was previously accepted as an inevitable consequence of living to a great age: 'senility' or 'senile dementia' has progressed to be re-designated 'Senile Dementia Alzheimer's Type' and lately simply Alzheimer's disease (of late onset). First changes occur in the cells of the hippocampus, which can be seen to be shrunken and atrophied, its cells cluttered with plaques and tangles. But the pathology spreads to include the cerebral cortex, particularly association areas of the parietal lobes. The cortex becomes thinned and the convolutions of the cerebral gyri more deeply ridged.

Argyrophillic plaques and tangles include amyloid deposits and the production of aberrant proteins, which form this amyloid, is implicated in the basic error that underpins many of the pathological changes. Careful clinico-pathological studies in the 1960s demonstrated a quantitative relationship between the severity of cognitive impairment in the last weeks of life and the number and concentration of argyropillic plaques identified at post mortem [10]. Advances in neuro-chemical techniques from the 1970s have demonstrated loss of neurotransmitters in AD, particularly acetylcholine, (leading to the 'cholinergic hypothesis'). Again there is a quantitative relationship between the severity of dementia in the last weeks of life and deficiency of acetylcholine found at post mortem [11]. There are changes in blood vessels in AD, and it seems probable that the absolute differentiation between AD and VaD which has become fashionable in recent decades will prove naïve. Certainly there is much greater willingness to accept the importance of a mixed (Alzheimer and vascular) aetiology.

Not surprisingly, given the complexity of the brain, as time has gone on the 'simple' cholinergic hypothesis has had to be adapted with the realization that numerous other neurotransmitters are implicated in AD, as in other forms of dementia [12]. Even the focus on plaques and tangles has been broadened as the significance of alternative pathological changes – e.g. the accumulation of hyperphosphorylated tau protein, β-amyloid deposits elsewhere than in plaques, or synaptic loss – have been noted [8].

Brain scanning techniques now allow the demonstration of structural and functional change within Alzheimer's and other dementias and contribute to their differential diagnosis [13]. Electro-encephalography (EEG) has never found a very great role in understanding Alzheimer's or the other dementias, but the technique can be useful in diagnosing Creutzfeldt-Jakob disease and delirium.

Vascular dementia

Optimal function of the brain is dependent upon a generous and competent blood supply Atherosclerotic obstruction to large or small vessels results in a range of neurological syndromes according to the site of obstruction and consequent infarction [14]. In addition, periods of hypo-perfusion of the brain may follow a heart attack, asystole, or systemic hypotension, with infarction in watershed areas. A smaller number (10%) of those whose dementia arises directly from circulation failure are survivors of intra-cerebral bleeds.

The clinical picture in VaD is described as 'patchy' with a mixture of preserved and lost functions. Overall the volume of cortex lost to infarction correlates with the severity of cognitive loss. Neurotransmitter changes occur in VaD but are less predictable and characteristic than in AD [12].

Dementia with Lewy bodies

Lewy bodies are inclusion bodies found within the basal ganglia neurones of people who have Parkinson's disease and, more widely, in the cerebral cortex of a subset of people with dementia identified for the first time in the 1980s [15]. Lewy bodies stain with ubiquitin, which only became available in the 1980s (making the diagnosis possible), and now with α-synuclein. The clinical picture in DLB includes periods of altered consciousness, vivid visual illusions, and hallucinations without (in the early stages) severe cognitive impairment. In DLB there is almost always some evidence of parkinsonism, and falls are not uncommon [16]. Parkinson's disease with dementia (PDD) is the term used for the substantial minority of people with idiopathic Parkinson's disease who go on to develop dementia [17].

Frontotemporal dementia

Malfunction of the frontal lobes, producing altered mood, disinhibition, or reduction of initiative, can occur within the spectrum of symptoms of dementia of any aetiology. Professor David Neary and others have characterized a condition that is based on atrophy of the frontal and temporal lobes, with relative preservation of the rest of the brain [18]. Clinical features are dominated by changes of behaviour, mood, and personality, with relative preservation of cognitive functions. The neuropathology is different from that seen in AD and this is probably a modern understanding of Pick's disease [19]. FTD is split into a frontal variant (mainly affecting behaviour and personality) and two main temporal variants (both affecting speech): progressive non-fluent aphasia and semantic dementia. A strong history of inheritance within the family is more marked than in the other common dementias.

Epidemiology

Dementia becomes progressively more common within old age as is demonstrated by calculations within the recent Dementia UK report (see Table 2.1).

A further 15,000 people in the UK have dementia under the age of 65 years, two thirds of these are aged 55–64 years (see Chapter 6). The Dementia UK study [1] estimated there to be 683,597 people with dementia in the UK in 2006. The number will increase dramatically over the next 45 years, as shown in Table 2.2.

Most of this increase will be in the age groups 75 years and above, largely because more people are expected to survive into these decades where the incidence and prevalence of dementia are greatest: prevalence rising from 1.3% (65–69years), 5.9% (75–79 years), and 20.3% (85–89 years) to over 30% (95+ years).

Maturation of the age profiles of countries in Europe has been a feature through the Twentieth Century [20]. The equivalent process is now occurring world wide with extraordinary implications for the number of people with dementia: 24.3 million in 2005 increasing at a rate of one new case every seven seconds to 81.1 million by 2040. Europe will see a doubling of numbers in that time span; India, China, and other South Asian and Western Pacific countries a fourfold increase [20].

Age is a major determinant of whether an individual will develop dementia. Genetic inheritance is another [21]. Particular gene loci are associated with very strong patterns within affected families with dementia of early onset. People with Down's syndrome, in which there is an extra chromosome 21 which carries a gene responsible for amyloid, develop Alzheimer pathology in their 30s and 40s. In addition, late onset AD is associated with the presence of Apo E in most, but not all populations studied.

Risk factors for vascular disease in middle age – hypertension, diabetes, smoking, obesity, and hyperlipidaemia – are all associated with the later incidence of both AD and VaD [22]. This offers hints towards a framework for early detection and possible prevention. For instance, some studies suggest that physical exercise and healthy diets, especially those higher in anti-oxidants, may be beneficial in terms of reducing the risk of dementia. As far as prevention goes, excessive use of alcohol has been recognized as a risk factor for dementia for some while [23]. However, social engagement and mental stimulation are said to have protective effects against AD. But the studies in many of these areas are on-going [24]. Interestingly, it seems likely that inflammation, stress or trauma of any sort may predispose to the development of dementia and may increase its rate of progression [25].

Table 2.1 Age and gender UK population with dementia 2005 [1]

Age (yrs.)	Male	Female	Total
65–69	19,593	14,058	33,651
70–74	33,599	30,096	63,695
75–79	42,795	72,026	114,821
80–84	57,573	121,682	179,255
85–89	42,796	117,624	160,420
90–94	21,586	67,942	89,528
95+	4,983	22,213	27,196
Total	222,925	445,641	668,566

Table 2.2 Predicted increases in numbers of people with dementia in the UK [1]

Year	People with dementia	% increase from 2006
2006	683,597	N/A
2021	940,110	38
2051	1,735,087	154

Living with dementia

It is difficult for individuals and even their closest family members to be sure when insidious changes herald a departure from the normal course of ageing. This is the situation for most people with AD or FTD. Sudden change associated with neurological symptoms of stroke can mean that the onset of VaD is easier to recognize – though recovery from each episode of cerebral insufficiency is welcomed, and the accumulative impact on cognition, mood, and personality may not be appreciated initially. The florid, fascinating, perceptual changes of DLB come early to attention. Both the patient and the family may fear that he or she is going mad.

Progress over time in all the dementias is variable [26, 27, 28]. What happens to an individual is a function of the underlying pathology, but is also influenced by their constitution, including their general health, and the way they respond to the progressive undermining of competence and accompanying loss of independence. Environmental factors are also important. The presence of sympathetic support, which adjusts to the changing needs of the individual, helps; but encouraging maintenance or recovery of other skills is the best of therapies [29]. Routines are helpful to all of us and carry added power within dementia; they should be encouraged and practised: rediscovered if recently lost. Robert Davis expressed relief and gratitude when people would walk with him rather than struggle to find intellectual reassurance with words [30]. Music, dance, poetry, and art can search out joy or peace [31, 32]. Involvement in the daily round of chores and shopping confirm a person's coordinates within the household. Acceptance and inclusion within the activities of a faith community, perhaps returned to in the face of difficulties, sustain a sense of spiritual identity and give strength [33, 34]. Thus people, places and activity have an influence.

Whilst most people, most of the time, will prefer to live in a private household, which has been 'home' for many years, this becomes rapidly hazardous if they are alone and muddled. Living with a long-term partner (spouse) or other relative is a more secure base. The health and wellbeing of carers, be they live-in or pop-in, therefore requires as much respect and attention as those of the individual with dementia [35]. If both remain well and supported, a very full and rewarding life may be sustained for many months or years, minimizing any potential feeling of entrapment or burden. Often the roles of main carer and cared for are accepted as naturally as hand in glove [36], but they may become taxing to either or both parties [37]. Periods of time apart, sharing the care with others, leavens the life with an alternative milieu. The legitimate aim of respite care is to extend time which can be spent in the health-giving fold of home-life. Nevertheless, at any one time 40% of people with dementia in the UK and similar countries are living in residential or nursing homes [2]. They would otherwise be living at unreasonable risk alone, or have demonstrated needs, or developed a behavioural profile, which could not be sustained elsewhere. Yet the apparent safety of life 'in care' comes at a cost. Relocation to any new environment is stressful and people with dementia are more at risk of this than people without dementia [38]. Life within a community of others, brought together by needs (often identified by someone else) rather than from positive personal choice, makes huge demands on individual resources. These having been subjugated by dementia, many people withdraw into a protective shell, not risking damage by engagement. Kitwood and others (see Chapter 25 in this volume) have championed the benefits of rediscovering the lost individual by careful personal research and re-orchestration of their main themes [39]. Quality of life and the maintenance of wellbeing and ability are acutely sensitive to the characteristics of the professional care environment.

Progression of cognitive impairment averages two points on the Mini-Mental State Examination annually but there is wide variation [40]. Physical frailty, loss of weight, loss of sphincter control, and vulnerability to recurrent falls and infections may eventually supervene in any setting as dementia shows itself as a terminal illness [41]. Life expectation in dementia is reduced in comparison with that of other people of the same age and birth cohort [42].

Dying with dementia

Survival from diagnosis of dementia ranges from a few months to more than ten years. Most people will die of intercurrent illness before experiencing the most debilitating dependency of end-state dementia [43]. Sudden death in a favoured, busy environment (as envisaged in McGough's poem [44]) is not common [45]. Falls, some associated with a fractured limb, an infection, or other organ failure, may mean that admission to a general hospital becomes appropriate or inevitable. Even for the *compos mentis*, general hospitals are difficult, often frightening, places. Staff too frequently feel uncomfortable with dementia and people with dementia and their families become frustrated [46]. Hospital stay may be prolonged and death via a period of acquired disability and secondary or tertiary complications may result. It is important that hospitals learn to appreciate the values by which the lives of their patients are metered. Survival may rate less in their hierarchy than peace, self-determination, or adventure [47]. Even at home or in a residential or nursing home, individuals may fade into a pre-death state of dependency [48] which may be sustained for weeks or months. Sensibility of thirst and hunger is lost, all aspects of homeostasis surrendered, and the body becomes dependent on external adjustments for its maintenance. Weight will decline in this catabolic state, partly through insufficient intake and perhaps through changes in metabolism of muscle and other organs [49]. There is then vulnerability to decubitus pressure sores, hastened by incontinence. Limbs may become contracted and potentially painful. The issue of pain perception and the communication of pain within dementia is complex, as discussed in Chapter 14. The concern is that individuals become distressed, yet are unable to communicate their experience. Treatment with analgesics, including narcotics, may be best practice in the face of behavioural or physiological changes that seem to be distress markers. Greatest difficulties arise when individuals are unable to cope with the oral intake of food or fluids. Swallow reflex may be lost acutely in conditions such as stroke – and a period of artificial feeding with tubes or drip is clearly indicated in anticipation of recovery. It is less clear that this is appropriate when the loss of this capacity is the product of slow progressive impairment from dementia. There are alternative views of the benefits of survival into more profound dementia courtesy of tubes and drips. All views have to be respected and a bespoke pattern of end-of-life care agreed for every individual, taking into account their own views when spoken or communicated in earlier days, with the interpretation of family, in discussion with responsible and well-informed medical and nursing staff. For the most part, people with dementia will be best served if they are enabled to die in settings common to all at the end of life. Yet there is need for a thoughtful and effective palliative care culture to be applied [50]. There are arguments for co-ordinating hospice-style centres to support such regimes in a modification of the hospices, which have added so effectively to the quality of life and death with cancer [51].

Life after dementia

For a time dementia throws a progressively darkening shadow over the life of an individual and those closest to them. Darkened, but never completely lost to shadow, the character of the individual is less available within the normal social round. Syndromes of anticipatory grief are recognized [52] and death may be felt as but a formalization of parting. Yet this period of altered being (dementia) is a short component of a whole life lived. The whole is what will be remembered in the future and for future generations. Traumas experienced and strengths gained during the caring process may lead to a more mature ordering of priorities and determination to share these with others. Dementia is a great teacher: testing and tempering philosophy and practice.

References

1. Knapp M, Prince M (2007). *Dementia UK*. London: Alzheimer's Society.

2. McCartney P (2007). *Memory almost full*. London: MPL Communications,.

3. Plemons J, Willis S, Baltes P (1978) Modiflability of fluid intelligence in ageing, *J Gerontol*. 33, 224–231.

4. Lishman W.A. (1978) *Organic psychiatry*, p. 9. Oxford: Blackwell.

5. Allen N, Burns A, Newton V, *et al.* (2003). The effects of improving hearing in dementia. *Age ageing*, **33**(2), 189–193.

6. Royal College of Psychiatrists (2005). Forgetful but not forgotten: assessment and aspects of treatment of people with dementia. *Council report CR119*. London.

7. Burns A, O'Brien J, Ames D (2005). *Dementia*, 3rd edn. London: Hodder Arnold.

8. Nagy Z, Hubbarb P (2008). Neuropathology, in Jacoby R, Oppenheimer C, Dening T, Thomas A (eds) *Oxford textbook of old Age psychiatry*, pp. 67–83. Oxford: Oxford University Press.

9. Maurer K, McKeith I, Cummings J, Ames D, Burns A (2006). Has the management of Alzheimer's disease changed over the past 100 years? *Lancet*, **368**(9547), 1619–1621.

10. Blessed G, Tomlinson B, Roth M (1968). The association between quantitative measures of dementing and senile change in cerebral grey matter of elderly subjects. *Br J Psychiatry*, **114**, 797–811.

11. Perry EK, Tomlinson BE, Blessed G, Bergmann K, Gibson PH, Perry RH (1978). Correlation of cholinergic abnormalities with senile plaques and mental test scores in senile dementia. *BMJ*, **2**, 1457–1459.

12. Piggott MA, Court J (2008). Neurochemical pathology of neurodegenerative disorders of old age, in Jacoby R, Oppenheimer C, Dening T, Thomas A (eds). *Oxford textbook of old age psychiatry*, pp. 85–101. Oxford: Oxford University Press.

13. Frisoni G (2001). Structural imaging in the clinical diagnosis of Alzheimer's disease. *J Neurol Neurosurg Psychiatry*, **70**, 711–718.

14. Desmond D (1996). Vascular dementia: a construct in evolution. *Cerebrovasc Brain Metabolism Revs*, **8**, 296–325.

15. McKeith I, Galasko D, Kosaka K, *et al.* (1996). Consensus guidelines for the clinical and pathological diagnosis of dementia with Lewy bodies (DLB). *Neurology*, **47**, 1113–1124.

16. McKeith IG, Dickson DW, Lowe J, *et al.* (2005). Diagnosis and management of dementia with Lewy bodies: third report of the DLB Consortium. *Neurology*, **65**, 1863–1872.

17. McKeith I (2000). Spectrum of Parkinson's disease, Parkinson's dementia, and Lewy body dementia. *Neurol Clin*, **18**(4), 865–902.

18. Neary D. Snowden S, Gustafson F, *et al.* (1998). Frontotemporal lobar degeneration: a consensus on clinical diagnostic criteria. *Neurology*, **51**, 1546–1554.

19. Sjogren M, Andersen C (2006). Fronto-temporal Dementia – a brief review. *Mech Ageing Dev*, **127**(2), 180–187.

20. Ferri C, Prince M, Brayne C, *et al.* (2005). Global prevalence of dementia: a Delphi consensus study. *Lancet,* **366**(9503), 2112–2117.

21. Holmes C (2008). The genetics and molecular biology of dementia, in Jacoby R, Oppenheimer C, Dening T, Thomas A (eds). *Oxford textbook of old age psychiatry*, pp. 103–117. Oxford: Oxford University Press.

22. Kivipelto M, Helkala E, Laakso M, *et al.* (2001). Midlife vascular risk factors and Alzheimer's disease in later life. *Brit Med J,* **322**, 1447–1552.

23. Oslin D. Atkinson R. Smith D and Hendrie H (1998). Alcohol related dementia: proposed clinical criteria. *Int J Geriatr Psychiatry,* **13**, 203–-12.

24. Breitner JCS, Albert MS. (2009). Prevention of dementia and cognitive decline, in Weiner MF, Lipton AM (eds). *The American psychiatric publishing textbook of Alzheimer disease and other ementias*, pp. 443–466. Washington DC: American Psychiatric Publishing Inc.

25. Perry VH, Cunningham C, Holmes C (2007). Systemic infections and inflammation affect chronic neurodegeneration. *Nat Rev Immunol,* **7**(2), 161–167.

26. Fitzpatrick A, Kuller L, Lopeez O, Kawas C, Jagust W (2005). Survival following dementia onset: Alzheimer's disease and vascular dementia. *J Neurol Sci,* **229–230**, 43–49.

27. Jellinger K, Wenning G, Seppi K (2007). Predictors of survival in dementia with Lewy bodies and Parkinson dementia. *Neurodegener Dis,* **4**(6), 428–430.

28. Grasbeck A, Englund E, Horstmann V, Passant U, Gustafson L (2003). Predictors of mortality in fronto-temporal dementia. *Int J Geriatr Psychiatry,* **18**(7), 594–601.

29. Marshall M (2005). *Perspectives on rehabilitation and dementia*. London: Jessica Kingsley.

30. Davis R (1989). *My journey into Alzheimer's disease*. Illinois: Tyndale House,.

31. Schweitzer P (2006). *Reminiscence theatre*. London: Jessica Kingsley.

32. Bryden C (2005). *Dancing with dementia*. London: Jessica Kingsley,.

33. Merchant R (2003). *Pioneering the third age: the church in an ageing population*. Carlisle: Paternoster Press,.

34. Jewel A (2004). *Ageing, spirituality and well-being*. London: Jessica Kingsley.

35. Woods R, Wills W, Higginson I, Hobbins J, Whitby M (2003). Support in the community for people with dementia and their carers. *Int J Geriatr Psychiatry,* **18**(4), 298–307.

36. Eagles J, Beattie J, Blackwood G, Restall D, Ashcroft G (1987). The mental health of elderly couples. *Brit J Psychiatry,* **150**, 299–303.

37. Gilhooley M (1984). The impact of care-giving on care-givers. *Brit J Med Psychol,* **57**, 35–44.

38. Hallewell C, Morris J, Jolley D (1994). The closure of residential homes: what happens to residents? *Age Ageing,* **23**(2), 158–161.

39. Brooker D (2007). *Person-centred dementia care*. London: Jessica Kingsley.

40. Clark CM, Sheppard L, Fillenbaum GG, *et al.* (1999). Variability in annual mini-mental state examination score in patients with probable Alzheimer's disease. *Arch Neurol,* **56**, 857–862.

41. Morrison R, Siu A (2000). Mortality from pneumonia and hip fractures in patients with advanced dementia. *JAMA,* **284**, 2447–2448.

42. Larson E, Shalden M, Wang L, *et al.* (2004). Survival after initial diagnosis of Alzheimer's disease. *Ann Intern Med,* **140**(7), 501–509.

43. Keane J, Hope T, Fairburn CG, Jacoby R (2001). Death and dementia. *Int J Geriatr Psychiatry,* **16**, 969–974.

44. McGough R (1967). Let me die a young man's death, in Henri A, McGough R, Patten B (republished 1983). *The Mersey Sound*, p. 105. Harmondsworth: Penguin.

45. Black D, Jolley D (1990). Slow euthanasia? The deaths of psychogeriatric patients. *BMJ,* **300**, 1321–1323.

46. Age Concern (2006). *Hungry to be heard*. London: Age Concern.

47. Downs M, Small N and Froggatt K (2006). Explanatory models of dementia. *Int J Palliat Nurs*, **12**, 209–213.

48. Isaacs B, Gunn J, McKechan A, McMillan I, Neville Y (1971). The concept of pre-death. *Lancet*, **1**(7709), 1115–1118.

49. White H, Pieper C, Schmader K (1998). The association of weight change in Alzheimer's disease with severity of disease and mortality. *J Am Geriatr Soc*, **46**(10), 1223–1227.

50. Hughes JC, Jolley D, Jordan A, Sampson EL (2007). Palliative care in dementia: issues and evidence. *Adv Psychiatr Treat*, **13**, 251–260.

51. Volicer L, Rheaume Y, Brown J, *et al.* (1986). Hospice approach to the treatment of patients with advanced dementia of the Alzheimer type. *JAMA*, **256**, 2210–2213.

52. Rudd M, Viney L, Preston C (1999). The grief experienced by spousal care-givers of dementia patients. *Int J Aging Hum Dev*, **48**(3), 217–240.

Chapter 3

The view of the person with dementia

Daphne Wallace

Introduction

For the past 25 years, in the National Health Service (NHS), I worked in psychiatry of older people, latterly as a consultant psychiatrist in Leeds for over 20 years. I looked after older people with many mental health problems, but inevitably a large number with dementia. I knew the implications of a diagnosis of Alzheimer's disease and of other types of dementia. As earlier diagnosis became more common, I had many opportunities to talk to people with dementia and their carers and families about the implications of such a diagnosis. After retirement from the NHS at 60, I continued with a private psychotherapy practice and had the privilege of continuing to support several people with dementia and their families.

Diagnosis

I was just 65 years old when I was diagnosed with early vascular dementia by a neurologist. I had talked to professional colleagues about some changes I had noticed and then went to my general practitioner (GP) to say that I felt I should see a specialist. I was referred to a local neurologist and, after a scan and neuropsychological tests, the diagnosis of small vessel vascular changes was confirmed.

Before the diagnosis was confirmed, I inevitably had anxieties that were in many ways intensified by my professional experience. Once the diagnosis was confirmed, there was a sense of relief. I had not been imagining things. It was not because I was 'doing too much' and should 'slow down' which was often other people's reaction to my anxiety about my symptoms. During the time of my assessment, I felt fairly alone, but I was fortunate that the whole process took only about two months. I know from many of the friends I have made since my diagnosis that the process of assessment can stretch for many months or even years.

Support after diagnosis

What support do I feel that I needed after diagnosis? The neurologist that I had seen emigrated to Australia, and I was not referred to anyone else. My GP has a good system for monitoring blood pressure and cardiovascular disease, but I was left with no specific follow-up for the dementia. I felt abandoned. Yes, in some ways, I was at an advantage because of my knowledge and professional experience, but I felt increasingly in limbo in the three years after diagnosis. Sometimes, I felt my condition was worsening; at other times, I felt it was static, but I could not be sure.

Another more practical type of support may be needed in the period shortly after diagnosis, namely help with management of resources. Has the person made a Will? I have, and my husband and I also signed mutual Power of Attorney forms, which need updating, especially in the light of the Mental Capacity Act 2005 [1], which governs such matters in England and Wales.

Some people have never had financial advice but may need it after diagnosis. These issues are best sorted out soon after diagnosis and may be vital both to the person with dementia and to their family. Financial arrangements are needed to ensure adequate provision and also to facilitate proper provision of care. With an early diagnosis, the person with dementia should be able to participate in planning and ensure that their wishes are complied with.

Because my symptoms are very specific, my problem is not obvious to people in general. I feel the changes and get distressed by them often. It is not pleasing to have been good at all maths and then finding that you are struggling to help a 6-year-old grandchild with basic arithmetic. Forgetting names is common, and I've always had difficulty remembering names of people I have just met. Now I can struggle to find the name of a lifelong close friend or even a relative. Words always came easily to me. Now I often struggle to find the word I want or come out with a completely wrong word. Cooking had always been a pleasure to me – for the family or for a large gathering. Now I have problems with working out quantities and cannot cope with interruptions. I still drive but have a sat-nav as a back-up to prevent using wrong exits off motorways or roundabouts. I can no longer listen to radio programmes while driving except for music as a background.

I cannot tell whether these specific things are static or changing. I need to feel that there is someone I can contact if I am worried and who is monitoring my mental state. I need someone with up-to-date knowledge whom I can trust to understand my needs and, while monitoring my condition, will also suggest any modification to treatment as appropriate. It would have helped me to have had that kind of support in the three years after diagnosis. I have now seen an appropriate consultant psychiatrist who will review me routinely twice a year, arrange for neuropsychological reassessment as indicated, and will be available if I feel the need for an expert opinion in between.

There are other benefits to this type of monitoring and support. I now have access to his team in the community if I (or my husband) feel in need of immediate support. At the time of greatest adjustment to the diagnosis, I was without professional support. Learning to live with a diagnosis of dementia involves loss, bereavement, adjustment, and revision of expectations. Depending on the specific diagnosis and likely rate of decline, this may need more changes than have been relevant to me. Coming to terms with such a diagnosis, for which there is no 'cure' and which will eventually lead to diminishment in day-to-day capabilities, is not simple or easy and support by informed professionals can help tremendously. Even though the support I now have is relatively low-key and infrequent, it has been an enormous relief to have the sense that there is someone there from whom to seek help and advice. Facing such a diagnosis can be a lonely and threatening experience. I know that the course of the illness is infinitely variable, but I still would wish to know what to expect. I used to be asked questions of that sort by my patients and their families, but this is predictable in only the most general way. Different people cope in different ways. I believe strongly that people need to know their diagnosis but also to be helped to find a continuing value in what they do and are. In my case, I wanted to make sure that I gave time to important leisure activities while I was coping. I sing and am now in a semi-professional choir, which involves a level of musical 'literacy', which I may lose as my illness progresses. My life is not less busy but definitely different from what it was when I was working in the NHS.

Living with dementia

Once I had got used to the fact that I have cognitive changes that are explained by pathological findings, I had to review my retirement plan. For some years, I had been very involved in both large and small charities concerned with aspects of dementia care. My role had often been one of leadership or management input and though I felt capable of continuing this for a while, I realized that it did not come as easily to me. Gradually, I came to realize that my professional background and experience, combined with the knowledge and experience of my own cognitive loss, gave me a particular perspective on the problems of living with dementia. I decided that any 'volunteer' time that I gave should perhaps be focussed on sharing this particular experience. As a result, I am as busy as ever, but I have to make sure I have enough rest as tiredness affects me more than it ever did in the past.

I have always believed in openness and, like several other people I now know who are also experiencing this illness, I feel it is important to share this experience as widely as possible in the hope that the fear and stigma can be reduced. Whether sharing with family and friends or in a more public way, I found I needed support because of the varied responses that I received. Some people were shocked and negative in response. Others could not accept what I was telling them and denied the possibility. Some friends even challenged the appropriateness of my continuing to work in certain capacities. Close friends were supportive and empathic. It is important that after diagnosis, the support is available to help to cope with the effects of such variable responses.

Person-centred care

Nowadays, people with a diagnosis of cancer are not usually shunned or feared. Unfortunately a diagnosis of dementia can evoke similar reactions to those to cancer in the past. In the developed world in particular, the importance of cognitive ability and an intellectual emphasis on life can cause neglect of the abilities and needs of those with dementia. This was pointed out by Kitwood [2]: 'For the greater part of the period in which dementia has existed as a clinical category, the subjectivity of those affected has been almost totally disregarded' (p. 70). Despite Tom Kitwood's work in identifying the need to see 'the **PERSON** with dementia rather than the person with **DEMENTIA**' [2, p. 7], this message is often a revelation to people responsible for providing or planning services. Even those I have known in the past with advanced dementia have revealed much of their underlying personality, which can inform carers with regard to the most appropriate care and response to their needs. Feelings do not need verbal expression to be significant.

Having promoted these ideas for much of my working life, I was pleased to be involved in the drafting of the UK Dementia Strategy in 2008 [3]. It is important to be involved with planners so that the experience of people with dementia can inform planners and professionals of the needs and wishes of those with dementia. During the discussions, the role of a 'Dementia Care Adviser' was proposed. This would be designed to ensure ongoing contact with one identified and informed person to provide just the sort of continuing informed support I found that I needed. This spurred me on to ask for the referral that has now filled this gap in my support.

Unfortunately, despite all this valuable work, many people with dementia still languish in institutions with little attention paid to their individual needs, wishes, and personalities. It is vital that, as well as attempts to ensure sufficient space, good food, privacy, and healthcare, the needs of the individual person are not ignored. Dementia does not destroy the ability to experience and appreciate the world about the person. For some time, concern has been expressed for those with dementia. The tendency to see people with advanced dementia as non-persons is still pervasive and, despite much work to change the situation, as a group, their individual personal and spiritual needs tend to be particularly neglected.

Fortunately, there are now many other people who are helping to spread the message. Killick [4], Killick and Cordonnier [5], Goldsmith [6], and Wallace [7] have spent much time looking at communication by people with loss of verbal ability and have written about their work (see Chapter 23 in this volume also). John Killick has developed his skills as writer and poet to help those with dementia communicate and has produced books of 'assisted' writings [4, 5], where he has written down things said to him in conversation when visiting as writer in residence to Westminster Health Care and the Stirling Dementia Services Development Centre. As Sue Benson, Editor of the *Journal of Dementia Care*, says in the Foreword to the collection published as *You Are Words* [4],

> John Killick's work has made two very special contributions to the cause of good practice in dementia care. Giving time and concentrated attention to an individual, listening carefully to what they say, tells each person with dementia that they are valued, that they are of interest and worth. The further step of writing down what is said powerfully underlines that statement of worth. (p. 5)

Killick's work has shown that even those who are severely affected by dementia, whom care staff believe to be incapable of communicating, can, with attention and confidence in the listener, communicate with great clarity and insight. Malcolm Goldsmith, during his time at Stirling, carried out research into communication with those with dementia, published as *Hearing the Voice of People with Dementia* [6]. I hope that in some small way, what I say and write expands people's understanding and knowledge of what it is like to have this diagnosis.

Spirituality

With the change towards the concept of whole person care, there is increasing awareness that spiritual well-being is relevant and important. Attention to spiritual needs leads to a better quality of life. Meeting them is not an add-on 'icing on the cake', but an integral part of whole person care. Recognition of the personhood of the individual is vital. In my chapter on spiritual care in *Practical Management of Dementia* [7], I have expressed my concern for the spiritual needs of those with dementia. Spirituality can be defined in many ways. I like the following: 'Spirituality can be described as a search for that which gives meaning and identity to a person's life and the wider world. Dementia does not destroy the ability to experience and appreciate the world about the person' [8, p. 2]. This is well illustrated by Paul Wilson writing in *Spirituality and Ageing* [9]. Despite the writing of Alison Froggatt in *Mental Health Problems in Old Age* [10], when she drew attention to this area, this was not really followed up, and if so, only with those having milder loss of cognitive ability [11]. In her own book, Shamy [12] gives a telling example of simple needs not met and Froggatt and Shamy [13] refer to the significance of the here and now:

> The Sacrament of the present moment has a particular poignancy in dementia, for most happenings may be forgotten soon afterwards. But the rose smells just as sweet **now,** and the birds on the table are squabbling **now**, and we can laugh. (p. 10)

For me an appreciation of my 'spirit' is part of me. The fact that this is expressed within the context of religious belief is how it is for me. For others, it may be more complex or less related to any concept of religion. I only know that for me supportive care will always include attention to this side of me as a person if it is to be truly person-centred.

Music is an integral part of my life. I am sure that it will always be important, wherever I am and whatever my mental state is. Relationships with friends and family are important, and I will need to have care that understands the significance of these things as well as my religious faith. If my care in the future is to be person-centred, these are three of the facets of my life which would have to be recognized as significant and be included in my care plan. With appropriate supportive care in the earlier stages, people are more likely to feel reassured that the important aspects of their personality will be known and appreciated. How do we make a care package that is individualized and relevant for the person and their particular needs?

I know that I will want individually tailored care. I will not want to be put into a 'category' with standardized solutions to my problems. My hope is that my care, and that of all the people with dementia, will be person-centred and responsive to need. What is perceived by management as needed may be different to the needs felt by those cared for; human beings are infinitely variable, and therefore, their needs are not easily predicted. Only individual packages are likely to be successful in achieving this goal. I shall want the care that I need in future to have these values.

I shall not want to be expected to accept care and attention that is uncongenial to me personally. But this type of provision has implications for costs and also for an ability to understand an individual's needs. Person-centred care may be intended, but to be given properly needs **staff** with **time.** Staff with time costs money. People need **relationships**, not just care, and continuity of staffing is part of building such relationships. To provide this sort of care, adequate training is essential.

Over the past few years, training in person-centred care has become available. The entire staff, from managers to care assistants, needs to have an understanding of this type of care and the ability to make it a reality. Besides the people I have already mentioned who have increased our understanding of these matters, two recent publications are worth mentioning. *State of the Art in Dementia Care*, edited by Marshall [14], gives a broad summary of work in the 1990s and includes contributions by some of those I have already mentioned. A more recent publication, looking particularly at person-centred care and building on the work of Tom Kitwood, is *Person-Centred Dementia Care* by Dawn Brooker [15]. These more academic books give a framework within which to base more practical training and increased understanding of the issues at stake. I certainly hope that this type of knowledge, combined with the insights of people like Bryden [16] and others who have written about their personal experience, will ensure that there is a generation of carers who understand that people with dementia are **PERSONS**.

Conclusion

As we get older, we are all increasingly likely to experience mental health problems – we may even become marginalized ourselves and socially excluded. We all want to be valued and treated as individuals. I, like all of you, will want the care that I need in future to manifest and respect these values. I do not want to be expected to accept care and attention that is uncongenial to me personally. I shall want my family to have appropriate, flexible help in meeting my needs.

I am only a short time into the journey of dementia (or, as Christine Bryden terms it, the dance of dementia [16]). Christine's description of her dance is poignant, informative, and at the same time, supportive. I would like to think that I could convey insights into my journey in some small but similar way.

To use an old Zulu saying: 'A person is a person through others' [17].

References

1. *The Mental Capacity Act 2005*. Norwich: The Stationery Office. Available at http://www.opsi.gov.uk/acts/acts2005/ukpga_20050009_en_1 [accessed on 29 March 2009].
2. Kitwood T. (1997). *Dementia reconsidered,* Buckingham: Open University Press.
3. Department of Health (2009). *Living well with dementia : a national dementia strategy*. London: Department of Health.
4. Killick J. (ed) (1997). *You are words.* London: Hawker Publications.
5. Killick J, Cordonnier C. (eds) (2000). *Openings.* London: Hawker Publications.

6. Goldsmith M. (1996). *Hearing the voice of people with dementia.* London & Bristol, PA: Jessica Kingsley Publishers.

7. Wallace D. (2004). Spiritual aspects of dementia, in Curran S, Wattis J P (eds) *Practical management of dementia – a multi-professional approach,* pp. 207–218. Oxford: Radcliffe Medical Press.

8. Hammond G, Moffitt L. (2000). *Spiritual care: guidelines for care plans.* Leeds : Christian Council on Ageing, Faith in Elderly People.

9. Wilson P. (1999). Memory, personhood and faith, in Jewell A (ed) *Spirituality and ageing,* p. 106. London: Jessica Kingsley.

10. Froggatt A. (1988). Self-awareness in early dementia, in Gearing B, Johnson M, Heller T. (eds) *Mental health problems in old age,* pp. 131–136. Maidenhead: Open University Press.

11. Keady J. (1996). The experience of dementia: a review of the literature and implications for nursing practice. *J Clin Nurs,* **5,** 1–13.

12. Shamy E. (1997). *More than body brain and breath,* p. 59. New Zealand : ColCom Press. (Edited version by Jewell A. (2003) under title *A guide to the spiritual dimension of care for people with Alzheimer's disease and related dementia.* London: Jessica Kingsley).

13. Froggatt A, Shamy E. (1998). *Dementia: a christian perspective.* Derby: Christian Council on Ageing Publications.

14. Marshall M. (ed) (1997). *State of the art in dementia care.* London: Centre for Policy on Ageing.

15. Brooker D. (2007). *Person-centred dementia care – making services better.* London: Jessica Kingsley.

16. Bryden C. (2005). *Dancing with dementia: my story of living positively with dementia.* London: Jessica Kingsley Publishers.

17. Battle M. (1997). Reconciliation – *The ubuntu theology of Desmond Tutu.* Cleveland, Ohio: The Pilgrim Press.

Chapter 4

The view of the family carer

Barbara Pointon

It was Christmas Eve, 1991. In a hospital concourse draped with glittering garlands and messages of good cheer, I sat at a table with my husband Malcolm, coffee going cold, stunned by the news that his diagnosis was probably Alzheimer's. He was 51 at the time, and I had no inkling that ahead of me lay 16 years of increasingly intensive care.

For two years he had been treated for endogenous depression, following a one-off night-time epileptic seizure, after which nothing was quite the same again. He made mistakes in his once-perfect piano playing, confused right and left (including driving the wrong way down the M11), and despite having built electronic music synthesizers from scratch, came to me one day for reassurance that he had wired up a three-pin plug correctly. Neither of us knew that Alzheimer's could affect younger people, nor that visuospatial problems could be early tell-tale signs. In addition, Malcolm, usually so patient, became uncharacteristically brusque with my mother.

When Malcolm said he could not do something he had always done, such as checking the oil level in the car, I now feel ashamed of my disbelief and tetchiness, for I thought he was winding me up. Early diagnosis is vital, for when we know, we can make allowances and protect the relationship. Things came to a head when Malcolm got completely lost, taking three hours to drive a familiar seven miles from our nearest town to home. He arrived in a cold sweat and pallid with fear. Our general practitioner (GP) promptly signed him off work and referred him to the hospital's memory clinic for a series of tests and scans.

At the diagnosis of a terminal illness, I was in shock and denial, and handing out an information leaflet is not enough. I would have preferred a friendly face, a brief chat, a telephone number to call for advice, and a promise of a visit in a few weeks' time. Supportive care begins at diagnosis: not so much hands-on care, but knowing how to help someone who is depressed, who is having problems with everyday tasks, who is losing their self-confidence. Feedback from the hospital concerning further tests and scans was helpful, but we really wanted strategies for everyday living. It was three years before a kind community psychiatric nurse (CPN) was allocated to us and a social worker came – and went again when he found we were self-funding. In that huge gap between diagnosis and starting to use services, I was left to re-invent the wheel.

Caring for someone with dementia is not the same as caring for the frail elderly; it demands special knowledge, skills, and approaches. I tried my best to spin it out of my hump but unintentionally made awful mistakes. What would have helped throughout the illness would have been a dementia care adviser, or a series of them, journeying alongside us, as a first stop for information of all kinds, practical advice and training, moral support and, when required, triggering services, equipment or higher levels of expertise. Whether rooted in health, social care, the Alzheimer's Society or Admiral nursing, such a person, in my opinion, would need to have a good backpack of practical knowledge about dementia care, local services, and counselling skills. As it was, I blundered on alone, neither knowing what belonged to where (even legal entitlements) nor knowing anything about dementia.

Meanwhile, Malcolm had retired early and I did the same a year later when he needed supervision. This had serious financial implications, but at least we could spend more quality time together. We took lots of walks, days by the sea, enjoyed concerts and theatre (making good use of the 'carer goes free' concession), visited friends, and kept the garden in better order – with Malcolm asking me to walk alongside him while he mowed the lawn because on the turns he couldn't work out where he had to go next. His diary is peppered with frustration, such as 'mental fog', 'head full of cotton wool', 'thoughts and actions slipping from my grasp', 'I can't go on like this', giving a flavour of the kind of psychological support he needed from me. It was hard to remain patient, especially when he kept on saying accusingly, 'It's all your fault!'.

Our CPN came and arranged daycare. I left Malcolm in a room full of people 20 years older and drove back, blinded with tears, feeling as though we had slipped a generation. Malcolm had been a talented amateur artist. At daycare, he was frequently given artwork to do, but retaining sufficient insight to know his pictures were now rubbish (thanks to his impaired visuospatial awareness), he would arrive home and throw his pictures in the bin, leaving me to contend with his frustration and self-loathing. He had always hated bingo, but by then had lost his sense of number, so when the apparatus was brought out he made for the door at great speed. I wish information concerning deficits shown up on an individual's tests and scans could flow from the hospital clinic to those providing daycare, so that activities likely to provoke distress could be avoided. Instead, when I went to collect him, I was told, 'Malcolm's been a bit difficult today', and I felt like the parent of a naughty boy being cautioned by the teacher.

Malcolm disliked dancing. At village dances, it was as much as I could do to get him to stagger round the floor to the last waltz, with him muttering, 'What idiot invented a dance in three-time when you've only got two feet?'. But one day I arrived at daycare to find him wiggling his bottom with the best of them. Alzheimer's had removed his inhibitions, his natural sense of rhythm as a musician came to the fore and dancing (or rather wiggling in time to the music) became our new shared pleasure. This suggests that we must be careful in making assumptions about what should constitute appropriate activities.

All of Malcolm's learning and skills gradually unravelled in the reverse order they had been acquired – until even following the thread of TV programmes became difficult, complicated by his belief that the people on the screen were actually in the room. This is where the family carer becomes desperate for ideas for suitable personalized activities, where being persistently shadowed becomes irritating and 24/7 vigilance wearing. I needed specific dementia care advice, and there was no local branch of the Alzheimer's Society. Friends and neighbours generously formed a rota to take Malcolm for long walks every day so that I could get on with my tasks uninterrupted.

Although Malcolm had lost his ability to remember, read, or write music, he continued to improvise lengthy virtuosic piano pieces. Much later (when he was scoring zero on the psychometric tests, his speech gobbledegook and his usual memory-span measured in seconds), his pieces still made perfect musical sense, and ideas set out at the beginning were recalled some twenty minutes later to give the piece form. This taught me to celebrate what Malcolm could still do (and indeed what many of us could not even begin to do), as opposed to mourning his losses, and the improvisations gave me both pleasure and an important insight into how he was feeling – angry, cheerful, wistful, or calmly resigned.

A darker side to the illness began to insinuate: perplexing behaviours, aggression, the beginnings of incontinence, and for me perhaps the most stressful period of caring. Malcolm took to hiding and hoarding. I would find my handbag in the washing machine, or car keys under cushions, and stoically accepted bucketfuls of fallen leaves and stones. It drove me crazy until a behavioural psychologist explained that, because people with dementia feel they are losing so much of themselves, if something important is left lying around, they will hide it 'safely' away, promptly forgetting where and who did it. Another example of light dawning – once we understand, we can make allowances and not make accusations. Yet many family carers, especially self-funders, do not automatically gain access to helpful dementia advice.

Then there was the incident of the new garden shredder – a red cylindrical machine with a domed top, standing about 1.5 metres high, with a round aperture in the middle to take the branches and two smaller circular white controls above it. Malcolm did not like the noise it made, so watched through the window. Afterwards, he met me at the door, said firmly, 'I've never done this to you and I don't want to do it, but you deserve it', and slapped me hard across my face. I burst into tears, shocked to the core, because Malcolm had never lifted a finger against me or our sons. That evening, his version slowly emerged. He thought the machine was a red devil, with eyes and an open mouth; to him, I was bowing as I offered it oblations, whereas it roared its approval. Devil worship! Having read *And Still the Music Plays* [1], I now appreciate that Alzheimer's patients can miscue environments and that reactions can stem from something in a person's history – maybe for Malcolm, as a youthful Primitive Methodist, hearing fire and brimstone sermons? If only I'd understood, and learned to go with the flow, however bizarre it seems, it would not have been so hurtful.

Similarly, Malcolm would shout and hit out at his image in the mirror. I thought he was just angry with himself, and not until much later realized he had time-travelled backwards, was probably 21 years old again in his head, did not recognize himself, and thought this stranger was 'Another Man' in the house. Was his wife being unfaithful? No wonder he became aggressive towards me. I have been held by my wrists against a wall, transfixed by a look that could literally kill, given karate chops in the back of my neck when I was helping to put his shoes on and much more. Nor did I appreciate that a very fine line lies between caring and controlling; I'm sure I was too bossy and frequently overstepped it, especially when helping with personal care. We began to have hourly paid careworkers for washing and dressing; Malcolm could not concentrate on two things at once, so I would hold his hands and talk or sing to distract him while the careworker got on with the business. Eventually, I received good advice from the new Alzheimer's Society's branch outreach worker, but she did not have the power to push Health or Social Care buttons and trigger services; that role could usefully be strengthened in the future.

As Malcolm's speech deteriorated he became even more aggressive – overturning the tea table, kicking in doors which I had locked to prevent him from leaving the house without me knowing (oh for an electronic device which would tell me which way he had gone!), resulting in my spending hours circling the countryside in the car, searching for him as it grew dark or began to rain. Our CPN was supportive, but confessed that his knowledge of mental health was too general, and he did not know enough about this stage of Alzheimer's. The same was true for our social worker. The answer from the medical profession was to prescribe anti-psychotics, which calmed Malcolm temporarily, but the anger came back in spades when it wore off. Once, when he went for a week's respite in a dementia ward, I had left a man who could walk for ten miles and on my return found him so overmedicated he could not stand and was pathetically confined to a wheelchair.

To cap it all, three sets of daycare collapsed (the staff not knowing how to deal with Malcolm, including refusing to help him aim properly to urinate in the lavatory bowl – that wretched visuospatial problem again) and so we began to have live-in carers from an agency. We were promised a rota of 3 or 4, but the reality was 14 in 8 months, none dementia-trained or having sufficient English knowledge to interpret Malcolm's fractured speech or understand the care plan. The promised respite for me never materialized, and the stream of new faces bewildered and angered Malcolm, who became increasingly violent, pulling down curtains and uprooting pot-plants. I was totally exhausted. For the first time in my life, the love I felt for Malcolm was being sorely tested – I just could not go on. I had to put him in a care home; it was for my sake, not his, and I still feel guilty about that.

What would have helped us most in that dark middle phase of the illness?

1 Properly trained care staff and continuity of personnel.

2 Practical and moral support at home, tailored to our situation, given by an expert in dementia care advice, helping me to understand the illness and enabling me to give better supportive care.

3 Ideas for suitable activities.

4 More opportunities to meet other carers who were a bit further along the road.

5 A 24-hour dementia helpline because once (when Malcolm had thrust his slippers down the loo and was rampaging round the bedroom), not knowing what to do and terrified, I phoned the out-of-hours GP service – only to learn that if he came out, he could only 'Section him' (i.e. compulsorily detain him under mental health legislation), or I could call the police. As if!

6 Flexible respite care would have helped us both. I thought the only respite available was for Malcolm to be cared for somewhere else. He disliked being away from familiar surroundings, for he always came back in a worse physical and psychological state. Some nights, I put Malcolm back to bed as many as 15 times, so instead of daycare, I would have appreciated some night cover so that I could get some sleep.

7 Replacement care at home, given by a consistent person, would have been less traumatic for Malcolm and would have given me peace of mind.

Perplexing behaviours, aggression, lack of trained and consistent staff, incontinence and loss of speech, together with a feeling of helplessness and being overwhelmed, lie at the heart of why many family carers give up at this point. Properly advised and supported, many could carry on caring for longer.

I looked at 14 nursing homes before finding one which met Malcolm's needs – room to pace about without bumping into objects, good natural light, colourful garden, and kindly staff with little turnover. For nearly two years, Malcolm was well cared for, but he became so rigid that he could not bend in the middle to sit in a chair and spent his days miserably lying on his bed. I just thought this was the next stage. His consultant had visited three times and recommended that his dosage of sodium valproate should be reduced, but it had not been actioned by the home's GP because the staff said that Malcolm was easier to manage now and was off his feet. Classic case of risk versus quality of life. And of the carer's dilemma: should we make waves or keep silent in case it has repercussions on the care and we gain a label of 'interfering relative'?

Supported by our social worker, and despite the senior nurse telling me, 'But you have handed the care over to us now', a meeting was called, resulting in Malcolm's dosage being gradually reduced. Within a week, he was walking about again, albeit gingerly, but with a smile on his face. Because once a carer, always a carer, we would like to be treated as partners in care when our relative is in a home. I believe those official bodies whose duty it is to inspect homes and set standards for them could help by requiring all care homes to have an active relatives' group. I decided to bring Malcolm home again, with a prediction of six months to live. It turned into seven years, and I do not regret it.

Determined not to have agency care again, I fought for Direct Payments (a system, whereby the person is given money to pay for care of his or her choice), which enabled me to choose who worked in our home, gave us more continuity of staff (who got to know Malcolm well and could spot small but significant changes in his condition), and regular replacement care at home.

Two live-in carers alternated one week on, one week off, working alongside me and sharing the night duties. I appreciated the support of The Rowan Organisation, employed by Social Services to help people on Direct Payments with all employment matters. Malcolm visibly improved.

But not long after coming home, Malcolm's mobility sharply declined, then suddenly went completely. We waited four months for a standing hoist, during which time we came near to injuring Malcolm and ourselves. When equipment is needed, it is needed *now*. We were grateful for the advice from the occupational therapist, a specially adapted wheelchair (because Malcolm's not knowing where he was in space, plus myoclonic jerking, made all transfers difficult), and for the early provision of a pressure-relieving mattress and cushion by our district nurses. Despite seven years of immobility and double incontinence, Malcolm never had a pressure sore. He was not bed-bound; several transfers each day between bed, wheelchair, recliner chair and armchair, plus scrupulous cleansing, incontinence pads of the correct absorbency and fit (no catheterization because of the danger of pulling at the apparatus) and pure aloe vera gel – all helped to keep the skin intact.

District nurses proved very supportive, but unfortunately did not know enough about how the overlay of dementia affects normal nursing procedures. For example, Malcolm's swallowing became compromised about four years before he died. The district nurses and GPs advised percutaneous endoscopic gastrostomy (PEG) tube feeding; I had to point to research which indicates that it is not usually recommended in dementia because there is an equal risk of choking on regurgitation.

The speech and language therapist advised that cold thickened drinks were more easily sensed and controlled in the mouth than tepid ones and the dietician advised on pureed food. Feeding requires time, patience, and continuity of staff. It is the most trustful thing in the world to open your mouth to be fed; Malcolm would refuse to take food from a new careworker for a couple of days. He ate the same amount of food almost until he died, yet he inexorably lost weight. I had to explain to the worried staff that weight loss is inevitable, for the brain gradually loses its capacity to control the digestive system's extraction of nutrients from food. Relatives of people in care homes (who might unfairly accuse the staff of neglect) need to know this too.

As for 'constipation', normal laxatives just caused faecal leakage; so together with the continence adviser, we devised a regimen which became similar to that used for paraplegics. The community dentist helped us to maintain good oral hygiene (including using aloe vera toothpaste to control thrush and gingivitis) and a paramedic recommended the use of oxygen in epileptic seizures; it worked like magic to decrease their severity or length. I had picked up from a conference that medication should be reduced in line with severity of dementia. Malcolm had episodes of Cheyne-Stokes breathing during the night, so with the permission of our GP we gradually reduced his dosage of clonazepam (used in epilepsy, but it can depress breathing) to a quarter of the usual dose, with excellent results.

These were some of the many professionals having to be called in for different aspects of supportive care. Sometimes, they saw only their bit of the jigsaw, and we received conflicting advice. In this severe stage, I believe the 'dementia care adviser' by our side should be an expert in dementia nursing care – such as an Admiral Nurse – and, as part of the community team, should see the holistic picture, give appropriate advice, and co-ordinate nursing care. They would be doing continuous assessment all the time, providing a firmer basis for applications for continuing care.

Over the years, I have developed a picture in my mind. Imagine an inverted pyramid with four layers. We enter the world at the point of that inverted pyramid as a baby with our own identity, essence, or spirit, if you like. We explore our immediate world in the second layer, using our five senses and experience emotions through them. As a toddler, we enter the third and learn to control our basic functions – standing, walking, talking, eye-hand co-ordination, feeding, washing, and dressing ourselves, becoming continent. Finally, we gain our primary-school skills, moving on to more abstract thinking, finer skills, and a wider view of the world, which form the top and largest layer. But Alzheimer's attacks that pyramid from the top until most of the two upper layers are destroyed, leaving the two lower ones – sensory, psychological, emotional, and spiritual needs – more exposed, and therefore, more important.

The greatest gift we can give to people with dementia is time. Supportive care, in all stages, but especially in the severe stage, is not just about physical tasks, but also means finding time to attend to other needs, through:

1 Sight: good light, bright colours (especially red/yellow), smiling faces, eye-contact

2 Taste: oral feeding, strongly flavoured food

3 Smell: of cooking, aromatherapy sessions

4 Hearing: continuing to talk, even if there is little response (we talk to babies, after all), laughter, and music of their taste (including our humming/singing)

5 Touch: the most important human need of all. We stroked Malcolm's hands and face, gave hugs, held him close when he awoke in fear at night.

The most important psychological need is to feel safe; emotional and spiritual needs are nurtured when people feel loved and cherished.

Family carers often feel helpless or unsure what to do when their loved one becomes mute, immobile, and expressionless, and this other side of supportive care also needs to be valued by professional caregivers. It is as important as physical care, whatever the setting, and time to give it should be factored into the careplan. I would love to see the phrase 'He/She's no trouble now' erased from our vocabulary.

As for supportive care in the dying phase, it begins with recognizing that the patient wants to let go. For years, Malcolm had recovered from numerous life-threatening chest infections with an almost primitive determination to survive, and I had to support him in that; but his last infection seemed intrinsically different. When his swallowing stopped altogether, his eyes and whole body exuded weariness and submission. Care staff needed reassurance that we were not 'starving him to death' and that he would feel neither hunger nor thirst provided we kept his mouth clean and lips moistened. I asked for the palliative care team to advise us in this last stretch. Sorry, only for cancer.

The family carer also needs emotional support in this last phase when making difficult decisions; I declined to have Malcolm admitted to hospital for intrusive intravenous treatment – he would have been terrified of unfamiliar, noisy surroundings – and instead chose to let nature take its course at home. As the subcutaneous syringe driver with a half-dose of morphine was set up, I knew in my heart it was the right decision, but it weighed heavily. I dissolved into tears and could not sleep. A week later Malcolm died peacefully and with dignity at home, tended by familiar hands and voices and, at the very end, physically cradled by his encircling family, including the young grandchildren.

The overwhelming sense of relief and release at Malcolm's death was tangible in all of us. But it actually got in the way of my grieving properly and it was over a year later that I hit rock-bottom, physically and emotionally, with bereavement shock. Commonly experienced by long-term carers, support for delayed bereavement should also be on our agenda.

My view in a nutshell? Holistic supportive care, given by properly trained family carers and/or staff with ready access to informed professional advice and offered with love, creates quality of life for both people with dementia and their carers.

Reference

1. Stokes G (2008). *And still the music plays*. London: Hawker Publications.

Chapter 5

Offering supportive care in dementia: reflections on the PEACE programme

Joseph W. Shega and Greg A. Sachs

Conceptual challenges and the US experience

With life expectancy in industrialized nations continuing to rise and age representing the biggest risk factor for the development of cognitive impairment, the prevalence of dementia is expected to increase to epidemic proportions [1]. In the US, an estimated 4 million persons have dementia and that number is expected to grow to 16 million by 2030 [2]. Dementia is a devastating illness that is characterized by gradual cognitive and functional decline as well as behavioural and psychological symptoms [3]. Since most etiologies of dementia are slowly progressive, with a median survival of 4 to 6 years after diagnosis, losses accumulate over time [4]. Also, multiple morbidities often co-exist, such as arthritis, heart disease, diabetes, and peripheral vascular disease, each of which can be associated with additional physical and psychological symptoms [5]. As the disease enters the end stage, patients are bed-bound, mostly non-verbal, and completely dependent upon others for care. Given the cognitive and functional changes along with a high symptom burden, ample opportunities exist to improve patient and family care through medical, psychological, social, and spiritual interventions. This approach is the cornerstone of supportive care, which through its integration into the ongoing medical management of persons with dementia, offers the opportunity to alleviate suffering and improve the quality of life of patients and caregivers.

Several barriers emerge to incorporating supportive care into the management of persons with dementia, particularly towards the end of life [6]. First, families and health-care providers experience difficulty viewing dementia as a terminal illness, which significantly reduces opportunities to discuss goals of care and treatment decisions for the underlying dementia as well as for comorbid conditions. Second, the time course of the disease is protracted, which compounds the difficulty of trying to identify when someone is 'dying.' Third, downturns in people with dementia, such as an infection, have treatments that are not viewed as burdensome and are usually effective. Physicians often struggle not to offer antibiotics as a 'curative' measure, whereas families have a difficult time declining 'standard' therapy. Fourth, as language and memory decline, the assessment and management of symptoms becomes less straightforward and necessitates additional input from families as well as direct observation. Fifth, caregivers face prolonged financial and personal strain as they care for loved ones with increasing needs. Finally, the reimbursement structure for US health care promotes hospitalization and acute care services, but offers little to no support for the management of chronic illness in a person's home. Taken together, these challenges are substantial, but not insurmountable. Clearly, the likelihood of incorporating a successful supportive care programme increases if these barriers are considered and addressed in advance.

In response to the these concerns, we sought to develop an interdisciplinary disease management model for persons with dementia and their family caregivers that integrated supportive care into the ongoing 'state of the art' management of dementia from diagnosis to the end of life [7].

The programme was initially conceptualized as a primary care model within a geriatrics clinic focussing on community-dwelling older adults with cognitive impairment. The objective was to enhance patient's and caregiver's quality of life through improved symptom assessment and management, mitigate functional decline, and delineate current and future health care wishes for patients. Caregivers benefited from: educational opportunities to understand the disease process better; attention to their psychological well-being; and connections being made to local, state, and federal resources, including services offered through community and professional organizations. The PEACE model, Palliative Excellence in Alzheimer Care Efforts, served as a demonstration project on the feasibility and preliminary efficacy of such an approach. While initially conceived and developed in the outpatient setting, we believe the concept is adaptable to other care settings (i.e. assisted living, nursing home, acute care, and health systems).

Description of the programme

The clinic setting and staff

The PEACE programme was conducted at a single clinical site, the Windermere Senior Health Center, located on the South side of Chicago approximately one mile from the University of Chicago Hospitals. At the time, the clinic provided primary care to approximately 2,200 older adults, of which about 500 patients had an underlying dementia diagnosis. The average age of the patient population was 80 years, about two-thirds were women and two-thirds were African–Americans. Caregivers, with patient's agreement, were strongly encouraged to attend clinic appointments.

The staff provided an interdisciplinary team approach to care. Clinic staff members consisted of nursing (a mid-level nurse practitioner, a full-time nurse, and two nursing assistants), social work (full-time on site), and nine geriatric fellowship-trained physicians. Physicians, acting as primary care providers, participated in the majority of routine clinic visits and were accessible by phone 24 hours a day. Other disciplines available onsite included neurology, geriatric psychiatry, a neuropsychologist, a nutritionist, ophthalmology, audiology, dentistry, and therapy services (physical, occupational, and speech). Patient care was co-ordinated mainly through the geriatricians, with close involvement of the other disciplines, particularly social work. This approach differs from many models of geriatric care in that nurse practitioners or physician assistants were not the 'gatekeepers' or designated co-ordinators of care. The advantages of this approach are that it is similar to how other primary care clinics operate, increasing the likelihood of programme transportability, as well as being more likely to lead to changes in the attitudes of physicians. The latter point is particularly relevant as one of the reasons often cited for the failure of the SUPPORT intervention was that it may have lacked sufficient strength to lead to changes in physician behaviour [8].

The health system was ideal to incorporate this model across care settings as it is confined to a limited number of facilities. Patients generally used the University of Chicago Hospitals for acute care needs and the geriatricians provide ongoing support and direction to patients, families, and hospital physicians during inpatient stays. Also, the geriatricians practised at two nearby nursing homes in the community so that patients who had needs requiring skilled attention post-hospitalization were able to continue their care with clinic physicians. Finally, we partnered with select home care agencies and home hospice programmes to further integrate the PEACE approach.

The PEACE intervention

The PEACE programme was initially funded through a grant by the Robert Wood Johnson Foundation as part of the Promoting Excellence in End-of-Life Care initiative. The project, a disease management model for persons with dementia, incorporated supportive care into ongoing medical management. Though the programme benefited from funding that provided research personnel to conduct patient and caregiver interviews every 6 months for 2 years, the basic principles of the programme can be integrated into any clinical setting (see Table 5.1). The PEACE programme was delivered concurrently with primary care in a geriatrics clinic. A formal control group was not included as PEACE was designed as a demonstration project examining the feasibility of integrating a supportive care approach as well as exploring the potential benefits of the programme. The data gathered from the patient and caregiver interviews also serve as benchmarks for quality care among persons with dementia.

Patient and family members were recruited by direct physician referral. Verbal consent was required and obtained from the patient and caregiver, or if the patient lacked decision-making capacity, caregiver consent with patient assent sufficed. Face-to-face interviews with trained research assistants were conducted at study entry, and every 6 months thereafter, for the duration of the study. The interviews with patients and caregivers occurred separately, and each encounter lasted between 15 and 30 minutes. To optimize continued participation of dyads, interviews were co-ordinated so that many occurred on the same day as routine clinic visits; some were conducted in the homes of patients at the request of patient or family. Target enrollment for the PEACE study was 150 patient-caregiver dyads. As part of the programme's evaluation, after-death interviews were conducted with caregivers of PEACE participants. Non-PEACE clinic patients with a

Table 5.1 Elements of a supportive care programme and potential role of interdisciplinary team (IDT) members

Domain	Approach to integration into routine care	Interdisciplinary team members
Physical and psychological symptoms	Automated telephone survey prior to clinic visit Symptom screen while waiting for an appointment	Nurse, Physician
Advance care planning	Periodic chart review Incomplete plans result in dedicated clinic visit to discuss options	Nurse Physician Social worker
Education on disease process	Identify and educate patient and family on observed deterioration Review anticipated changes over time Provide relevant stage-specific reading material	Nurse Physician Social Worker
Community resources	Review of caregiver needs Assessment of strain and depression Identify relevant social networks	Nurse Social Worker
Coordination of care	Develop relationships with dependable agencies (i.e. home care, nursing home, hospice) Educate dyads on potential events (i.e. falls, incontinence, pneumonia, feeding tube)	Nurse Physician
Patient-family centred care	Encourage caregivers to attend clinic appointments Promote shared decision making when appropriate	Nurse Physician Social Worker
Hospice Services	Aware of enrollment guidelines for dementia Encourage families to consider hospice	Nurse Physician Social Worker

clinical diagnosis of dementia, who received care at the clinic and died during the study period, were also interviewed and used as a comparison group.

During the routine clinic visits, all clinicians were asked to continue to provide ongoing comprehensive primary care, but also to incorporate a palliative care philosophy for patients with dementia. Attempts were made to incorporate the following domains:

1 Physical and psychological symptoms (patient's most bothersome symptom, pain, depression, agitation, depression, and strain in the caregiver)

2 Advance care planning with family and patient (if still capable)

3 Education about disease process, including that dementia is a life-defining, eventually fatal illness for which supportive and palliative care takes on increasing roles with disease progression

4 Connections to community resources for both direct care and structured programmes (formal caregiver programmes, senior centre day programmes, support groups for patients and families, Alzheimer's Association programmes, and other services)

5 Co-ordination of care with an interdisciplinary team led by a clinical nurse specialist

6 Patient-family-centered care

7 Encouragement to use hospice services for end-stage patients.

Again, this approach was provided for all patients with a diagnosis of dementia at all stages of the disease. The emphasis of individual domains varied depending upon stated and uncovered needs during the clinical encounter with patients and caregivers.

The data collection elements for patient and caregiver research interview are summarized in Table 5.2. In addition, basic demographic information was gathered for patients and caregivers, and questions asked about the use of psychoactive medication in the caregivers, the quality of medical care, and about advance directives for patients.

Table 5.2 Data collection elements for patient and caregivers in the PEACE study

Domain	Data Collection Elements	Reference Number
Patient Pain	7-point verbal descriptor scale: right now and average day	9
	Checklist of non-verbal pain indicators	19
Patient most bothersome symptom	In the past week what symptom has been the most bothersome	10
Patient depression	Geriatric Depression Scale	11
Patient behaviours	Cohen-Mansfield Agitation Inventory	15
	Revised Memory and Behavioral Problem Checklist	16
Patient function	Katz Activity of Daily Living	17
	Instrumental Activity of Daily Living	18
	Functional Assessment Staging of Alzheimer's Disease	21
Patient cognition	Folstein Mini-mental state exam	12
Quality of medical care	Dartmouth atlas	10
Patient comorbidity	Charlson's weighted index of comorbidity	20
Caregiver depression	Beck Depression Inventory	14
Caregiver strain	Caregiver Strain Index	13

Directly after the clinical interview with the patient, interviewers completed the checklist of non-verbal pain indicators [19]. Patient chart review provided additional demographics, a current medication list, a weighted index of comorbidity, [20] a medical complications checklist, and the Functional Assessment Staging (FAST) scale [21].

For patients who died during the study period, structured after-death interviews were conducted with caregivers over the telephone. The conversation typically lasted 20 to 25 minute and used an interview instrument adapted from the Toolkit of Instruments to Measure End-of-Life Care [10]. Information collected during the interview included patient and caregiver demographics (for non-PEACE patients where these were not collected previously), patient preference for location of death, actual location of death, caregiver satisfaction with patient care, caregiver assessment of the patient's pain and of the most bothersome symptom in the last 2 weeks of life, and whether the patient was enrolled in hospice at the time of death.

Soon after the research interviews, the nurse specialist reviewed the information gathered by both the patient and the caregiver encounters to identify care needs. The medical record was also reviewed to determine if the needs uncovered in the research interview were addressed in the clinical encounter. Through this process, unmet needs were identified and discussed with the interdisciplinary team. The team subsequently developed a revised plan of care, which was executed by the appropriate discipline. For example, if the patient reported a high level of depression during the research interview and it was not uncovered during the clinical encounter, the nurse specialist would identify this as an unmet need that would be discussed in the interdisciplinary team. The team recommendations, such as starting an anti-depressant, would be followed up by a phone call to the patient and/or caregiver. In this case, the clinical nurse specialist would talk about the patient's depression and review treatment options. Alternatively, caregivers reporting higher levels of strain would lead to a referral to the social worker to explore some of the reasons for elevated stress, offer a tailored approach to improve coping skills and self-health, and facilitate referrals to local support groups and agencies to assist with patient care needs.

Given that one goal of the programme was to match patient and caregiver needs with available resources, lack of insurance coverage is one barrier that often precludes potentially helpful palliative interventions. Since one needed to be over the age of 65 to receive care at the clinic, all patients were Medicare eligible, the federally sponsored health-care programme for older adults. Health-care providers used available Medicare benefits, but incorporated supportive care principles as much as possible. For instance, an older adult with dementia who fell and developed an acute painful vertebral fracture might be admitted to the hospital for pain control. Patients could access Medicare to cover hospital expenses, where clinic physicians worked with hospital specialists to provide pain control, without sacrificing cognition or further functional decline. Subsequently, the patient could be transferred to a skilled care facility also covered under Medicare. These facilities provide intensive rehabilitative services, wound care for multiple high stage sores, parenteral therapies such as antibiotics, and the care of new feeding tubes. Given that our clinic physicians were on staff at the two most frequently used local nursing homes, we had direct oversight of most patient's care plans and were able to ensure ongoing symptom control as well as physical and occupational therapy to maximize patient independence. Lastly, once the patient was ready for discharge to home, home care services could be initiated. For a typical patient, it might include a home nurse coming in twice a week for several weeks to monitor the patient on a new medication regime and rehabilitative therapy to ensure patient safety and appropriate use of devices intended to assist the person at home.

Medicare also covers outpatient services, such as practitioner clinic visits (physician, nursing, and social work), outpatient therapy services (physical, occupational, and speech therapy), and some adaptive equipment. At the time, Medicare did not yet cover prescriptions. In addition to

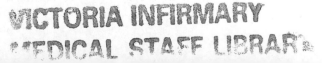

routine or urgent care visits with physician and nurses, patients and families were encouraged to meet with social workers to explore advance care planning further or discuss the availability of community resources.

Better utilization of community resources represented another focus of PEACE. These programmes offered opportunities for formal and informal education, socialization, and direct patient care if eligibility requirements were met. The PEACE programme was initially implemented in the Chicagoland area and benefited from the availability of city, county, state, federal, and private agency programmes. For patients that met income eligibility, formal caregivers were available for several hours a week Monday to Friday. Adult day care programmes provided a more structured and social venue for dementia patients. The local chapter of the Alzheimer's Association offered support groups for patients and caregivers with content reflective of the patient's stage of illness. Community centres and local churches provided additional resources and opportunities for socialization for patients and families.

Another goal of the programme was to improve end-of-life care through greater use of hospice services. In the United States, persons enrolled in hospice programmes must have an estimated life expectancy of 6 months or less. Two physicians must certify that a patient meets the prognosis criteria, usually the patient's primary care physician and hospice physician. Guidelines have been developed to help physicians determine when patients with a non-cancer diagnosis such as dementia have a life expectancy of 6 months or less. The criteria are as follows: functional dependency (unable to walk, bathe, or dress without assistance, urinary and faecal incontinence, and inability to speak more than 6 intelligible words a day) and a severe comorbid condition within the last 6 months (aspirations pneumonia, urinary tract infection, sepsis, recurrent fever after antibiotics, or multiple progressive stage 3 or 4 pressure ulcers) [22]. Hospice provides interdisciplinary care (nursing, social work, chaplains, therapy, nutrition, and physicians) in the patient's home (or nursing home) with the support of family. The benefit also includes medical equipment, medications for symptom control, and periodic respite services. A person can remain on hospice for longer than 6 months as long as the patient continues to meet prognostic eligibility criteria and decline is evident from the previous certification period, 90 days for the first 6 months and every 60 days thereafter.

Findings from PEACE

General results

Target enrollment of 150 patient-caregiver dyads was obtained and two years of follow-up was completed. Almost all patient-caregiver dyads approached to enter the study agreed to participate. The average age of the patient was 82.1 years with 75% being female and 82% being African-American. The majority of participants lived with another person, usually a spouse or close relative with only 16% living alone. The majority of caregivers were female (77%) and African-American (79%).

At the baseline interview, 97% of the patients and 93% of the caregivers reported receiving the best medical care possible. Approximately 75% of the patients report overall care as excellent or very good, compared to 81% of caregivers. All patients and 96% of the caregivers reported confidence in the health care team. These findings persisted throughout the subsequent research interviews. Taken together, patients and caregivers were positive about incorporating a supportive care approach to their health care.

Medication use

One important outgrowth of the PEACE study was the development of an approach to medication management. The model sought to provide clinicians with a framework to evaluate the appropriateness of medication in persons with advanced illness [23]. Consideration of the following domains helped providers to determine whether to recommend to continue or discontinue a specific pharmacologic therapy: a patient's remaining life expectancy, time until actual therapeutic benefit, the goals of medical care, and treatment targets (symptom management, life prolongation, prevention of morbidity or mortality, maintenance of function or cure from an acute illness). This approach provides a practical method to guide patients and families on whether to stop pharmacologic therapies that are no longer congruent with the established plan of care.

This model was subsequently incorporated into a project aimed at identifying appropriate medication use for patients with advanced dementia [24]. Each geriatrician in the PEACE study evaluated a comprehensive list to determine the appropriateness of each pharmacological agent in this population. Through a modified Delphi process, consensus was reached on which category each therapy fitted into: never appropriate, rarely appropriate, sometimes appropriate, and always appropriate. The results were subsequently applied to a small sample of 34 nursing home patients to evaluate medication use relative to the panel's recommendations. Patients were taking an average of 6.5 medications with 6 patients taking 10 medications or more daily. Consensus was reached on 69 of 81 therapies taken by patients. Of the 222 total medications prescribed, 46% were in a category other than always appropriate. Also, 29 % of the patients (10/34) were taking a medication classified as never appropriate. This preliminary study suggests consensus on medication appropriateness can be reached and that interventions are needed to decrease polypharmacy in patients with advanced illness.

Non-cancer pain

One major focus of PEACE was physical and psychological symptoms. Given this, PEACE provided an opportunity to understand non-cancer pain better in patients with dementia. In fact, this was one of the first studies to examine the prevalence of pain in community-dwelling persons with dementia comprehensively [25–27]. All PEACE patients and their caregivers were asked about patient pain 'right now' and 'on an average day.' We found that over a third of patients in PEACE reported pain 'right now' and almost half reported pain 'on an average day.' This study also examined the congruence between self and caregiver reports of patient pain and identified factors associated with non-congruence of reports. Similar to the cancer literature, caregivers report more pain than patients. Importantly, few caregivers overlooked moderate or greater patient pain.

The PEACE study also recorded the use of over-the-counter and prescription medication based upon caregiver report and chart review. As a result, we were able to examine pain management in this vulnerable population. We found that over half of persons who reported pain 'on an average day' did not report analgesic use. Of those patients who reported moderate intensity pain or higher, few patients were taking the medications currently recommended by the American Geriatrics Society guidelines for the evaluation and treatment of persistent pain [9]. Importantly, patients defined as having insufficient analgesia were more likely to have severe cognitive impairment and functional impairment. This highlights the importance of the need for quality improvement initiatives aimed at improving pain assessment and treatment in persons with dementia (see Chapter 14 in this volume).

Caregiving experience

The PEACE programme provided an opportunity to examine the predictors of strain experienced by caregivers of community-dwelling patients with dementia while enrolled in a palliative care programme. Identifying and managing caregiver strain has recently become more important as studies have found higher levels of strain associated with higher mortality compared to less strained caregivers. In our study, caregiver strain was measured overall and consisted of three factors: adjustment or role strain, personal strain, and emotional strain [28]. The identification of patient behavioural problems was associated with all types of caregiver strain. The caregiver's perception of lack of support from the health care team was associated with personal and emotional strain, whereas higher income predicted greater role strain. Finally, functional limitations of patients were associated with role and personal strain. Taken together, caregivers experienced substantial strain. Clinicians ought to try to identify sources of strain to intervene more effectively.

Symptom assessment

Given that research interviews with dementia patients and caregivers were conducted around the same time (usually the same day), we could elicit whether concerns identified in the research interview were actually discussed during the clinical encounter [29]. We chose to focus on the caregiver's report of the most bothersome symptoms in advanced dementia patients to serve as an initial benchmark to the programme's overall success in addressing care concerns. Through chart review we established that geriatricians documented 84% of the most bothersome symptoms and 70% of the second most bothersome symptoms during the clinical encounter. While we cannot assume documentation of an issue that equates to improvements in care, acknowledgement of a symptom is a necessary first step in the process. The most frequent bothersome symptoms were those related to pain, memory problems, behavioral problems, changes in mood, functional dependency, and gait impairment.

Hospice enrollment

Another outcome of the PEACE study was a better understanding of the role of hospice in the care of persons dying of dementia in the community [30]. A total of 31 (or 21%) of PEACE participants died during the two-year study period and an after-death interview was conducted two to six months later. In addition to caregivers of PEACE patients, caregivers of non-PEACE patients who died with a diagnosis of dementia during the same period completed an after-death interview. A total of 152 PEACE and non-PEACE dementia patients died during the study period; caregivers of 135 patients (89%) agreed to participate in the study. Of the 135 caregivers who participated in the telephone interview, 58 (43%) reported that the patient had been enrolled in a hospice programme in the last weeks of life, while 77 (57%) were not. The high rate of hospice participation in our clinic contrasts to the estimated 10% enrollment rate nationally for patients dying from dementia. Notably, this occurred in a predominately African-American population that has historically low rates of hospice use.

Persons enrolled in hospice were significantly more likely to die in their location of choice and less likely to die in the hospital compared to non-enrollees. This is particularly noteworthy because studies that have examined patients' wishes about end-of-life care consistently report dying at home and out of the hospital as an important goal. Also, compared to non-enrollees, caregivers of hospice enrollees were more likely to rate patient care as excellent or very good. However, approximately 50% of caregivers of hospice enrollees and non-enrollees reported patient pain, on average, at a moderate intensity or higher in the last two weeks of life. In short, patients dying with dementia in hospice care had improvements in several meaningful outcomes compared to those with routine care.

In summary, the PEACE programme integrated supportive care into the ongoing management of persons with dementia and their families. Through the process, supportive care facilitated dialogue about medication appropriateness, attention to physical symptoms, and promoted hospice utilization. Also, the project underscored the importance of monitoring the caregiver's well being and developing interventions to improve his or her condition.

Lessons learned

Reflecting on the PEACE programme, the lessons we learned fell into the following broad categories: patient, caregiver, and health system issues.

Occasionally, participants would grow impatient during the research interview owing to the length of the instruments used to assess the domains of interest. Many of the tools currently available for patient and caregiver assessment come from specific disciplines, such as geriatrics, dementia care, or palliative care. Even though they have been extensively validated for research purposes, many of these instruments are often too narrow in focus and lengthy for use in routine clinical care. If such assessments are going to be integrated into busy clinical practice, other than using measures that lack established validity, researchers need to determine if shortened versions or select subscales of standard instruments might be suitable.

We believe the PEACE approach improved patient care through the identification and management of unmet needs. However, our process depended heavily on the expertise and judgment of the clinical nurse specialist. No uniform standard was developed to determine when a symptom or need reached a threshold to warrant a team intervention. We strongly advocate that future attempts to integrate this model of care delineate clinically relevant cut-off points to trigger an action plan. Using this approach, 'triggers' could be activated in real time so that the team can address the issues and modify the care plan during the clinical encounter. In the example of caregiver stress, a trigger could be initiated once scores on the screening tool reached a predetermined threshold or displayed a meaningful change from the previous visit. This approach is particularly attractive with the increasing availability of the electronic medical record; so that once a threshold is reached, an automatic message could be generated and forwarded to care providers. Similar approaches have been incorporated into other settings. Many cancer centres conduct automated telephone interviews with patients days before their scheduled appointment. The results of the survey are transmitted to the health-care team so that they have a 'heads up' on some of the issues that will need to be addressed during the clinical encounter.

Another lesson concerned the importance of the inclusion of protocols. The care provided to PEACE subjects was fairly uniform as two nurse specialists worked side by side in one geriatric primary care clinic. Also, as described in the clinic setting section, patients benefited from ongoing contact with clinic care providers in other care settings, including the acute care hospital and nursing home. As such, care was generally provided in a uniform and co-ordinated fashion. However, the lack of inclusion of protocols limits the reproducibility of the programme and its direct dissemination. While the principles of the model can still be incorporated into any health system, the specific details of the interventions implemented by the nurse specialists remain ill-defined and not easily replicated. Future work will develop protocols and educational materials that incorporate the domains of interest. These protocols need to be rigorously tested to determine the feasibility of their actual use and effectiveness in clinical care. For example, patients identified with under-treated pain might prompt the use of a pain management protocol. This protocol could be developed in line with the American Geriatrics Society's pain management guidelines, but in order to ensure the appropriateness of its use, its effectiveness would need to be evaluated in an actual clinical setting in persons with dementia.

Family caregivers frequently reported high levels of strain and depression. The team worked hard to match caregiver needs with available resources, including educational efforts, support groups, community services, and respite care. One roadblock occasionally encountered was the unavailability of formal caregiver hours sponsored by local agencies owing to income requirements. Families of moderate means may have too many resources to qualify for these programmes, but not enough actually, to afford to pay for the necessary hours privately. At the same time, families qualified for services such as respite care, but despite repeated attempts, were unwilling to take advantage of the benefit.

Finally, the health system itself limited our ability to integrate supportive care better into the ongoing management of persons with cognitive impairment and their families. For instance, to be eligible for hospice services in the United States, a person must have a life expectancy of six months or less. Hospice programmes usually determine eligibility by applying the National Hospice and Palliative Care Organizations 1996 Medical Guidelines for Determining Prognosis in Select Non-cancer Diseases [22]. The adopted criteria for dementia do a poor job of predicting a survival of 6 months or less so that a notable number of enrollees live longer than six months [31]. While hospice enrollment beyond this point provides needed support for patients and caregivers, as the proportion of enrollees that survive beyond six months increases, so does the likelihood of regulatory scrutiny. As a result, hospices feel pressure to discharge patients who live longer than six months, yet meet eligibility criteria. At the time of discharge, families are left scrambling trying to replicate the comprehensive services provided by hospice. Innovative federally sponsored programmes are needed to try to care for this population better. For instance, a benefit may be created that if the patients and families goals are comfort care and one's life expectancy is less than two years, a hospice is paid a slightly lower daily rate. As such, overall resource utilization would in all likelihood be less (compared to cancer patients), yet lengths of hospice stays (and their benefits) would be considerably longer. Using this approach, the goals of care and health care needs would be better matched, hopefully resulting in improved care and decreased total costs.

Future directions

Additional efforts are needed to develop supportive care models that can be effectively integrated into health systems. At the same time, research is critical to evaluate the effectiveness of these models compared to routine care in improving the outcomes of persons with dementia and their caregivers. These models need to be easily replicable and feasible for integration in an array of health care settings. Additional approaches might include the evaluation of a resource line, case managers, or collaborative care between specialty clinics and primary care. In the end, we believe the further integration of supportive care into the ongoing management of persons with dementia can reduce symptom burden, increase advance care planning, heighten patient and caregiver awareness of the disease process, strengthen the coordination of care, and enhance the use of hospice programmes. These steps serve to mitigate some of the burden persons with progressive cognitive loss and their loved ones face over many years.

Acknowledgements

Funding for this book chapter came in part from a career development award from the National Palliative Care Research Center and the National Institute on Aging K23AG029815 (P.I. Joseph Shega).

References

1. Evans DA, Scherr PA, Smith LA, Albert MS, Funkenstein HH (1990). The east Boston Alzheimer's disease registry. *Aging*, 2(3), 298–302.

2. Leisi H, Scherr P, Bienias J, Bennett D, Evans D (2003). Alzheimer's disease in the US population: prevalence estimates using the 2000 census. *Arch Neurol*, **60**(8), 1119–1122.

3. Dubois B, Feldman HH, Jacova C, *et al.* (2007). Research criteria for the diagnosis of Alzheimer's disease: revising the NINCDS-ADRDA criteria. *Lancet Neuro.*, **6**(8), 734–746.

4. Walsh JS, Welch HG, Larson EB (2000). Survival of outpatients with Alzheimer-type dementia. *Ann Intern Med*, **113**, 429–434.

5. Bynum JP, Rabins P, Weller W, Niefeld M, Anderson GF, Wu AW (2004). The relationship between a dementia diagnosis, chronic illness, medicare expenditures, and hospital use. *J Am Geriatr Soc*, **52**, 187–194.

6. Sachs GA, Shega JW, Cox-Hayley D (2004). Barriers to excellent end-of-life care for patients with dementia. *J Gen Int Med*, **19**, 1057–1063.

7. Shega JW, Levin A, Hougham GW, *et al.* (2003). Palliative excellence in Alzheimer care efforts (PEACE): a program description. *J Palliat Med*, **6**, 315–320.

8. SUPPORT Principle Investigators (1995). A controlled trial to improve care for seriously ill hospitalized patients: the study to understand prognosis and preferences for outcomes and risks of treatments (SUPPORT). *JAMA*, **274**, 1591–1598.

9. AGS Panel on Persistent Pain in Older Persons (2002). The management of persistent pain in older persons. *J Am Geriatr Soc*, **50**, 1–20.

10. Center to Improve the Care of the Dying, Toolkit of Instruments to Measure End of Life. Available at: http://www.gwu.edu/~cicd/toolkit/toolkit.htm. [Accessed on February 14, 2009].

11. Yesavage JA, Brink TL, Rose TL, *et al.* (1982). Development and validation of a geriatric depression screening scale: a preliminary report. *J Psychiatr Res*, **17**, 27.

12. Folstein M, Folstein S, McHugh P (1975). Mini-mental state: a practical method for grading the cognitive state of patients for the clinician. *J Psychiatr Res*, **12**, 189–198.

13. Robinson BC (1983). Validation of a caregiver strain index. *J Gerontol*, **33**, 344–348.

14. Beck, AT, Steer RA. (1984). Internal consistencies of the original and revised Beck Depression Inventory. *J Clin Psychol*, **40**(6), 1365–1367.

15. Cohen-Mansfield J. (1986). Agitated behaviors in the elderly: II. Preliminary results in the cognitively deteriorated. *J Am Geriatr Soc*, **34**, 722–727.

16. Teri L, Traux P, Logsdon R, Uomoto J, Zarit S, Vitaliano (1997). Assessment of behavioral problems in dementia: the revised memory and behavioral problems checklist. *Psychol* Aging, **7**(4), 622–631.

17. Katz S, Ford AB, Moskowitz RW., *et al.* (1963). Studies of illness in the aged. The index of ADL: a standardized measure of biological and psychological function. *JAMA*, **185**, 914–919.

18. Lawton MP, Brody EM. (1969). Assessment of older people: Self-maintaining and instrumental activities of daily living. *Gerontologist*, **9**, 179–186.

19. Feldt K. (2000). The Checklist of Nonverbal Pain indicators. *Pain Manag Nurs*, **1**(1), 13–21.

20. Charlson ME, Pompei P, Ales KL, MacKenzie CR (1987). A new method of classifying prognostic comorbidity in longitudinal studies: development and validation. *J Chronic Dis*, **40**, 373–383.

21. Reisberg B (1988). Functional assessment staging (FAST). *Psychopharmacol Bull*, **24**, 653–659.

22. Stuart B (1999). The NHO medical guidelines for non-cancer disease and local medical review policy: hospice access for patients with diseases other than cancer. *Hosp J*, **14**, 139–154.

23. Holmes HM, Hayley DC, Alexander GC, Sachs GA (2006). Reconsidering medication appropriateness for patients late in life. *Arch Int Med*, **166**(6), 605–609.

24. Holmes HM, Sachs GA, Shega JW, Hougham GW, Cox-Hayley D, Dale W (2008). Integrating palliative medicine into the care of persons with advanced dementia: identifying appropriate medication use. *J Am Geriatr Soc*, **56**(7), 1306–1311.

25. Shega JW, Hougham GW, Stocking CB, Cox-Hayley D, Sachs GA (2004). Pain in community dwelling persons with dementia: frequency, intensity, and congruence between patient and caregiver report. *J Pain Symptom Manag*, **28**(6), 585–592.

26. Shega JW, Hougham GW, Stocking CB, Cox-Hayley D, Sachs GA (2005). Factors associated with self and caregiver report of pain among community dwelling persons with dementia. *J Palliat Med*, **8**(3), 567–575.

27. Shega JW, Hougham GW, Stocking CB, Cox-Hayley D, Sachs GA (2006). Management of non-cancer pain in community-dwelling persons with dementia. *J Am Geriatr Soc*, **54**, 1892–1897.

28. Diwan S, Hougham G, Sachs GA (2004). Strain experienced by caregivers of dementia patients receiving palliative care: findings from the palliative excellence in Alzheimer care efforts (PEACE) program. *J Palliat Med*, **7**(6), 797–807.

29. Garrett S, Cox-Hayley D, Hougham G, Sachs GA (2006). To what extent do geriatricians document the most bothersome symptoms of patients with advanced dementia. *J Am Geriatr Soc*, **54**, 1563–1566.

30. Shega JW, Hougham GW, Stocking CB, Cox-Hayley D, Sachs GA (2008). Patients dying with dementia: experience at the end of life and impact of hospice care. *J Pain Symptom Manag.*, **35**(5), 499–507.

31. Luchins DJ, Hanrahan P, Murphy K (1997). Criteria for enrolling dementia patients in hospice. *J Am Geriatr Soc*, **45**, 1054–1059.

Chapter 6

Services for younger adults with dementia

Bob Barber and Helen Cooper

Introduction

This chapter focusses on the impact of dementia on working age adults and their families. Dementia at any age has a significant impact on life expectancy, health, functioning, and family life. Each generation and age group will experience the illness from a different perspective. Correspondingly, needs will vary and ideally this will be reflected in the planning and provision of services, though arguably the core elements of good clinical care in dementia are ultimately independent of age.

There is a limited evidence base to draw upon to evaluate the components of good clinical practice and supportive care. The main focus of services to date has been to address the diagnostic needs of patients and their community-based management, with palliative care and end-of-life issues being less well developed and researched.

The chapter is organized in two parts. The first part aims to provide an overview of the clinical and service issues facing younger patients, their carers, and professionals as highlighted in the literature, particularly where these deviate from those faced by older people. The second part draws upon the local experience of a service and its evaluation, supplemented by personal comments, to try to identify the aspects valued by patients and their family, which in turn could contribute to a model of supportive care. This section has been co-written by Dr. Helen Cooper, the wife and carer of a patient who developed dementia.

Overview of clinical and service issues

Epidemiology and dementia sub-types

Young onset dementia accounts for just over 2% of all people with dementia in the UK [1]. There are at least 15,000 people with young onset dementia, compared to around 700,000 with late onset dementia (i.e. onset after the age of 65 years). Dementia before the age of 40 years is rare and the majority of younger patients will be in the age range of 50 plus at onset. Compared to older patients, young onset dementia is relatively more common in men and people from black and ethnic groups.

The aetiology of dementia can differ in younger people compared to older people. As summarized in Box 6.1, the diversity of illnesses causing dementia can make the diagnostic assessment and management complex and at times uncertain and prolonged. Genetic risk factors, though not common, are relevant in a number of the conditions listed in Box 6.1, but routine genetic counselling and testing is primarily reserved for patients at risk of Huntington's disease. Individuals will require a great deal of support and information in order to be able to consent to presymptomatic, confirmatory or preimplantation genetic testing for the disease.

Box 6.1 Diagnoses in younger people with dementia [2]

Diagnosis	Frequency
Alzheimer's disease	34%
Frontotemporal dementia	12%
Vascular dementia	18%
Alcohol-related dementia	10%
Dementia with Lewy bodies	7%
Heterogeneous mix including: progressive supra-nuclear palsy, cortico-basal degeneration, multiple sclerosis, HIV-related, prion diseases, Huntington's disease, dementia related to learning disability such as Down's syndrome	19%

Dementia occurring at an earlier age will shorten life and those with severe cognitive impairment have a greater risk of institutionalization and death compared with older individuals with the same degree of dysfunction [3]. The median duration of survival after diagnosis for the commonest forms of degenerative dementia in younger people - notably Alzheimer's disease (AD) and frontotemporal dementia (FTD) - is between 4 to 5 years, possibly shorter in FTD [4, 5]. Dementia as the root cause of death may not always be evident from death certificates. As regards the immediate cause of death, in a longitudinal sample pneumonia was the most common cause (73%), followed by malignancy (20%) and heart disease (7%) [6]. Male gender, early disease onset, concurrent physical illness, and a low mini-mental state examination score increased the likelihood of death in patients with early-onset Alzheimer's disease.

Clinical aspects

There has been a debate about whether dementia occurring at an earlier age is 'not simply different but worse' [7], but any differences between younger and older people with dementia are more likely to be a matter of degree or intensity rather than one of nature or substance. Consistent with this standpoint, certain concerns and issues have regularly featured in the literature on younger people with dementia. These issues are summarized below along with their implications for supportive care.

Diagnosis

Delays accessing a diagnostic assessment have been widely reported, with numerous accounts of patients and their families moving from 'pillar to post' before accessing the relevant services [8]. Aside from causing delays in diagnosis, it can hinder the implementation of treatment and support, adding further stress. Services have been experienced as fragmented and lacking continuity, and the provision of a specialized service has been advocated as the preferred service model to address these concerns, as discussed later.

Even where specialist clinics operate, there will be occasions when it is prudent to monitor further before making a diagnosis in order to reduce the risk of making a premature false positive diagnosis of dementia. Occasionally 'delays' in assessment can be more indicative of patient or family related factors: for example initially it can be difficult to decipher the nature of emerging changes; or some patients may defer an assessment 'fearing the worst'.

Finding the right pace and approach to facilitate diagnostic disclosure and subsequent engagement is important. Furthermore, though the diagnostic assessment is a crucial step, (helping to explain the changes and to plan treatment), it is rarely an end point, as many practical, emotional, ethical, and legal issues lie ahead.

Family

Dementia in younger people is untimely and unexpected. Patients and their families are not usually prepared for the diagnosis and its consequences, such as early retirement, loss of role, and the wider impact on future opportunities. Preparing for what follows often raises complex issues for individuals with cognitive impairment, their families and professionals. Proactive planning for the future, using for example advance directives, has intuitive and practical appeal, but gauging the timing and extent of these discussions can be difficult: ensuring people have as much ownership over their future care is clearly important, but it can take a 'crisis' for the factors that will shape the future to be revealed and experienced.

Each family will have their own practical and emotional needs. These feelings may be raw, open, and expressed; other times reactions relating to equity, justice, and blame are important but may be more masked [7].

Seeing the patients' family as a resource is essential. Invariably solutions work best when those closest to the patient are involved in plans from start to finish, especially when this allows families to retain as much control as possible.

Carers can experience high levels of stress, isolation, and at times stigma [9]. Financial and personal problems can be compounded by a carer's need to reduce or stop employment. Transitions of care from home to respite or permanent care are often times of heightened emotional stress. The tailored provision of information as well as practical and emotional support for carers will be central to management. This may be via individual sessions and/or attendance at carer groups (e.g. as provided by non-statutory services such as the Alzheimer's Society in the UK).

The illness has an impact at a different phase of the family life cycle compared to older people and individuals are more likely to have younger children. The emotional, psychological, and practical ramifications for the children are often significant and multi-layered. They may feel anxious, fearful, and distressed whilst struggling to make sense of the changes, eventually experiencing the loss of their parent. Staff can feel uncertain how best to respond, and at times liaison with child and adolescent psychiatric services can be helpful. Where risks are apparent, child protection issues will also need addressing. A framework for managing family caregiving has been proposed by Keady and Nolan [10].

Work and independence

The illness leads to underperformance at work and ultimately loss of employment. This will adversely affect current and future income and potentially increase the risk of isolation, boredom, frustration, and loss of self-esteem and role. Where necessary, advising and supporting patients on employment rights and risks as well as benefit entitlement can lead to a more satisfactory financial and personal outcome. Charitable organizations such as the Citizens Advice Bureau can be helpful (www.citizensadvice.org.uk/). Unfortunately, sometimes individuals will have been dismissed before a formal diagnosis or due process. Decline in driving skills will also need managing. In-car driving assessments can help all concerned reconcile whether it is safe to continue driving.

Clinical features

Compared to older people, younger people may experience a higher occurrence of behavioural and psychological symptoms, a more rapid progression and higher levels of dependency at an earlier stage [2, 11, 12]. Conversely, some studies suggest younger people have a greater level of insight. Generally, younger people will be more active and fitter.

Age-appropriate services

Concerns about the lack of 'age-sensitive' or 'age-appropriate' services have consistently featured in the literature. Services that are prominently used by older people, such as day care or residential care, are often seen as inappropriate and potentially stigmatizing, especially in the early stages of the illness. This can reduce their acceptability to carers who may feel an added pressure to extend the time they provide care at home.

Palliative care

The majority of younger patients with advanced dementia are likely to be cared for in settings primarily designed for and used by older people with dementia. In the UK, only a small percentage of people will remain at home until death; this will require close collaboration between the person's family and statutory services, including social, specialist, primary, and palliative care services. Most people, however, will spend the last months or years of their life in private nursing homes or a NHS continuing care facility, with varying standards of staff experience, training, and building design. It can be difficult to gauge whether a person is affected positively or negatively by being cared for in an environment predominantly shared with older patients.

Most palliative care services developed for younger patients have focused on the needs of patients with progressive neurological disorders such as motor neurone disease, multiple sclerosis, and most notably Huntington's disease (HD). To date, the end-of-life care in younger people with HD provides one of the closest parallels with conditions like AD and FTD. In relation to HD, a working group from the USA [13] highlighted the importance of advance directives and the anticipation of end-stage care needs, with disease progression, denial, family conflict, and clinician blind-spots potentially impeding implementation. The group advocated several priority areas for patient care in HD: autonomy; dignity; meaningful social interaction; communication; comfort; safety and order; spirituality; enjoyment, entertainment, and well-being; nutrition; and functional competence. It is highly likely that patients with other forms of advanced dementia, such as AD, will share similar issues. Indeed, it is conceivable that age-related differences diminish as dementia progresses and it follows that many of the issues facing younger people with advanced dementia will be shared with older people, as explored in this book.

Specialized services for younger people with dementia

The development of community-based dementia services for older people from the 1970s and 80s exposed the gaps in provision for younger people with dementia [2]. During the early 1990s there was growing concern regarding the quality and availability of services for younger people with dementia. Importantly, patients and their families, expressing their voice through organizations such as the Alzheimer's Society, were advocating access to a comprehensive, integrated, specialist service from diagnosis to long-term care or death [14]. This service framework, now endorsed by many national and international bodies, is essential for the delivery of supportive care and offers a number of advantages [15]:

1 Improved co-ordination, effectiveness, and age-appropriateness
2 Clearer referral and care pathways improving access and continuity
3 Framework providing diagnostic, treatment, and research clinics
4 Closer links between statutory and voluntary organizations
5 Facilitation of staff training, supervision, development, and expertise.

Most, but not all, specialized services are provided by old age psychiatry services. Their availability has increased over the last 10 years [15, 16], but provision is patchy and challenges remain.

Services for patients with co-morbidities such as learning disability, substance misuse and people from minority groups continue to be underdeveloped [16, 17], and the relatively low prevalence of dementia in younger people in general creates challenges for the commissioning and provision of local services. Furthermore, although a specialized service can provide a 'single gateway to information, advice, expertise, and appropriate care' [8], the very nature of the disorders that can cause cognitive impairment in younger patients means other medical and surgical specialities will need to be involved. As argued by Larner [18]:

> Dementia is neither a neurological nor a psychiatric disease: it is a brain disease that does not respect traditional professional boundaries. Therefore, there can be no argument that it should be managed solely by neurologists or psychiatrists. Nor is dementia a unitary, or uniform condition, as seems to be the implication of the NICE/SCIE guidance. Therefore, a truly integrated care pathway must acknowledge the input from both these disciplines, and possibly others: neuroradiology, neuropsychology, neurosurgery, geriatric medicine, clinical genetics, occupational therapy, speech and language therapy.

Services from the perspective of patients and their carers

The most valuable aspects of a service for younger people with dementia are explored further by reviewing the findings from a qualitative evaluation of a service and reflecting on a more personal account of the experiences of a carer whose husband developed Alzheimer's disease, as recorded in Box 6.2.

Evaluation of a local service

As indicated, the number of dedicated services for younger people with dementia has increased and some services are now well established [8, 11, 12]. In Newcastle upon Tyne, a service has been operating for over 10 years. The team, originally set up as a pilot service in response to local concerns raised by patients and carers, consisted of a community psychiatric nurse (CPN), occupational therapist (OT), and a social worker. Its initial aims were to provide age-sensitive care packages and intensive support for carers, to determine existing resources, to develop a future model, and to raise awareness amongst service providers.

An independent evaluation of the service was conducted over 18 months using qualitative research methodology involving clients, carers, staff, and other stakeholders [19, 20]. Overall, the service was viewed positively, but exploring insights into the reason for this appraisal by patients and their relatives revealed the central importance of the 'therapeutic relationship'. The team was perceived as trustworthy, credible, and reliable, and this essential ingredient allowed patients and their carers to feel more secure and able to share concerns. It appeared the most valuable asset of the team lay not in the provision of a specific type of intervention or therapy, but in being able to foster a therapeutic relationship: though this can take time to develop, once established it became the cornerstone for what followed. Accessibility and continuity of support was also valued and it is important not to downgrade the importance of practical support. Community teams like the one in Newcastle often only provide a limited number of services themselves, but will have a crucial role in networking, either linking families to established services or trying to source innovative, personalized care packages. The conclusion reached by the evaluation was [19, 20]:

> The model is not based on distinct pathology but on socio-cultural responses to untimely dementia. In a society that has certain expectations of people at certain ages, early onset dementia, in the way that it prevents people meeting these expectations, has a number of social and personal implications. These implications include physical, social and psychological dimensions and the corresponding model of response and care is similarly complex and broad. There is no reason why it should be exclusive to this group . . . and not extended to older people with dementia too.

Box 6.2 A carer's view on what helped most after Alzheimer's disease was diagnosed (by Helen Cooper)

In the terrible journey that life becomes helping a dear partner cope with dementia, I had more luck than most carers. Though both medical, we had ignored the early signs and B, exhausted, retired early at 61, looking well and youthful, financially secure and with children educated and independent. He was a great reader and poetry lover and soon began to write a memoir of his wartime childhood and could still enjoy all his cultural activities – but soon could do no practical things like lay the table, cook or do gardening. It took more than a year and a half to get him to a doctor, but then the investigation was full and fast with the diagnosis 'likely Alzheimer's disease'.

The team for younger people with dementia was crucial to our next years. It was close-knit, well organized, and able to share information regarding clients. But what services helped most after diagnosis?

1 Early introduction to the CPN to monitor drug treatment who was then able to visit really regularly to get to know and win the trust of patient and carer, both of whom would benefit from her expertise in the years to come.

2 Educational sessions – highly informative and introduced the social worker (who helped with finances, benefit advice, and later finding a suitable care home), Alzheimer's Society, and a carers' group, which allowed carers to meet and feel less isolated – hugely important as the illness progressed.

3 The OT ran a men's weekly day club: patients could be monitored while they had fun and it gave carers support or a break.

4 The speech therapist was only with us for a short time but important when there was early speech loss. She arranged combined sessions with another patient and we used this contact to ease B into the men's group. She also helped us gain an Enduring Power of Attorney by giving us printed advice on how to interview a patient with cognitive and speech problems for our solicitor, who then used it wisely and well.

5 The Support Group – this allowed informal feedback of what was going on with the carer and family. I benefited, as later he developed increasing visuo-spatial and mobility problems, incontinence, probably delusions, and hallucinations, leading to nightly dramas, aggression, and exhausting lack of sleep.

After hospital admission and assessment, he was admitted to a nearby five-bedroom supported living home where I could be fully involved in his daily care, in line with their ethos of client-centred support, active understanding of attachment, and the need for continuity of care. After a successful year or so there, B had a major seizure with significant after-effects, in that he had acute back pain and was 'off his feet'. Eventually, physiotherapy helped to remind B's brain how to stand. His own drive then got him walking fast! Sadly, other fits followed with the emergence of unexplained fears, making him insist on getting up at night. Loud disturbing behaviour, with his strength and insistence that he avoid the stairlift, made matters dangerous for him and the staff.

After a sad re-admission to hospital, B was admitted to a continuing care NHS home. From the outside this was a paint peeling building, but inside the care was excellent. Over one single

Box 6.2 A carer's view on what helped most after Alzheimer's disease was diagnosed *(continued)*

weekend B's named nurse achieved a relaxed, comfortable, glowing patient who was confident that he was going to be well looked after. Here are some reflections from this time:

1 While in hospital (having a posture problem with dystonia, perhaps also poor positioning in the chair that was available, as well as pain and other unknown fears) he would writhe until he was hanging over the side of the chair and clinging to its under parts – escaping from something or seeking what? Luckily, a comfortable chair was found on the first day.

2 His beard, present for over two years because of difficulty in shaving him, and now unkempt, matted, and dirty with food, was lovingly removed without leaving a mark on his skin. I wept at his 'return'.

3 His days were spent in a small lounge with two older ladies where he could listen to classical music and avoid TV soaps and jingles, which he hated.

4 Ambulant patients called in to visit or listen quietly before moving off, perhaps to the big safe garden to which they had free and easy access. Patients could be found sitting by the secretary as she worked in her office or with the cleaner in the corridor, feeling busy but safe because every staff member was part of the watchful, caring team which could allow such planned freedom. The quiet buzz of work and chat and bursts of laughter, even when things were really busy, demonstrated the stability, quiet pride, and team spirit there, where many had worked for several years.

5 The individual patient monitoring and attention to detail on the part of nursing staff, who maintained a level of 'hands-on' care in the face of burdens in the office, was obvious in the level of information shared with visiting carers and at regular patient medical reviews, where their expertise was acknowledged by the medical staff. Sadly, such exceptional teams are not valued enough. The building was to be given up, so the team was dispersed.

It was, therefore, a sad move to the modern building deemed more suitable for the palliative care of patients with dementia. The much-vaunted en-suite rooms seemed of little value and appeared to be an actual problem or danger to some ambulant patients. More important was the rapidly demonstrated excellent nursing which continued to manage his skin care, feeding, incontinence, and severe, long-standing constipation; tasks made difficult because of his neck torsion, posture problems, sometimes excessive drooling, and recurrent urinary tract infections. It was difficult to interpret facial expressions: was he in pain caused by reflux, colic, or musculoskeletal problems, or was he hallucinating or delusional? Yet still there was recognition and even moments of apparent lucidity. His seizures required ongoing control – 23 tablets per day, while also needing speech therapy for a variable swallowing impairment. Finally, distressing, prolonged, myoclonic jerks were the most difficult problem to control, but we were lucky and grateful to have the support of two of his long-term care workers at the end.

Since the initial pilot, further developments of the team and the supportive care pathway have included:

1 Involving a dedicated consultant (old age psychiatrist) to assist with medical diagnosis and treatment as well as team identity, training, continuity, integration, and inter-professional liaison

2 Creating a single point of referral to the service and linking this with a memory clinic with involvement from clinical psychology

3 Involvement of team members in the assessment clinic and a widening of roles, such as assisting in the reviews of patients receiving antidementia medications

4 Setting up additional supports including a memory support group, men's day group and carers' information group

5 Using novel forms of respite care: for example by forming links with voluntary organizations to provide short breaks at activity centres designed for people with disabilities

6 Linking with supported living homes to provide alternative forms of 24-hour care

Many challenges remain, including improving the interface between the team and other medical and psychiatric services and the development of a palliative care pathway that proactively provides greater opportunities to formulate advance decisions.

Conclusion

Younger people with dementia will inevitably share many of the same experiences as older people. But they also experience the illness in, and indeed from, a different context and perspective. Prevailing attitudes, expectations, emotions, and social beliefs will affect how the illness is experienced [7]. Services should strive to reflect these issues, and a key variable to success appears to be the quality and continuity of the 'therapeutic relationship' between staff, patients, and families. Further research and service development are required so the end-of-life issues facing younger people with dementia can be better understood and managed.

References

1. Dementia UK (2007). A report into the prevalence and cost of dementia prepared by the Personal Social Services Research Unit (PSSRU) at the London School of Economics and the Institute of Psychiatry at King's College London, for the Alzheimer's Society UK.

2. Harvey RJ (1998). *Young onset dementia: epidemiology, clinical symptoms, family burden, support and outcome.* London: Dementia Research Group.

3. Heyman A, Wilkinson WE, Hurwitz BJ, *et al* . (1987). Early-onset Alzheimer's disease: clinical predictors of institutionalization and death. *Neurology, 37*(6), 980–984.

4. Claus JJ, van Gool WA, Teunisse S *et al.* (1998). Predicting survival in patients with early Alzheimer's disease. *Dement Geriatr Cogn Disord, 9*(5), 284–293.

5. Roberson ED, Hesse JH, Rose KD *et al.* (2005). Frontotemporal dementia progresses to death faster than Alzheimer disease. *Neurology, 65*(5), 719–725.

6. Ueki A, Shinjo H, Shimode H, Nakajima T, Morita Y (2001). Factors associated with mortality in patients with early-onset Alzheimer's disease: a five-year longitudinal study. *Int J Geriatr Psychiatry, 16*(8), 810–815.

7. Tindall L, Manthorpe J (1997). Early onset dementia: a case of ill-timing. *J Mental Health, 6*(3), 237–249.

8. Williams T, Cameron I, Dearden T (1999). *From pillar to post. Early onset dementia in Leeds: prevalence, experience and service needs.* Leeds Health Authority.

9. Freyne A, Kidd N, Coen R, Lawlor BA (1999). Burden in carers of dementia patients: higher levels in carers of younger sufferers. *Int J Geriatr Psychiatry, 14*(9), 784–788.

10. Keady J, Nolan M (1999). Family caregiving and younger people with dementia: dynamics, experiences and service expectations, in Cox S, Keady J (eds). *Younger people with dementia,* pp. 203–223. London: Jessica Kingsley Publishers.

11. Ferran J, Wilson KCM, Doran, M *et al* . (1996) The early onset dementias: a study of clinical characteristics and service use. *Int J Geriatr Psychiatry*, **11**, 863–869.

12. Baldwin R, Murray M (2005). Services for younger people with dementia, in Burns A, O'Brien J, Ames D (eds). *Dementia,* pp 316–322. third ed. London: Hodder Arnold.

13. Klager J, Duckett A, Sandler S, Moskowitz C (2008). Huntington's disease: a caring approach to the end of life. *Care Manag J*, **9**(2), 75–81.

14. Alzheimer's Society (2005). Younger people with dementia an approach for the future. London: Alzheimer's Society.

15. Barber R (1997). A survey of services for younger people with dementia. *Int J of Genriatc Psychiatry*, **12**, 951–954.

16. Cantley C, Fox P, Barber R (2002). Better services for younger people with dementia? *Findings from a regional survey of service planning and development.* NHS Northern and Yorkshire Regional Office.

17. Royal College of Psychiatrists (2006). Services for younger people with Alzheimer's disease and other dementias. *Council Report CR135.* UK: Royal College of Psychiatrists.

18. Larner AJ (2007). Integrated care pathways in dementia: a challenge to National Institute for Health and Clinical Excellence/Social Care Institute for Excellence guidance. *J Integr Care Pathw,* **11**, 95–99.

19. Cantley C, Reed J, Stanley D, Clarke CL, Banwell L (2002). Services for younger people with dementia. *Dementia*, **1**(1), 95–112.

20. Reed J, Cantley C, Stanley D (2007). Younger people with dementia, in Keady J, Clarke CL, Page S (eds). *Partnerships in community mental health nursing and dementia care: practice perspectives,* p. 152–166. Buckinghamshire: Open University Press/McGraw Hill Publications.

Chapter 7

Huntington's disease and dementia

Belinda Bilney and Meg E. Morris

Introduction

Huntington's disease (HD) is an inherited neurodegenerative disorder for which there is currently no known cure. The disease is caused by an abnormally long CAG sequence on the IT15 gene on the short arm of chromosome 4 [1] which is passed to the next generation with a 50% penetrance. Disease onset usually occurs around 35–45 years of age and may be signalled by early cognitive changes that progress to dementia, voluntary and involuntary movement disorders such as bradykinesia, akinesia, postural instability, chorea, dystonia, and dysphagia, and emotional changes such as depression, aggression, apathy, and anxiety [2]. HD can be challenging for people with the disease and their families owing to the combination of dementia, movement disorders, and emotional changes. Cognitive impairments of executive function such as initiating, planning, and sequencing tasks may occur early in the disease, however orientation and insight usually remain intact. Neuropsychiatric symptoms such as anxiety, irritability, and agitation can also be early symptoms [2]. These impairments are thought to be due to early changes in the sub-cortical circuit projections of the prefrontal cortex to the caudate and thalamus. As the disease progresses and the medial prefrontal circuits are affected, symptoms of depression and apathy may present. These difficulties can adversely affect the ability to participate in work, family, and leisure activities. As HD progresses over 15–20 years, people typically become reliant upon others to assist them with self-care activities, with some people requiring residential care at a relatively young age [3].

There is currently no evidence that the rate or level of progression of HD can be altered, and there is only limited evidence to support the effectiveness of pharmacological interventions to manage symptoms such as chorea and depression [4]. Therefore, the mainstay of management of people with HD and their families is supportive care. Supportive care is an inter-professional approach to the management of the physical, cognitive, and emotional aspects of HD, providing assistance for the person with HD and their family throughout the disease. There is a growing body of research that identifies the supportive care needs of people with HD and their families [3, 5–7]. Although the supportive care needs for many individuals are high, there is little evidence of a definitive model of care that addresses needs throughout the duration of the disease. Furthermore, there is limited evidence to confirm the effectiveness of some supportive care interventions used by therapists such as gait, balance, and activity of daily living retraining [8]. This chapter synthesizes the current evidence relating to the supportive care needs for people with HD and considers how the unique aspects of HD, such as the effects on families caused by the autosomal dominant nature of disease transmission, the relatively early onset of the disease, and long disease duration, affect the provision of supportive care.

Supportive Care in HD

The supportive care needs for people with HD are complex, in part on account of the variable onset of dementia, movement, and behavioural disorders which can occur when the person is relatively young and more likely to be raising a family or working [9]. Dementia associated with HD has the potential to have a negative impact on relationships between an affected parent and their children, changing the family dynamics and increasing the likelihood of conflict within the family unit [10]. Because of dementia, movement disorders, and fatigue, the person with HD may need to reduce their work hours or discontinue paid employment [6]. As the disease progresses, the person's partner may also need to reduce their paid working hours in order to take on the role of primary carer [11]. Evaluation of the care needs for people with HD and their families highlights the challenging financial difficulties that many families with HD experience [6, 10].

Because of the autosomal dominance of HD, the effects of a family member being diagnosed with the disease can be felt across several generations [12]. People at risk of HD may have first-hand experience with dementia and other symptoms through observation of the neurological deterioration of a grandparent, parent, sibling, or other relative. Parents may be concerned about their children inheriting the disease or have feelings of guilt related to the risk of inheritance. Sometimes, unaffected siblings can experience guilt in relation to their relatives affected by HD. Offspring may have increased anxiety related to providing care for an affected parent.

Family members often take on the role of primary caregiver for people with HD [9, 12]. Because of the early onset of symptoms in comparison to other dementias, caregivers of people with HD are often young adults. The prolonged time course of the disease also means that some family members can be required to provide care for extended periods of time (15–20 years) [9]. The burden associated with caring for a person with HD can be high owing to the considerable number of hours required to provide care. For example, Pickett, Altmaier and Paulsen [9] reported caregivers spent an average of 6.9 hours per day providing care for dependents with HD. Cognitive changes that impair the person's problem-solving skills and memory, behavioural changes such as apathy and the presence of depression, can also contribute to the perception of increased caregiver burden [5, 9, 12, 13]. Some caregivers report that the presence of cognitive and behavioural changes are more likely to prevent them from continuing to provide care than symptoms related to movement disorders [14].

Some caregivers of people with HD have reported significant psychological distress, anxiety, depression, and loss of independence associated with their caring role [9]. The substantial caregiving provided by the family of a person with HD is recognized in a supportive care model, which also acknowledges that resources need to be allocated to support caregivers. Dawson *et al.* [3] described two broad areas of support for caregivers: practical and psychological support. Practical support includes access to home care and respite care provided by knowledgeable and reliable workers, the provision of equipment to assist in activities of daily living, assistance with transport to appointments and financial support [5, 6]. Psychological support includes counseling and the provision of accurate information about HD. Many caregivers also value support provided by the HD Associations and easy access to health care workers including allied health professionals.

Models of supportive care

There is limited evidence evaluating the effectiveness of supportive care for people with HD, and an absence of published guidance for standards of care [7]. Nevertheless, several authors have identified the important elements in a supportive care model [3, 5, 7]. A supportive care model needs to be flexible enough to accommodate the broad range of impairments that contribute to disability, as well as the varying levels of coping in individuals and caregivers. Ideally, the priorities for supportive care would be set by the person with HD together with their family [6]. Flexibility is also required to accommodate differences in the age of disease onset and speed of disease progression [7]. The supportive care needs of the person with HD and their family vary according to the duration and severity of the disease, for example, in the early phases of the disease care may be based on a rehabilitation model, whereas in the later stages of the disease a palliative care model may be more appropriate [3]. An inter-professional team can be beneficial for addressing the cognitive, emotional and physical impairments associated with HD [15, 16]. Comprehensive team management is argued to minimize the effects of disability, impairment, and participation restrictions on the persons' ability to participate in work, family, and social life. The team is sometimes large because of the complexity of the symptoms. Moreover, the composition of the team typically changes given that the primary impairments affecting activity and participation vary throughout the disease. The team may, for example, include a neurologist or psychiatrist with specialist knowledge of HD [17], the patient's general medical practitioner, a neurogeneticist, case manager, nurse, physiotherapist, occupational therapist, speech pathologist, dietitian, psychologist, neuropsychologist, respite care service team and staff of a long-term residential care facility [17, 18]. The team should be knowledgeable about the consequences of the disease and must be able to anticipate the changes in function that occur over the time course of the disease. They should also have a good understanding of the issues that effect people with HD and their families [19]. It can be advantageous for care to be coordinated by a case manager because the supportive care needs of people with HD usually involve many different health professions over the duration of the disease. It is essential that care does not become fragmented [7]. The case manager is responsible for initiating timely referrals, coordinating services, ensuring that the patient and the family receive timely and accurate information about the disease throughout its progression and when appropriate advocating for the patient and their family [3, 5].

Ideally, a model of supportive care for people with HD and their families should span the continuum of the disease and include care for people who are at risk of the disease yet do not know their disease status through to those at the end stages of the disease.

Supportive care for people who are at risk or pre-symptomatic

Specialized counselling from a team that could include a geneticist, neurologist, social worker, or psychiatrist is recommended for people who are at risk of HD due to the challenges around testing and potentially disclosing test results to other members of the family [20]. After the test results have been provided, counselling may continue as appropriate.

People who are pre-symptomatic may benefit from the input of a case manager or social worker to provide information about HD in both a timely and sensitive manner [3, 7]. Although it is important that health professionals provide accurate information about the disease, people with HD have identified that too much information provided soon after diagnosis can be stressful [3]. Therefore, it is important that information provided by health professionals matches the needs of the individual.

Although there is no evidence in humans yet that the progression of the disease can be altered, evidence from the HD mouse model suggests that environmental enrichment may delay the onset of cognitive and motor decline [21]. It may, therefore, be important to assist people who are pre-symptomatic to establish or maintain a healthy lifestyle. This may include assistance from a dietician to plan a healthy diet and input from a physiotherapist or exercise physiologist to design a fitness programme that includes elements of strength, endurance and balance training.

Supportive care early in the disease

In the early phase of disease progression the person with HD may have noted the onset of cognitive changes such as impairments of planning, organizing, problem solving, new learning, and attention [22, 23]. Movement disorders can also be apparent such as mild postural instability, bradykinesia, chorea, and dystonia that may affect the speed, timing, and accuracy of movements such as walking and handwriting [24–26].

The primary aim of supportive care in the early phase of HD is to continue to support a healthy lifestyle and maximize activity and participation by addressing primary and secondary impairments that may limit the persons' activity [27]. The ideal supportive care model would facilitate early access to allied health professionals for baseline assessments, intervention as required and reassessment triggered by a change in functional status [7]. The team involved in the early phase of disease progression could include a case manager responsible for the initiation and coordination of referrals, education related to the early phase of disease progression, and advocacy for the person with HD and their family. The purpose of physiotherapy in the early phase is to provide a baseline assessment of all movement disorders and identify how they affect activities including gait and balance, upper limb function, and other sport or leisure activities that may be important to the person [19, 28, 29]. The physiotherapist can also initiate a programme to prevent the secondary impairments of decreased muscle strength and cardiovascular fitness due to inactivity and encourage a healthy lifestyle programme which may include general endurance training, strengthening and balance exercises. Deficits in gait such as reduced speed, step length and cadence should be addressed with gait retraining that has an emphasis on increasing step size using attentional strategies [29] or step frequency using auditory cues [30, 31]. Postural instability during walking or turning may occur owing to delayed and prolonged latency response to postural perturbation [32, 33]. Instability can be addressed with balance retraining that includes exercises to increase readiness to respond to postural perturbations, increasing the person's attention to identify threats to balance, and education regarding falls prevention strategies such as avoiding dual tasks and reducing environmental hazards [15, 28].

Occupational therapists can also complete baseline assessments of function, including ability to carry out activities of daily living, domestic tasks, work, and driving. The assessment typically includes an evaluation of the effect of both the movement disorders and cognitive deficits on the ability to complete activities. In the early phase of the disease a home assessment may be helpful to provide advice on modifications and equipment that may be required in the future to maximize safety and independence [34]. A workplace assessment may also be useful to identify if work can be restructured to maintain meaningful paid employment for as long as possible. Capacity to drive may be impaired by cognitive deficits such as reduced attention and speed of processing, movement disorders including hypokinesia and chorea and occulomotor deficits such as impaired tracking [4]. The occupational therapist may be required to conduct on-road and off-road driving assessments so that they can make recommendations about driving capacity [35].

Assessment by the speech pathologist may include evaluation of speech intelligibility, comprehension, confrontational naming, and swallowing [36–38]. They may also work with the occupational therapist or neuropsychologist to complete a detailed assessment of cognitive function including problem solving and memory. If the person with HD or their family has noted any difficulty with swallowing, such as coughing when drinking or eating, the speech pathologist will conduct a swallowing assessment to determine their capacity to swallow food and drinks of different consistencies safely. Impairments of language and comprehension may be addressed using a rehabilitation approach [15].

Several studies have indicated that people with HD have a lower body mass index than matched healthy controls [39]. Although the pathogenesis of weight loss in people with HD is not yet clear, one possible explanation is that the daily energy requirements of a person with HD are increased due to additional energy expended during involuntary movements such as chorea [40]. Therefore, it is important that a dietitian works with the persons with HD and their families to calculate energy requirements and establish a plan to ensure that weight is maintained within a healthy range. Additional kilojoules may be required if the person with HD is participating in a strengthening or endurance exercise programme.

Because HD affects families, the person with HD may have experienced the deterioration of a close relative as the disease progresses. Counselling can be offered to support the person as they come to terms with their own disease and, if appropriate, to work with the person to make some informed decisions on how they would like their care managed in the future. Communicating how they wish their care to be managed in the future may provide some relief to families who otherwise will need to make difficult management decisions, particularly towards the end of life [3]. It is optimal to assess the person regularly to monitor for depression and, if appropriate, their medical practitioner should initiate treatment.

Supportive care for people in mid-stages

In the mid-stages of HD, the person may no longer be able to continue activities such as work and driving and may find domestic and self-care tasks such as cooking, cleaning, and dressing more difficult owing to cognitive impairments and movement disorders. Balance can be impaired during walking, turning, and reaching and falls during activity may become more frequent [41]. Walking speed may continue to slow and the walking pattern may be characterized by increased variability in both the step length and step timing [26, 42, 43]. Reach and grasp may also become more difficult due to hypokinesia and incoordination caused by the intrusion of choreic movements on normal movement [25, 44]. Cognitive changes such as impaired memory, slowed processing and inflexibility of thought may begin to impair everyday activity such as managing a budget or planning and preparing a meal. Emotional changes such as apathy, depression, or difficulty coping with change in routine may further impair the person's ability to complete everyday activities of daily living [14].

The focus of supportive care during the mid-phase of HD is on maintaining function and safety through the use of compensatory strategies and, where appropriate, regaining function using a restorative approach [27]. Caregivers may begin to find the cognitive deficits associated with HD increasingly difficult to cope with [14]. Therefore, it is essential that there are sufficient and coordinated resources provided to people with HD and their caregivers to ensure that the person with HD can continue to live in the community and not be prematurely admitted to residential care [45]. Resources may include home support services such as assistance with activities of daily living and respite services. Strategies to compensate for cognitive deficits such as a structured daily routine with written cues to prompt each task may also be of assistance and can be established with the assistance of an occupational therapist in conjunction with a speech pathologist and neuropsychologist. Fatigue may also begin to affect the person's capacity to function and this could also be addressed by structuring the daily routine to ensure that important tasks are completed before fatigue impairs performance. The occupational therapist may provide advice regarding additional equipment or home modifications that may be required to maintain independence and safety. Physiotherapy continues to address changes to gait and balance and treatment may begin to have a greater emphasis on a compensatory approach [27], such as teaching the person with HD and their caregivers how to reduce the likelihood of falls. The speech pathologist will continue to monitor the safety of swallowing and introduce strategies to reduce the risk of aspiration such as modifying the consistency of the food and providing education on behaviours to increase safety when eating [46]. They continue to monitor and initiate treatment for changes in communication due to dysarthria, pharaphasic errors, and word finding difficulty and impairment of comprehension [37, 38]. The dietitian continues to monitor weight and work in conjunction with the speech pathologist to recommend changes to diet including the use of supplements to maintain a healthy weight [47]. Supportive care during the mid-phase of the disease continues to have an emphasis on timely and appropriate education about HD and counselling as required for the person with HD and their family.

Supportive care for people in late stages

The late stages of disease progression are characterized by increasing dementia, dysphagia, weight loss, hypokinesia, and incontinence [17, 27, 47]. The focus of supportive care in the late phases of the disease is on prevention and management of complications such as chest infections and weight-loss due to dysphagia, muscle contractures and pain due to dystonia, rigidity, or immobility, injuries caused by falls, and skin breakdowns due to pressure caused by abnormal postures and immobility [17]. The occupational and physiotherapist continue to work with caregivers to ensure that the person with HD can be safely transferred and mobilized which may require a hoist and wheelchair. Physiotherapists at this stage may direct more of their time towards educating the caregivers about programmes of passive movements or positioning to maintain muscle length. They also work with the speech pathologist to achieve a posture that facilitates a safe swallow. If safe swallowing can not be maintained, then dependent on the person's advance directive percutaneous endoscopic gastrostomy (PEG) feeding may be considered [3]. However, in advanced dementia the evidence (at least in Alzheimer's and other generally late onset dementias) suggests that tube feeding does not improve nutritional status or prevent aspiration (see Chapter 28 for further discussion of this point). It is possible that tube feeding may reduce quality of life by preventing the opportunity to taste food or experience intimate human contact that occurs during hand-feeding.

As disability progresses, caregivers may find it is no longer possible to care for the person with HD at home. Ideally residential care would be provided by a team that is knowledgeable and skilled in caring for people with HD [5]. Unfortunately, there are few specialized residential care facilities for people with HD [3]. For example, Paulsen and Robinson [48] reported that many residential care facilities were reluctant to care for people with HD, which may have been due to a poor understanding of the disease and a belief that people with HD require excessive levels of care because of the cognitive and emotional deficits associated with the disease. It is important that residential care services develop their skills in managing people with HD and that consideration is given to providing an environment that is appropriate for younger people.

In the final phases of the disease, supportive care is usually directed towards a palliative care model that manages the process of dying and provides psychological support to the family [6]. Health professionals continue to work with the person with HD and their family to ensure that their prior wishes in relation to the continuation or withdrawal of treatment are carried out.

Conclusion

The needs of people with HD and their families vary throughout the duration of the disease and supportive care must be tailored to individual needs, as indicated in Table 7.1. At times, the supportive care needs are high and may require intensive input from many health professionals to ensure an appropriate level of care. The model of care for people with HD needs to be flexible so that in the early phase of the disease there is an emphasis on a functional restorative approach, which may change to a compensatory approach as the disease progresses, and to a palliative approach towards the end of life. It is essential that additional research is conducted to evaluate the effectiveness of many of the treatment strategies used by health professionals, and that this evidence is used to inform guidelines for best practice in the management of people with HD.

Table 7.1 Summary of supportive care needs through the progression of Huntington's disease

	Pre-symptomatic	Early stages of HD	Mid stages of HD	Late stages of HD
Focus of supportive care	Counselling Healthy lifestyle	Functional restorative approach	Compensatory approach	Palliative care
Cognitive impairments		Memory Planning Problem solving Organizing New learning Attention	Slowed processing Impaired memory Inflexibility of thought Difficulty with sequencing Impaired attention Verbal fluency	Increased severity of cognitive impairments
Emotional impairments		Depression Lack of motivation Fatigue	Depression Anxiety Irritability Impulsiveness Delusions	Cognitive impairments may mask emotional impairments
Motor impairments		Chorea Postural instability Hypokinesia Dystonia Occulomotor deficits	Postural instability & falls Hypokinesia Dystonia Dysarthria	Bradykinesia/akinesia Rigidity Dysphagia Dysarthria Incontinence Contractures
Activity	No deficits	Slowing or decreased accuracy of upper limb function Postural instability during walking	Some difficulty with personal and domestic activities of daily living	May no longer be able to mobilize, requiring hoist and wheelchair
Participation	No deficits	Working Sport/Leisure Driving	Reduced work hours or unable to continue paid employment Modified leisure or sporting activities May no longer be able to drive	Reduced participation in social and leisure activities

Table 7.1 (continued) Summary of supportive care needs through the progression of Huntington's disease

	Pre-symptomatic	Early stages of HD	Mid stages of HD	Late stages of HD
Education	Implications of testing for patient and family	Maintaining healthy lifestyle Likely disease progression and implications	Falls prevention Communication strategies Strategies to compensate for cognitive deficits Decision making about end of life care	Education to caregivers for safe transfers or mobilization, pressure care, chest care, safe swallowing
Family	Education and counselling about the implications of genetic testing or the test result	Change in family dynamics Adjusting to the effects of the disease	Change in family roles Psychological support Support with respite, equipment, home services, transport Financial support	Psychological support Support for transition into care or assistance to manage person with HD at home Financial support
Disciplines involved in care	Genetics counsellor Neurologist General practitioner Exercise therapist Dietitian HD Association	Case Manager / Social Worker Neurologist Neuropsychiatrist General practitioner Physiotherapy Occupational therapy (OT) Speech pathologist (SP) Dietitian Counselling HD Association	Case Manager / Social Worker General practitioner Neurologist Home support services Respite care OT/SP/neuropsychologist Physiotherapy Dietitian Counselling neurologist HD Association	Case manager/social worker General practitioner Neurologist Home support services Respite care Residential care Nursing Occupational therapist Physiotherapist Speech pathologist Dietitian HD Association

References

1. Huntington's Disease Collaborative Research Group (1993). A novel gene containing a trinucleotide repeat that is expanded and unstable on Huntington's disease chromosomes. *Cell*, **72**, 971–983.

2. Kirkwood SC, Su JL, Conneally PM, Foroud T (2001). Progression of symptoms in the early and middle stages of Huntington disease. *Arch Neurol*, **58**(2), 273–278.

3. Dawson S, Kristjanson LJ, Toye CM, Flett P (2004). Living with Huntington's disease: need for supportive care. *Nurs Health Sci*, **6**(2), 123–130.

4. Bonelli RM, Wenning GK, Kapfhammer HP (2004). Huntington's disease: present treatments and future therapeutic modalities. *Int Clin Psychopharmacol*, **19**(2), 51–62.

5. Aoun S, Kristjanson L, Oldham L (2006). The challenges and unmet needs of people with neurodegenerative conditions and their carers. *ACCNS J Comm Nurse*, **11**(1), 17–20.

6. Kristjanson LJ, Aoun SM, Yates P (2006). Are supportive services meeting the needs of Australians with neurodegenerative conditions and their families? *J Palliat Care*, **22**(3), 151–157.

7. Travers F, Jones K, Nichol J (2007). Palliative care provision in Huntington's disease. *Int J Palliat Nurs*, **13**(3), 125–130.

8. Bilney B, Morris ME, Perry A (2003). Effectiveness of physiotherapy, occupational therapy and speech pathology for people with Huntington's disease: a systematic review. *Neurorehabil Neural Repair*, **17**(1), 12–24.

9. Pickett T, Jr, Altmaier E, Paulsen JS (2007). Caregiver burden in Huntington's disease. *Rehab Psych*, **52**(3), 311–318.

10. Luscombe G, Brodaty H, Freeth S (1998). Younger people and dementia: diagnostic issues, effects on carers and use of services. *Int J Geriatr Psychiatry*, 13, 323–330.

11. Kristjanson L, Aoun S, Oldham L (2005). Palliative care and support for people with neurodegenerative conditions and their carers. *Int J Palliat Nurs*, **12**(8), 368–377.

12. Aubeeluck A, Moskowitz CB. (2008). Huntington's disease. Part 3: family aspects of HD. *Br J Nurs*, **17**(5), 28–31.

13. Shakespeare J, Anderson J (1993). Huntington's disease—falling through the net. *Health Trends*, **25**(1), 19–23.

14. Bourne C, Clayton C, Murch A, Grant J (2006). Cognitive impairment and behavioural difficulties in patients with Huntington's disease. *Nurs Stand*, **20**(35), 41–44.

15. Zinzi P, Salmaso D, De Grandis R, Graziani G, Maceroni S, Bentivoglio A, *et al* . (2007). Effects of an intensive rehabilitation programme on patients with Huntington's disease: a pilot study. *Clin Rehab*, **21**(7), 603–613.

16. Aubeeluck A, Wilson E (2008). Huntington's disease. Part 1: essential background and management. *Br J Nurs*, **17**(3), 146–151.

17. Nance MA (2007). Comprehensive care in Huntington's disease: a physician's perspective. *Brain Res Bull*, **72**(2–3), 175-178.

18. Klimek ML, Rohns G, Young L, Suchowersky O, Trew M (1997). Multidisciplinary approach to the management of a hereditary neurodegenerative disorder: Huntington disease. *Axone*, **19**(2), 34–38.

19. Imbriglio S. (1992). Huntington's disease at mid-stage. *Clin Manag*, **12**(5), 62–72.

20. International Huntington Association (IHA) and the World Federation of Neurology (WFN) Research Group on Huntington's Chorea (1994). Guidelines for the molecular genetics predictive test in Huntington's disease. *Neurol*, **44**, 1533–1536.

21. Hockly E, Cordery PM, Woodman B, Mahal A, van Dellen A, Blakemore C, *et al* . (2002). Environmental enrichment slows disease progression in R6/2 Huntington's disease mice. *Ann Neurol*, **51**(2), 235–242.

22. LoGiudice D, Hassett A. (2005). Uncommon dementia and the carer's perspective. *Int Psychogeriatr*, **17**(Suppl 1), S223-S231.

23. Snowden JS, Craufurd D, Thompson J, Neary D (2002). Psychomotor, executive, and memory function in preclinical Huntington's disease. *J Clin Exp Neuropsychol*, **24**(2), 133–145.

24. Tian JR, Herdman SJ, Zee DS, Folstein SE (1991). Postural control in Huntington's disease (HD). *Acta Otolaryngol*, Suppl 481, 333–336.

25. Phillips JG, Bradshaw JL, Chiu E, Teasdale N, Iansek R, Bradshaw JA (1996). Bradykinesia and movement precision in Huntington's disease. *Neuropsychol*, **34**(12), 1241–1245.

26. Bilney BE, Morris ME, Churchyard A, Chiu E, Georgiou-Karistianis N. (2005). Evidence for a disorder of locomotor timing in Huntington's disease. *Mov Disord*, **20**(1), 51–57.

27. Dal Bello-Hass V (2002). A framework for rehabilitation of neurodegenerative diseases: planning care and maximising quality of life. *Neurol Rep*, **26**(3), 115–129.

28. Bilney BE, Morris ME, Denisenko S (2003). Physiotherapy for people ith movement disorders arising from basal ganglia dysfunction. *NZ J Physiol*, **31**(2), 94–100.

29. Churchyard A, Morris M, Georgiou N, Chiu E, Cooper R, Iansek R. (2001). Gait dysfunction in Huntington's Disease: Parkinsonism and a disorder of timing, in Ruzicka E, Hallett M, Jankovic J (eds). *Advances in neurology*. Philadelphia: Lippincott Williams & Wilkins.

30. Thaut MH, McIntosh GC, Rice RR, Miller RA, Rathbun J, Brault JM (1996). Rhythmic auditory stimulation in gait training for Parkinson's disease patients. *Mov Disord*, **11**(2), 193–200.

31. Thaut MH, Miltner R, Lange HW, Hurt CP, Hoemberg V (1999). Velocity modulation and rhythmic synchronization of gait in Huntington's disease. *Mov Disord*, **14**(5), 808–819.

32. Huttunen J, Hömberg V (1990). EMG responses in leg muscles to postural perturbations in Huntington's disease. *J Neurol*, **53**, 55–62.

33. Tian J, Herdman SJ, Zee DS, Folstein SE (1992). Postural stability in patients with Huntington's disease. *Neurology*, **42**, 1232–1238.

34. Huntington's Disease Society of America. *Physical and occupational therapy for Huntington's disease*. Available at: http://www.had.org/edu/therapy.html [accessed 20th November 2008].

35. Rebok GW, Bylsma FW, Keyl PM, Brandt J, Folstein SE (1995). Automobile driving in Huntington's Disease. *Mov Disord*, **10**(6), 778–787.

36. Kagel MC, Leopold NA (1992). Dysphagia in Huntington's disease: a 16-year perspective. *Dysphagia*, **7**(2), 106–114.

37. Murray LL (2000). Spoken language production in Huntington's and Parkinson's diseases. *J Speech Lang Hear Res*, **43**(6), 1350–1366.

38. Murray LL, Lenz LP (2001). Productive syntax abilities in Huntington's and Parkinson's diseases. *Brain Cogn*, **46**(1–2), 213–219.

39. Farrer LA, Yu PL (1985). Anthropometric discrimination among affected, at-risk, and not at-risk individuals in families with Huntington's disease. *Am J Genet*, 21, 307–316.

40. Pratley RE, Salbe AD, Ravussin E, Caviness JN (2000). Higher sedentary energy expenditure in patients with Huntington's disease. *Ann Neurol*, **47**, 64–70.

41. Koller WC, Trimble J (1985). The gait abnormality of Huntington's disease. *Neurology*, **35**(10), 1450–1454.

42. Hausdorff JM, Cudkowicz ME, Firtion R, Wei JY, Goldberger AL (1998). Gait variability and basal ganglia disorders: stride-to-stride variations of gait cycle timing in Parkinson's disease and Huntington's disease. *Mov Disord*, **13**(3), 428–437.

43. Hausdorff JM, Mitchell SL, Firtion R, Peng C-K, Cudkowicz ME, Wei JY, *et al*. (1997). Altered fractal dynamics of gait: reduced stride-interval correlations with aging and Huntington's disease. *J Appl Physiol*, **82**(1), 262–269.

44. Phillips JG, Chiu E, Bradshaw JL, Iansek R (1995). Impaired movement sequencing in patients with Huntington's disease: a kinematic analysis. *Neuropsychologia*, **33**(3), 365–369.

45. Moskowitz CB, Marder K (2001). Palliative care for people with late stage Huntington's disease. *Neurol Clin*, **19**(4), 849–865.

46. Klasner ER (1990). *Managing swallowing difficulties associated with Huntington's disease*. Cambridge: Huntington Society of Canada.

47. Trejo A, Boll M-C, Alonso ME, Ochoa A, Velasquez L (2005). Use of oral nutritional supplements in patients with Huntington's disease. *Nutrition*, **21**(9), 889–894.

48. Paulsen JS, Robinson RJ (2001). Huntington's disease, in Hodges JR (ed). *Early onset dementia. A multidisciplinary approach*, pp.338–366. Oxford: Oxford University Press.

Chapter 8

Patients with HIV-associated dementia

Mary Ann Cohen and Charles E. Schwartz

Introduction

Supportive care of persons with HIV-associated dementia (HAD) presents clinicians, caregivers, families, and loved ones with special biopsychosocial challenges posed by the infectious nature of HIV, the specific modes of HIV transmission, the particular way HIV affects the brain, the age of onset, and the complex stigma of HIV superimposed on the stigma associated with all dementias. These challenges differentiate HAD from dementia of other causes, have significant clinical and public health implications, and necessitate early recognition and treatment as well as early supportive care. The multifactorial nature of these challenges is summarized in Table 8.1, and some unique aspects of HAD are briefly summarized in Box 8.1.

AIDS psychiatrists, psychosomatic medicine psychiatrists, physicians trained in both medicine and psychiatry, and other mental health clinicians can play a vital role in recognition and care of HAD, in the prevention of HIV transmission, and in training of other clinicians to alleviate distress, reduce ongoing high risk behavior and non-adherence, provide support for patients and families, and improve quality of life. In this chapter, we shall review the biopsychosocial aspects of HAD and suggest strategies to address the unique challenges of this devastating and complex illness.

HIV dementia: special considerations

Background and scope

Over the past 28 years, an estimated 25 million people have died of AIDS, and over 33 million people are living with AIDS worldwide [3]. The remarkable advances in HIV treatment since the introduction of protease inhibitors and combination antiretroviral therapy (CART) in 1996 have transformed AIDS from a rapidly fatal illness into one that is chronic and progressive for individuals with access to both HIV-experienced clinicians and to CART. In some areas of resource-rich countries and in many resource-limited countries and continents, persons with HIV and AIDS do not have the benefits of access to HIV medical and mental health care or treatment with CART. Even in areas with available care and medication, untreated psychiatric disorders such as HAD, substance use, anxiety, depression, mania, and psychosis can prevent persons with risk behaviours from getting HIV tested, obtaining results if tested, getting medical care, and changing behaviour to reduce risk and facilitate adherence with treatments.

CART has had a remarkable impact on HAD, cutting its incidence by half, and dramatically reducing its severity. CART may prevent HAD in HIV-infected adults without cognitive impairment and may prevent cognitive and motor developmental delay and deterioration in children. Thus, it is important to diagnose HIV infection early and begin CART, since there is evidence that HIV begins to damage the brain within months of infection, causing subtle neurocognitive

Table 8.1 Biopsychosocial aspects of HIV-associated dementia

Biological aspects	Psychological aspects	Social aspects
Constitutional (pain, fatigue, weakness, insomnia, anorexia, cachexia/wasting, fevers, diaphoresis, disfigurement, lipodystrophy)	Cognition (confusion, memory impairment, executive dysfunction, impaired concentration)	Family (stigma, rejection, abandonment, isolation, loss of role functioning, dependence, family psychosocial and financial stress)
Neurologic (pain, apathy, psychomotor slowing, dementia, delirium, peripheral neuropathies, myelopathies, paralysis, neuropsychiatric disorders, malignancies, PML)	Mood (adjustment disorder, dysthymia, major depressive disorder, mania, bereavement, demoralization)	Community (stigma, rejection, abandonment, isolation, loss of social support, loss of community resources)
Ophthalmologic (CMV/other retinitis, blindness)	Anxiety (PTSD, generalized anxiety disorder, panic disorder, agoraphobia)	Religion (stigma, rejection, abandonment, isolation, moral judgment)
Dermatologic (dry skin, pruritus, decubitus/pressure ulcers, Kaposi's Sarcoma)	Psychosis (hallucinations, delusions, psychotic disorders)	Economics (loss of job, income, home, finances, other resources; impoverishment)
Cardiac (dyspnoea, tachypnoea, cardiomyopathy, pulmonary hypertension, coronary artery disease, congestive heart failure)	Impulse control (disinhibition, agitation, inappropriate sexual behavior, unsafe sex, accidental firesetting, taking of other peoples' property, violence, suicidality)	Function (loss of ability to perform: complex learned tasks, instrumental and other activities of daily living, live independently, manage financial affairs)
Respiratory (pneumonias, dyspnea, hiccups)	Substance Misuse (intoxication, withdrawal, alcohol and other substance abuse/dependence, sharing of needles and drug paraphernalia in injection drug use)	Loss of Capacity (decisional incapacity, inability to: participate in discharge planning, manage financial affairs, and make future plans for partner and children)
Gastrointestinal (nausea, vomiting, dysphagia, diarrhea, candidal/other stomatitis/ esophagitis, gastritis, colitis, hepatitis and end-stage liver disease)	Spirituality/Meaning (existential anxiety; fear of: illness, physical/ mental disability, isolation, failure, dependence, burdening others, abandonment, death; loss of: faith, meaning, dignity, self esteem; guilt)	
Genitourinary (STDs, renal disease, incontinence, end-stage renal disease, genital infection, and cancers)		
Infections (opportunistic and non-HIV-related)		
Malignant (Kaposi's Sarcoma, lymphomas, non-HIV- associated cancers)		
Endocrinopathies (thyroid, adrenal, gonadal)		
Myopathies		

(1; 2)

(Key: CMV=cytomegalovirus; PML=progressive multifocal leukoencephalopathy; PTSD=post-traumatic stress disorder; STDs=sexually transmitted diseases)

Box 8.1 How HIV-associated dementia differs from most other dementias

Infectious aetiology

Modes of transmission: unsafe sex, sharing of needles in injecting drug, perinatal

Both HIV and HAD are preventable currently

Disinhibition and subsequent behavior can lead to HIV, Hepatitis B and Hepatitis C viruses, and STD transmission

Stigma heightened owing to both dementia and HIV status

Age of onset from young to old age

Treatment, reversibility, or stabilization with anti-retrovirals is possible (though exacerbation by treatment with anti-retrovirals can occur)

Multiple infections and complex medical comorbidities are common

High prevalence of psychiatric disorders including substance use and its consequences

High prevalence of delirium caused by respiratory, cardiac, metabolic illnesses, and end-stage renal and liver disease

Unique neurological deficits, such as paresis, paralysis, pain

Unique behavioral manifestations

deficits that increase the risk of HAD. When HAD develops, CART reduces its severity, and slows progression, inducing full recovery in some people [4, 5]. Though CART has improved life expectancy, overall prevalence of HAD has risen [6] and 60% have pathologic changes consistent with HAD at autopsy [7, 8].

The majority of patients with HAD are left with persistent, albeit milder neuropsychiatric deficits despite CART [7]. In some instances, CART actually appears to accelerate HAD, perhaps through an immunologically mediated cerebritis associated with the immune reconstitution inflammatory syndrome, (IRIS) [9, 10].

HAD is said to be the most common and treatable cause of dementia in those under 50 years of age and along with age and functional impairment, continues to be a powerful predictor of AIDS progression and death [7, 11].

Age

The young comprise almost half of all new HIV infections worldwide, and account for the vast majority of AIDS deaths [3]. Young women of childbearing age now represent more than half of all HIV-infected persons [3]. Young persons with HIV dementia present special challenges as they face shortened lives, unachieved hopes and dreams, and are especially prone to agitation and disinhibition [12].

The prevalence of HIV in older adults is increasing [13], and the elderly have significantly higher incidence and greater severity of HAD [14]. Both HIV and CART are risk factors for comorbid atherosclerosis and stroke [15] and Alzheimer's disease [9, 16, 17].

Stigma

Early in the epidemic, persons with AIDS were shunned and ostracized, and even quarantined as a result of irrational fears of contagion and death from simple touching, and non-intimate proximity [18, 19]. 'AIDSism' or discrimination against persons with AIDS is based on homophobia, addictophobia, misogyny, and fear of contagion. AIDSism led to rejection by families, friends, and communities and exclusion from churches, classrooms, jobs, homes, homeless shelters, nursing homes, long-term-care facilities, hospices, and even funeral homes and cemeteries.

Today, most physicians provide compassionate care for persons with AIDS, but AIDSism and denial still persist in society at large.

Socioeconomic disadvantage

HIV disproportionately affects vulnerable and disenfranchised populations throughout the world, including gay men, women, children, elderly, intravenous drug users, minorities, people of colour, and socioeconomically disadvantaged, mentally ill, and incarcerated individuals. Two thirds of all people with HIV live in poverty in sub-Saharan Africa [20].

Poverty leads to malnutrition, which directly increases HIV brain vulnerability to HAD [21], and indirectly leads to HAD through decreased access to HIV treatment [22, 23, 24]. Sadly, poverty is associated with both increased HIV morbidity and mortality [26], as well as diminished access to palliative care [25].

HIV-associated dementia – pathology and diagnosis

HIV infects and destroys subcortical white matter, disrupting neural networks, signal transmission, and frontal lobe function [27]. HAD is a subcortical dementia with cognitive and psychomotor slowing, and impaired attention, concentration, judgment, impulse control, and executive function. This may leave persons with HAD unable to live independently [8], adhere to CART, and in need of substantial support services surprisingly early in their illnesses [2].

HIV affects both the central and peripheral nervous systems superimposing neurological symptoms on HAD. Although CART has reduced their incidence and severity, HIV continues to cause motor deficits resulting in impaired coordination and ambulation, and peripheral neuropathy resulting in pain, particularly in older persons [28].

All persons with HIV should be evaluated for HAD with a thorough and comprehensive psychiatric evaluation including a full assessment of cognitive function [19]. Neuropsychological testing, while considered to be the gold standard in the diagnosis of HAD, is costly, available primarily in research programmes, and difficult to obtain in clinical settings. Screening tools developed to assess for cortical dementias are not useful for the diagnosis of HAD. A screening device adapted from neuropsychological testing, Oral Trailmaking Part B (also called the Mental Alternation Test), is an effective 60-second test for HAD that has been validated [29] but is applicable only in early stages of dementia. The HIV Dementia Scale (HDS) [30, 31] is useful throughout the course of HAD. No screening test can substitute for complete psychiatric examination and cognitive assessment [19].

HAD medical treatment

CART can stabilize or slow down the progression of HAD and can sometimes substantially reverse cognitive impairment [2, 27]. Adherence to the sustained CART regimen that is necessary to have an impact on HAD may be difficult and requires substantial support and supervision. In addition, patients should be treated for ongoing alcohol or drug use as well as comorbid medical illnesses (such as hepatitis C virus (HCV)) since these can exacerbate and accelerate cognitive and functional impairment. No other adjunctive pharmacologic treatment has proven to be effective for HAD [11].

HAD-associated co-morbid medical disorders

In the CART era, hepatitis C, organ system failures, and malignancies have replaced CNS opportunistic illnesses (OIs) as the most common and lethal HIV medical comorbidities [32]. These disorders can also cause or exacerbate cognitive impairment and other neuropsychiatric symptoms and are summarized in Table 8.1. Hepatitis C infection is associated with fatigue, depression, and subcortical cognitive dysfunction [33], and the resulting liver disease can cause impaired concentration and delirium [34]. Patients with comorbid HIV and hepatitis C are at even higher risk of HAD. HIV can also be associated with endocrinopathies and nephropathies that can compound HAD dysfunction.

Cardiac disease, including pulmonary hypertension, cardiomyopathy, and coronary artery disease can occur in association with HIV and HIV treatments, but also be unrelated to HIV. Similarly, neurologic, haematologic, pulmonary, and gastrointestinal illnesses cause considerable morbidity and suffering.

Disinhibition and psychomotor agitation

HAD impairs judgment and impulse control and causes disinhibition and agitated behavior. HAD patients who smoke cigarettes or have access to kitchen appliances may accidentally start fires because of HAD-associated lapses in attention, impaired judgment, motor incoordination, sensory neuropathies, and impaired vision [2]. Persons with HAD may also impulsively take things that do not belong to them [35], speak or act inappropriately, expose genitals, use obscenities, or engage in high risk sexual behaviour [36].

Delirium superimposed on dementia

The multiplicity of HIV comorbid illnesses and complex medication regimens make persons with HAD very vulnerable to delirium [37] and agitation [12].

Unless the condition precipitating the delirium is treatable, delirium is a harbinger of death in HIV-infected individuals [38], leaving those who survive with accelerated dementia progression [39].

Agitated delirious patients need rapid behavioural stabilization to ensure safety, facilitate neuromedical workup and treatment, and alleviate patient and family distress [40]. Second generation antipsychotic medications are the treatment of choice for agitation in HAD patients, who are exquisitely sensitive to antipsychotic extrapyramidal side effects of first generation agents. Benzodiazepines, antihistamines, and anticholinergics are contraindicated in HAD because they can oversedate, increase cognitive dysfunction, or precipitate disinhibited, 'paradoxical' excitation and agitation [40].

Other HAD-associated psychiatric disorders

Psychiatric disorders, are highly prevalent in patients with HIV/AIDS, add significant burden, and can exacerbate HAD. They are aetiologically complex (see Table 8.1), and require comprehensive biopsychosocial diagnostic assessment [4, 19].

Alcohol, substance use, and adverse effects of medications

Alcohol and other substance misuse occur in as many as 50% of the patients with HIV [20, 41]. CNS side effects of medications and drug–drug interactions are the leading causes of reversible

HIV-associated psychiatric disorders. Neuropsychiatric side effects may occur with HIV CART medications, treatments for hepatitis C, and antibiotics. For example, efavirenz, a non-nucleoside reverse transcriptase inhibitor, may cause neuropsychiatric symptoms, especially in persons with HIV and mood disorders.

Depression, desire for death, and suicide

One third of persons with HIV may have depression [20, 41, 43]. HAD increases suicide risk [44, 45], with depression compounded by impaired judgment and impulse control [46], and/or substance abuse. Furthermore, HAD increases desires for hastened death as quality of life declines [47, 48]. Desire for death that is the result of end-of-life thinking has to be differentiated from pathological suicidal ideation.

Psychiatric treatment

Persons with HAD have a high prevalence of psychiatric disorders including mood disorders, anxiety disorders, and psychotic disorders and require psychotherapeutic interventions such as psychotherapy, crisis intervention, couple therapy, family therapy, and group therapy, in addition to psychopharmacologic intervention [19]. Medications recommended for persons with HAD are summarized in Table 8.2.

Medical decision-making and advance directives

HIV and HAD present special life challenges. Ongoing dialogue with patient and family about advance directives should begin early in the clinician–patient relationship, when the individual is in good physical and mental health [49], emphasizing the importance of maintaining autonomy and control over medical decisions [50]. Appointing a health care agent who can convey the patient's previously expressed wishes concerning artificial hydration and nutrition when all other medical care becomes futile maintains dignity and control at the end of life. With HAD and superimposed delirium, capacity to make informed decisions may fluctuate over hours or days.

Permanency planning for children

People with HAD are disproportionately younger adults, and those who are parents face the difficult task of planning for those who will be left behind. By 2010, 25 million children will be AIDS orphans [51] and in sub-Saharan Africa an entire generation of children (some 18 million) will be

Table 8.2 Psychopharmacologic recommendations for HAD

Class	Preferred Agents	Indications	Comments
Antidepressants	Citalopram, escitalopram	Depression, anxiety disorders	Relatively free of drug interactions with HIV medications
Anxiolytics	Lorazepam, clonazepam	Anxiety disorders, insomnia	Not effective for panic disorder, may be added to antipsychotic for agitation
Antipsychotics	Quetiapine, olanzapine	Psychosis, agitated delirium, bipolar disorder, mania	Monitor for extrapyramidal side effects (EPS), HIV patients are very sensitive to EPS
Mood Stabilizers	Valproic acid	Bipolar disorder	Few drug interactions, monitor for drug-induced hepatitis, encephalopathy

affected [52]. Grandmothers, often impoverished and without spouses [53], are overwhelmed by the sheer volume of orphaned grandchildren, some of whom are HIV-infected as well [54, 55].

HAD's unpredictable course raises many challenging questions. When should patients acknowledge impending mortality and that they will not be around for those who have depended on them? When should they disclose to their children, and select future parents for them? And when is it too late?

In the US, fewer than 50% of the parents with AIDS ever discuss their diagnosis with their children, leaving them vulnerable to more severe subsequent psychological distress [56]. Fewer than 50% make advance custodial decisions [57].

Family support

Clinicians should establish an alliance with the family early in the course of illness, providing ongoing emotional support, concrete management suggestions, and facilitating needed support services. As HAD worsens and burden increases, home care provided by teams including physicians and mental health specialists and day care can help maintain patients at home. Although more than 90% of the HIV-infected individuals wish to die at home [58], most are unable to do so. In-patient hospices and other residential facilities geared to the needs of individuals with advanced HAD provide alternatives to homes and hospitals, permit respite, and integrate families in terminal care [59].

The burden of caring for progressively disabled loved ones, exacerbated by poverty, minority ethnicity, stigma, and social isolation, may cause or worsen medical and mental health problems in families [60, 61]. Families need help with reconciliation and mourning for one or more years after the individual dies, as families face new psychosocial challenges and vulnerability to psychiatric and medical illness [62].

Role of the physician in the care of HIV-associated dementia at the end of life

Physicians can provide continuity and support to patients and families, who often feel lonely, stigmatized, and abandoned as HIV and HAD advance. Regular visits are essential. Palliation of distressing symptoms is important throughout the entire course of severe and complex illnesses such as AIDS and HAD.

At the end of life, palliative care becomes the most important therapeutic modality. Physicians may have to overcome their own feelings of helplessness and sorrow in order to remain with the patient and family throughout the course of the dying process, treating patients and families with worth and dignity [63]. This is the time for physicians to perform their time-honoured role, 'holding the hands of the dying' patient and family [49], listening and empathically witnessing the patient's and/or family's struggle with spiritual issues in light of illness, disability and untimely mortality, reinforcing meaning, dignity, and legacy [63]. Holding the hand of a person with HAD at the end of life is an especially significant antidote to stigma and fear of abandonment.

Conclusions

From the onset of illness to the end of life, supportive care plays a significant role in the care of persons with HIV-associated dementia. Loss of memory, loss of key roles, and loss of ability to function independently can be overwhelming to patients and loved ones. When the cause of dementia is infectious and associated with stigma and stigmatized risk behaviours, the burden of both bereavement and stigma can become unbearable. A biopsychosocial approach can help to lighten this burden and meet the challenges of this devastating illness with optimism and dignity.

References

1. Selwyn PA, Forstein M (2003). Overcoming the false dichotomy of curative vs. palliative care for late-stage HIV/AIDS: 'Let me live the way I want to live, until I can't.' *JAMA,* **290**, 806–814.

2. Cohen MA, and Alfonso CA (2004). AIDS psychiatry: psychiatric and palliative care, and pain management, in GP Wormser (ed). *AIDS and other manifestations of HIV infection*, fourth edition, pp. 537–576. San Diego: Elsevier Academic Press.

3. UNAIDS (2008). *Report on the global AIDS epidemic*. Geneva Switzerland: United Nations Joint Programme on HIV/AIDS.

4. Cohen MA, Jacobson JM (2000). Maximizing life's potentials in AIDS: a psychopharmacologic update. *Gen Hosp Psychiatry*, **22**, 375–388.

5. Cysique LAJ, Maruff P, Brew BJ (2006). Variable benefit in neuropsychologicalfunction in HIV infected HAART treated patients. *Neurology*, **66**, 1447–1450.

6. McArthur JC, McDermott MP, McClernon D, *et al.* (2004). Attenuated central nervous system infection in advanced HIV/AIDS with combination antiretroviral therapy. *Arch Neurol*, 2004, **61**, 1687–1696.

7. Tozzi V, Balestra P, Bellagamba R, *et al.* (2007). Persistence of neuropsychologic deficits despite long-term highly active antiretroviral therapy in patients with HIV-related neurocognitive impairment: prevalence and risk factors. *J Acquired Immune Def Syndr JAIDS*, **45**(2), 174–182.

8. Boisse L, Gill MJ, Power C (2008).HIV infection of the central nervous system: clinical features and neuropathogenesis. *Neurologic Clin*, **26**(3), 799–819.

9. Alisky JM (2007). The coming problem of HIV-associated Alzheimer's disease. *Med Hypotheses*, **69**(5), 1140–1143.

10. Nath A, Schiess N, Venkatesan A, Rumbaugh J, Sacktor N, McArthur J (2008). Evolution of HIV dementia with HIV infection. *Int Rev Psychiatry*, **20**(1), 25–31.

11. Uthman OA, Abdulmalik JO. Adjunctive therapies for AIDS dementia complex. Cochrane Database of Systematic Reviews 2008, (3). (Art. No.: CD006496). DOI:10.1002/ 14651858.CD006496.pub2.

12. Peterson JF, Pun BT, Dittus RS, *et al.* (2006). Delirium and its motoric subtypes: a study of 614 critically ill patients. *J Am Geriatr Soc*, **54**(3), 479–484.

13. Simone MJ, Appelbaum JS (2008). HIV in older adults. *Geriatrics*, **63**(12), 6–12.

14. Valcour V, Yee P, Williams AE, *et al.* (2006). Lowest ever CD4 lymphocyte count (CD4 nadir) as a predictor of current cognitive and neurological status in human immunodeficiency virus type 1 infection—the Hawaii Aging with HIV Cohort. *J Neurovirol*, **12**(October (5)), 387–391.

15. Modi G, Modi M, Mochan A (2008). Is stroke a HIV-related neurologic manifestation? *Exp Rev Neurotherap*, **8**(8), 1247–1253.

16. Xu J, Ikezu T (2009). The comorbidity of HIV-associated neurocognitive disorders and Alzheimer's disease: a foreseeable medical challenge in post-HAART Era. *J Neuroimmune Pharmacol*, **4**(2), 200–212.

17. Sacktor N, Skolasky R, Selnes OA, *et al.* (2007). Neuropsychological test profile differences between young and old human immunodeficiency virus-positive individuals. *J Neurovirol*, **13**(3), 203–209.

18. Anderson MEG, Gerver SSI, Fenton K, Easterbrook P (2008). HIV/AIDS-related stigma and discrimination: accounts of HIV-positive Caribbean people in the United Kingdom. Soc Sci Med, **67**(5), 790–798.

19. Cohen MA, Gorman JM (2009). *Comprehensive textbook of AIDS psychiatry*. New York: Oxford University Press.

20. Adewuya AA, Afolabi MO, Ola BA, Ogundele OA, Ajibare AO, Oladipo BF (2007). Psychiatric disorders among the HIV-positive population in Nigeria: a control study. *J Psychosomatic Res,* **63**(2), 203–206.

21. Fein G, Di Sclafani V (2004). Cerebral reserve capacity: implications for alcohol and drug abuse. *Alcohol*, **32**(1), 63–67.

22. UNDP (2005). *Human Development Report*. New York, NY: United Nations Development Programme.

23. Hardon AP, Akurut D, Comoro C, *et al.* (2007). Hunger, waiting time and transport costs: time to confront challenges to ART adherence in Africa. *AIDS Care*, **19**(5), 658–665.

24. Weiser SD, Frongillo EA, Ragland K, Hogg RS, Riley ED, Bangsberg DR (2009). Food insecurity is associated with incomplete HIV RNA suppression among homeless and marginally housed HIV-infected individuals in San Francisco. *J Gen Int Med*, **24**(1), 14–20.

25. Kutzen HS (2004). Integration of palliative care into primary care for human immunodeficiecy virus-infected patients. *Am J Med Sci*, **328**, 37–47.

26. Chu C, Selwyn PA (2008). Current health disparities in HIV/AIDS. *AIDS Reader*, **18**(3), 144–146, 152–158, (C3).

27. Reynolds A, Kammogne G, Kadiu I, Gendelman HF (2008). HIV and the Central Nervous System, in Cohen MA, Gorman JM (Eds). *Comprehensive textbook of AIDS psychiatry*, pp. 207–253. New York: Oxford University Press.

28. Robinson-Papp J, Byrd D, Mindt MR, Oden NL, Simpson DM, Morgello S. Manhattan HIV Brain Bank (2008). Motor function and human immunodeficiency virus-associated cognitive impairment in a highly active antiretroviral therapy-era cohort. *Arch Neurol*. **65**(8):1096–1101.

29. Jones BN, Teng EL, Folstein MF, Harrison KS (1993). A new bedside test of cognition for patients with HIV infection. *Ann Int Med*, **119**(10), 1001–1004.

30. Power C, Selnes OA, Grim JA, and McArthur JC (1995). HIV Dementia Scale: a rapid screening test. *J Acquir Immune Def Syndr Hum Retrovirol*, **8**, 273–278.

31. Ganasen K A, Fincham D, Smit, J, Seedat S, Stein D (2008). Utility of the HIV Dementia Scale (HDS) in identifying HIV dementia in a South African sample. *J Neurologic Sci*. **269**(1–2), 62–64.

32. Selwyn PA. Rivard M (2003). Palliative care for AIDS: challenges and opportunities in the era of highly active anti-retroviral therapy. *J Palliat Med*, **6**(3), 475–487.

33. Crone C, Gabriel GM (2003). Comprehensive review of hepatitis C for psychiatrists: risks, screening, diagnosis, treatment and interferon-based therapy complications. *J Psychiatr Pract*, **9**, 93–110.

34. Ferrando SJ, Lyketsos CG (2008). HIV-Associated Neurocognitive Disorders, in Cohen MA, Gorman JM (eds). *Comprehensive textbook of AIDS psychiatry*, pp. 439–454. New York: Oxford University Press.

35. Murrough J and Cohen MA (2008). Unique Manifestations of HIV-Associated Dementia, in Cohen MA, Gorman JM (eds) *Comprehensive textbook of AIDS psychiatry*, pp. 189–194. New York: Oxford University Press.

36. Brewer-Smyth K, Bucurescu G, Shults J, *et al.* (2007). Neurological function and HIV risk behaviors of female prison inmates. *J Neurosci Nurs*, **39**(6), 361–372.

37. Margiotta A, Bianchetti A, Ranieri P, Trabucchi M (2006). Clinical characteristics and risk factors of delirium in demented and not demented elderly medical inpatients. *J Nutr, Health Aging*, **10**(6), 535–539.

38. Uldall KK, Ryan R, Berghuis JP, Harris VL (2000). Association between delirium and death in AIDS patients. *AIDS Patient Care Stds*, **14**(2), 95–100.

39. Fick DM, Agostini JV, Inouye SK (2002). Delirium superimposed on dementia: a systematic review. *J Am Geriatr Soc*, **50**(10), 1723–1732.

40. Breitbart W, Alici Y (2008). Agitation and delirium at end of life—we couldn't manage him. *JAMA*, **300**, 2898–2910.

41. Bing EG, Burnam MA, Longshore D, *et al.* (2001). Psychiatric disorders and drug use among human immunodeficiency virus-infected adults in the United States. *Arch Gen Psychiatry*, **58**, 721–728.

42. Bartlett JA, and Ferrando S (2004). Identification and management of neurologic and psychiatric side effects associated with HIV and HAART. *Medscape*. Retrieved April 25, 2007, from http://www.medscape.com/viewarticle/470017.

43. Gaynes BN, Pence BW, Eron JJ Jr, Miller WC (2008). Prevalence and comorbidity of psychiatric diagnoses based on reference standard in an HIV+ patient population. *Psychosom Med,* **70**(May (4)), 505–511.

44. McKegney FP, O'Dowd MA (1982). Suicidality and HIV status. *Am J Psychiatry,* **149**, 396–398.

45. Perry S, Jacobsberg L, Fishman B (1990). Suicidal ideation and HIV testing. *JAMA,* **263**, 679–682.

46. Alfonso CA, Cohen MA (1994). HIV dementia and suicide. *Gen Hosp Psychiatry,* **16**, 45–46.

47. Pessin H, Rosenfeld B, Burton L, Breitbart W (2003). The role of cognitive impairment in desire for hastened death: a study of patients with advanced AIDS. *Gen Hosp Psychiatry,* **25**(3), 194–199.

48. Rosenfeld B, Breitbart W, Gibson C, *et al.* (2006). Desire for hastened death among patients with advanced AIDS. *Psychosomatics,* **47**(November–December(6)), 504–512.

49. Brendel RW, Cohen MA (2008). End-of-life issues, in Cohen MA, Gorman JM. *Comprehensive textbook of AIDS psychiatry,* pp. 567–576. New York: Oxford University Press.

50. Schwartz CE, Dubler N, Steimuller R (1998). The medical psychiatrist as a physician for the chronically Ill. *Gen Hosp Psychiatry,* **20**, 52–61.

51. Sherr L, Varrall R, Mueller J, *et al.* (2008). A systematic review on the meaning of the concept 'AIDS Orphan': confusion over definitions and implications for care. *AIDS Care,* **20**(5), 527–536.

52. Andrews G, Skinner D, Zuma K (2006). Epidemiology of health and vulnerability among children orphaned and made vulnerable by HIV/AIDS in sub-Saharan Africa. *AIDS Care,* **18**(3), 269–276.

53. Howard BH, Phillips CV, Matinhure N, Goodman KJ, McCurdy SA, Johnson CA (2006). Barriers and incentives to orphan care in a time of AIDS and economic crisis: a cross-sectional survey of caregivers in rural Zimbabwe. *BMC Public Health,* **6**, 27.

54. Heymann J, Earle A, Rajaraman D, Miller C, Bogen K (2007). Extended family caring for children orphaned by AIDS: balancing essential work and caregiving in a high HIV prevalence nations. *AIDS Care,* **19**(3), 337–345.

55. Bock J. Johnson SE (2008). Grandmothers' productivity and the HIV/AIDS pandemic in sub-Saharan Africa. *J Cross Cult Gerontol,* **23**(2), 131–45.

56. Wood K, Chase E, Aggleton P (2006). 'Telling the truth is the best thing': teenage orphans' experiences of parental AIDS-related illness and bereavement in Zimbabwe. *Soc Sci Med,* **63**(7), 1923–1933.

57. Rotheram-Borus MJ, Lester P, Wang PW, Shen Q (2004). Custody plans among parents living with human immunodeficiency virus infection. *Arch Pediatr Adolesc Med,* **158**(4), 327–332.

58. Goldstone I, Kuhl D, Johnson A, Le R, and McLeod A (1995). Patterns of care in advanced HIV disease in a tertiary treatment centre. *AIDS Care,* 7(Suppl 1), S47–S56.

59. Pratt R, Washer P (1998). HIV-related encephalopathy. *Nurs Stand,* **13**(7), 38–40.

60. Flaskerud JH, Lee P (2008). Vulnerability to health problems in female informal caregivers of persons with HIV/AIDS and age-related dementias *J Adv Nurs,* **33**(1), 60–687.

61. Ssengonzi R (2007). The plight of older persons as caregivers to people infected/affected by HIV/AIDS: evidence from Uganda. *J Cross Cult Gerontol,* **22**(4), 339–353.

62. Kissane DW, McKenzie M, Bloch S, Moskowitz C, McKenzie DP, O'Neill I (2006). Family focused grief therapy: a randomized, controlled trial in palliative care and bereavement. *Am J Psychiatry,* **163**(7), 1208–1218.

63. Dickerman AL, Breitbart W, and Chochinov HM (2008). Palliative and spiritual care of persons with HIV and AIDS, in Cohen MA, Gorman JM (eds). *Comprehensive textbook of AIDS psychiatry,* pp. 417–438. New York: Oxford University Press.

Chapter 9

Down's syndrome and dementia: a framework for practice to support people with Down's syndrome and dementia living in generic care homes

Heather Wilkinson and Karen Watchman

Introduction

Despite the recognized longevity of people with Down's syndrome, the age-related long-term care needs of this population have yet to be fully understood and addressed. Owing to an increase in medical and social interventions, people with Down's syndrome are living longer. This has led to the current awareness that there are a number of illnesses in later life that people with Down's syndrome are susceptible to, one of which is dementia. Since the shift from institutionalization to community care [1,2], models of provision specifically for people with Down's syndrome who are growing older now range across a continuum: from the most segregated specialist provision specifically for older people to services for older people with a learning disability, either as part of general services for older people or in the context of more individualized routes of care [2]. The focus of this chapter is specifically on generic care provision and, in particular, the use by people with Down's syndrome and dementia of mainstream care home provision for older people when they are moved from other services or need a placement when home or family care structures break down.

The majority of adults with Down's syndrome live in the family home, often with older parents [3]; statistics suggest that 63% of all adults in the UK with a learning disability live in private households, usually with their own family [4]. As health and social care needs increase, it is often difficult for older parents to continue in this caring role, yet until this point many families are not known to local authorities or social services. This increasingly leads to an emergency change in accommodation, often to a generic nursing or care home. This chapter will present a framework to support staff and people with Down's syndrome in a care home setting, a setting that is currently under-researched with little recording of evidence-based practice. There are particular challenges associated with providing residential care for people with Down's syndrome who can develop dementia at a significantly younger age than the general population.

Using recent qualitative, longitudinal research in Scotland a framework of questions to support care is proposed that is centred on the individual with Down's syndrome and dementia. Within this framework, there are three specific areas included: staffing issues, communication, and mealtimes. These three areas have been identified in research as flash points leading to staff experiencing difficulty in caring for a person with Down's syndrome [5]. The areas for key questions are presented in Figure 9.1 and are used to highlight ways in which quality of life can be developed and improved throughout the progressive deterioration associated with dementia in people with Down's syndrome. A case study of Michael (see Figure 9.2), a man with Down's syndrome and

Questions to be developed reviewed and shared with all staff:

✓ After diagnosis as the basis for future care
✓ Regardless of accommodation, as the questions and answers move with the person
✓ Before every change of accommodation

To be included in decisions made:

✓ Person with Down's syndrome using appropriate communication
✓ Carer
✓ Family
✓ Friends
✓ Key staff that the person is familiar with

Staffing issues

✓ Identify who will give information to staff and family about early signs of dementia and the different stages
✓ Record the signs or words used when a diagnosis or explanation was given to the person
✓ Identify who is taking the lead on future health and dental screening
✓ Record who is leading communication between agencies
✓ Confirm all staff speak English when working
✓ Note the person's favourite colour
✓ Note the clothes that they like to wear
✓ Record the music, TV, sport and movies the person likes now and when they were younger
✓ Note the time of day that TV is watched
✓ Record who will give information about the end stages including funeral wishes

Mealtimes

✓ Record the average time that a mealtime usually takes
✓ Note what food was preferred when younger, and now, and how it was cooked
✓ Record how much is usually eaten
✓ Record what kind of help is needed at mealtimes
✓ Record if tea, coffee or something else is preferred to drink with and between meals
✓ If the person buys their own food note the support for menu planning and shopping
✓ Confirm that coloured dishes are available for pale coloured food
✓ Record if finger food is eaten
✓ Note how much background noise is preferred during mealtimes
✓ Record if the person likes staff to talk to them during mealtimes
✓ Note if a napkin, bib or apron is wanted
✓ Confirm meals are eaten in a dining area

Communication

✓ Record the communication method used when younger
✓ Note the communication method that is currently used between carers and people with Down's syndrome
✓ Record the activities the person enjoyed when they were younger
✓ Record the activities they enjoy presently and who supports this
✓ Note who is taking lead responsibility for coordinating life story work
✓ If person has a life story book confirm that people in photographs are identified
✓ Note if the person likes to be touched or hugged
✓ Note if the person likes to sing and, if so, which kind of music
✓ Note their favourite songs
✓ Record how the person shows pain, both verbally and non verbally

Fig. 9.1 Framework of support – taking a questioning approach.

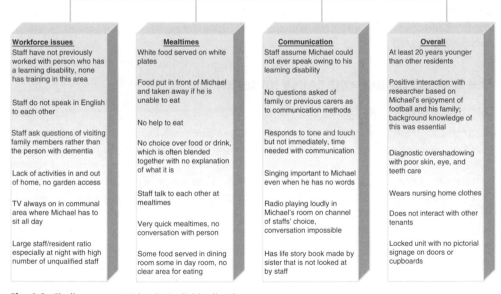

Michael
For 50 years lived with older sister, who is now ill

No social work involvement

Admitted to hospital aged 49 with chest infection. Seven week stay in hospital ward as sister too ill for Michael to return home

Admitted to care home after psychiatrist intervention

Diagnosed with dementia aged 48 although believed to have had this for a while with sister not seeking help

Has not been given a diagnosis or explanation of changes he is experiencing

Workforce issues
Staff have not previously worked with person who has a learning disability, none has training in this area

Staff do not speak in English to each other

Staff ask questions of visiting family members rather than the person with dementia

Lack of activities in and out of home, no garden access

TV always on in communal area where Michael has to sit all day

Large staff/resident ratio especially at night with high number of unqualified staff

Mealtimes
White food served on white plates

Food put in front of Michael and taken away if he is unable to eat

No help to eat

No choice over food or drink, which is often blended together with no explanation of what it is

Staff talk to each other at mealtimes

Very quick mealtimes, no conversation with person

Some food served in dining room some in day room, no clear area for eating

Communication
Staff assume Michael could not ever speak owing to his learning disability

No questions asked of family or previous carers as to communication methods

Responds to tone and touch but not immediately, time needed with communication

Singing important to Michael even when he has no words

Radio playing loudly in Michael's room on channel of staffs' choice, conversation impossible

Has life story book made by sister that is not looked at by staff

Overall
At least 20 years younger than other residents

Positive interaction with researcher based on Michael's enjoyment of football and his family; background knowledge of this was essential

Diagnostic overshadowing with poor skin, eye, and teeth care

Wears nursing home clothes

Does not interact with other tenants

Locked unit with no pictorial signage on doors or cupboards

Fig. 9.2 Challenges to Michael's individualized support.

dementia, is used to illustrate how the framework can in practice work better to support people with Down's syndrome and dementia in care home settings. The process of asking the key questions and recording and sharing responses with other professionals is part of effective care planning. It is also fundamental to providing effective person-centred care and to future planning. Answers to the questions can be updated as necessary, for example, to share information and understanding with new carers if a change in accommodation is needed in the future. In this way, previous and present preferences are recorded – essential for continuing care as dementia progresses.

It will be seen that the questions suggested by the framework are equally applicable, and indeed recommended, for those in the general population who have dementia, but are needed specifically for people who have Down's syndrome owing to the history of 'diagnostic overshadowing' [6], whereby staff and carers often provide care in ways that respond to the learning disability rather than the person themselves. This is a recurring theme throughout the chapter; it is essential for care to be provided in a way that does not assume that the person is unable to communicate as a result of having Down's syndrome. This common assumption, especially among staff that are not experienced in the learning disability field, can result in few or no attempts being made to interact using other methods, particularly non-verbal methods of communication (see Chapter 23 for further discussion of communication in dementia). People with Down's syndrome can often have less contact with family members [7], so may lack the support network to give background information and family history. As a direct consequence people with Down's syndrome are not routinely asked the kind of questions that many of us take for granted, resulting in a lack of inclusion in their own future planning, including planning for their end-of-life care.

As a group of people already experiencing marginalization, the failure to address health and social care needs of people ageing with Down's syndrome adds to the process of their exclusion [8]. If residential providers are committed to providing a lifetime of community care, then a more detailed understanding of the practices that support people as they grow older is urgently required. In this chapter, we provide an overview of the demographics and policy imperative in developing stronger policy and practice responses to the needs of people growing older with Down's syndrome and dementia. We, then, focus on the proposed framework using a case study to illustrate the urgent requirement for more detailed research evidence and policy responses to this underserved area of practice.

The demographics and policy imperatives

Demographics

With significant advances in medical and social support, better living conditions, and improved nutrition, people with a learning disability are now living into older age [9]. For a person with Down's syndrome life expectancy has increased dramatically from an average of only 9 years in the early 1900s to an average of 45 years in the 1990s [10], and to over 60 for many today. In predicting forthcoming trends, it is expected that the number of people with a learning disability will continue to grow by over 1% a year over the next 10 years [4,11]. It is expected that 25% of the learning disability population will be aged over 60 by 2040 in Scotland, although the life expectancy of a person with Down's syndrome is still significantly lower than the life expectancy of the general population.

With this longer life expectancy, increasing numbers of people with a learning disability will encounter associated illnesses and conditions of older age, such as dementia. Although dementia generally affects people with learning disability in the same manner as it does other older people, this is not the case for individuals with Down's syndrome [12]. Adults with Down's syndrome are at greater overall risk of being affected by dementia, often but not exclusively Alzheimer's disease, and are usually affected at an earlier age with a precipitous decline and loss of skills within a shorter period of time. Early signs are different to the general population including the withdrawal of spontaneous communication, apathy, lack of interest in previously enjoyed activities, and loss of road sense. Further examples of differences include earlier difficulty with thresholds such as stepping between rooms or across different flooring and the higher onset rate of epilepsy. The loss of daily living skills is more apparent than memory loss in the early stages, often leading to late diagnosis or misdiagnosis of dementia in people with Down's syndrome. Other treatable conditions common in people with Down's syndrome that are often mistaken for dementia include urinary tract infections causing acute confusional states, lack of sleep, depression, or hypothyroidism[13].

Estimates of incidence of dementia in people with Down's syndrome vary from 75% for the individuals aged 60 years and over [14], to 54.9% for the people aged 60–69 down to only 36% for the age group 50–59 years [13]. Elsewhere, an average age of dementia onset of 54.7 years has been recorded [12]. Although statistics are not consistent, this is clearly a specific health issue for the people with Down's syndrome as they age, and a matter of concern for their carers who need to be aware of different presentations and issues associated with dementia in people with Down's syndrome.

Policy

Dementia is of particular concern for service planners and practitioners as the increased likelihood of the rapid progression of dementia in the individual places considerable extra demands on services [15,16]. Despite the clear demographic imperative for understanding the needs of people with Down's syndrome and dementia, there is a dearth of policy guidance for this group in the UK [17]. For example, in England, the National Service Framework for Older People [18] does not discuss the needs of older people with a learning disability. Policies specific to people with a learning disability (Valuing People (in England) [4] and The Same as You (in Scotland) [11] are significant in their lack of discussion of ageing issues. Thus there is a lack of useful information and evidence on how best to provide services that are needs-led, multi-disciplinary, and supportive [19]. Any models of care and proposed frameworks for people with Down's syndrome and dementia have to pay attention to these different and changing needs, which require differently trained staff, programming, as well as attention to environmental issues [20].

Current practice responses

Accommodation

One of the fundamental challenges in providing appropriate care for people with Down's syndrome and dementia is making accommodation choices. The choice of accommodation will have a major impact on the ensuing model of care. Although there are no comprehensive statistics available as to where people with Down's syndrome and dementia are being cared for since deinstitutionalization and the major shift to community care, people tend to live within a continuum of accommodation types. This ranges from learning disability specific group homes to care homes for older people in general.

There is debate [9,17] within research as to whether the preferred option should be to keep a person with Down's syndrome in their own accommodation with additional supports, move to dementia specific accommodation, or move to a generic care provision. Providing appropriate care is simply about enabling a person with Down's syndrome to age and die in an appropriate place, but also concerns how the process of caring can best be supported, bearing in mind the complex staffing, service, and resource implications [19]. The most common description of current models of care for someone with Down's syndrome and dementia is based on the potential pathways that an individual may follow post diagnosis:

1 'Ageing in place' where the person will remain in their own accommodation with appropriate supports provided

2 *'In place progression'* where the staff and environment are continually developed and adapted to become increasingly specialized to provide long-term care for the person with dementia within the residential (learning disability) service, but not necessarily in their own accommodation

3 *'Referral out'* where the person is moved out of the learning disability service to a long term care home or nursing home facility, or similar type of provision [9].

In order to address the planning process associated with best meeting the needs of people with Down's syndrome, we suggest the following framework as a means to maintain quality of life.

Framework of support – taking a questioning approach

This framework of support has evolved from the analysis of qualitative longitudinal data gathered over 2 years as part of wider research into the experience of dementia in people with Down's syndrome living in three different accommodation settings.

In this section, we build on these foundations of care to provide a series of key questions focussing on central issues in providing care to someone with Down's syndrome and dementia in a care home setting. Each set of questions suggested by Figure 9.1 relates to staffing issues, mealtimes, and communication. This gives scope for a number of crucial answers, each needing to be known by family, carers, and professionals. The questions should be answered where possible by the person who has Down's syndrome rather than for them, using their preferred method of communication before moving onto the next set of questions. Each set consists of simple yet essential questions that are often neglected in day-to-day care. It is important to challenge the mistaken assumption that people with Down's syndrome will not have these preferences because of their learning disability or will not have the means to communicate them either verbally, non-verbally, or through an advocate.

Here, we demonstrate a framework that suggests topics for appropriate questions to ask in order to provide support. In addition to asking questions, the answers must be recorded.

Having presented the framework, we shall now discuss how it would work in practice using the example of Michael, a person with Down's syndrome and dementia living in a care home. A crucial point is that the quality of the care provided as a result is more important than the accommodation setting in which it takes place.

Michael – referral out to generic nursing home

This section will examine some of these issues in more detail and discuss the impact that staffing, communication, and mealtime issues have on Michael's quality of life (see Figure 9.2). This illustration is based on data gathered through 2 years of observation and one-to-one meetings mostly using non-verbal communication. It highlights the areas of poor practice or challenges in providing care for Michael within his particular care home and is intended to demonstrate the individualized support that must be put in place until further research identifies a preferred model of care.

The example of Michael is not intended as a critique of care homes, it is acknowledged that many may have considered all of the above factors in advance and may be carrying out appropriate and high quality care provision when working with a resident with a learning disability. However, such evidence is consistently lacking in research. Michael's situation shows how the care received will impact on his quality of life. The use of this framework based on asking questions about staffing issues, communication, and mealtimes is a starting point. It encourages thought and planning to develop support alongside a person who has Down's syndrome and dementia.

By asking Michael appropriate questions based on this framework, we may see a different experience of dementia for him in this generic care home. Could his placement have been successful if the staff knew more of his wishes and preferences before and after his admission? Would he have a better understanding of the changes that were happening to him if he were given an explanation or a diagnosis? What do the staff need to do to support Michael better when he reaches the end stages of dementia? Such questions are crucial if future care is to encompass all areas of support. Yet it is important to stress that the questions are not accommodation specific. If they remain relevant from the time of diagnosis and through the course of dementia in a supportive way, there is a greater likelihood of a positive quality of life being maintained whatever the care setting.

The core areas of questioning – staffing issues, mealtimes, and communication – will now be expanded upon. Although research evidence is limited, these three issues are recurring themes in care homes [5].

Staffing issues

Michael's situation illustrates the impact that lack of training and experience of working with people who have a learning disability has in generic care homes. Research focussing on the support of people with Down's syndrome as they age suggests that practitioners do not feel well-equipped and that older people's services do not always have the opportunity to share experiences and skills [15]. Particularly in supporting people with high support and health needs, as in the case of individuals with dementia, the intersection between health- and social-care services is not clear, leading to a problematic agenda for new service demands [21]. Generic care services exist for older people with dementia in the general population along with specific learning disability services with very little overlap between the two. Hussein and Manthorpe [22] highlight the potential for integrated health and social care sectors to make the most of staff by acknowledging and building on their transferable experience and expertise.

Michael is an example of many people with Down's syndrome and dementia who move out of family homes and into residential care when their needs increase. Thompson and Wright [23] concluded that, just as in Michael's case, care homes generally lack suitable staff training, have inadequate staffing levels and people with a learning disability do not mix socially with other residents. Many of the people had entered homes for reasons other than their health; most had moved because of the death of the primary caring relative or because their previous service was closed or reorganized.

Any proposed framework for someone with Down's syndrome has to have the central goal of enhanced quality of life for the person. There is also a need to recognize the importance of the following points:

1 Flexible and comprehensive day and night caring services [15]

2 Staff will require additional training and support to be able to provide the care for someone with Down's syndrome and dementia; such support can often be drawn from the community learning disability team, or from previous learning disability care staff, and from relatives and friends who know the person well [24]

3 Staff whose first language is not English should be required to speak clear English whilst working to avoid confusion for the person with dementia, unless they are also able to speak the same language, and can therefore, communicate

4 Staff from different cultures may have different previous experiences of working with people with a learning disability [25], just as residents' perceptions of their carers may be based on cultural differences and stereotypes [26].

Beyond responding to these staffing issues, care homes will also need to begin to address key areas such as eating, drinking, and communicating, which are essential for physical and emotional health and well-being.

Mealtimes

Mealtimes, and generally ensuring adequate nutritional and fluid intake, are central elements of both basic care and quality of life [27]. Regulatory bodies that inspect care homes should routinely ensure nutritional content of meals is adequate. However, even this does not show how much food is actually being eaten and often family members are not aware of this either. Diagnostic over-shadowing was illustrated in the case of Michael's experience through his undiagnosed difficulties with swallowing, eating, and drinking as shown by weight loss, dry skin, food avoidance, dehydration, and choking [27]. In Michael's case, these signs were attributed to his learning disability rather than to dementia, despite this being a recognizable area for speech and language therapy intervention.

Mealtimes can be a starting point for communication [28] resulting in physical comfort for the person with dementia plus comfort for the carer in being able to do something of practical use. A home-like atmosphere in the kitchen and dining room contributes to social relationships [29], with the benefits of food going beyond mere nutrition. Key questions around mealtimes are part of the framework to ensure that recognition is given to the changing needs of the person with Down's syndrome whose preferences and recognition of different foods may change as dementia progresses.

Attention to mealtimes, not only meets nutritional needs, it helps to include the person with Down's syndrome in the social aspects of eating. Without the information gained from each set of questions, carers cannot begin to know the person and will not have enough background knowledge to make mealtimes a pleasurable, social experience.

Communication

Evidence indicates that many people with a learning disability living in care homes for older people are there because of a breakdown in their caring networks, both family and formal [23]. This suggests the imperative for services to take greater account of service-users' views [21]. In order to do this the preferred method of communication must be known and understood by the carer.

The move by a person with Down's syndrome to a care home for older people is generally considered unsatisfactory [23]. This is due to a lower level of support in providing individualized programmes and failure to adapt communication methods. The importance of non-verbal communication in people with Down's syndrome and dementia has not been fully researched. Although care homes are often assessed as meeting the minimum standards required, this does not include basic skills in interaction and kindness as a routine part of communication in day-to-day work [30]. Using this framework should ensure carers' familiarity with the preferred communication methods of the person with Down's syndrome and their more subtle communication needs relating to pain, hunger, personal choice, and preferences. Just as children with Down's syndrome have difficulty in interpreting the emotions of others [31] the same can apply to adults. If there are no explanatory words to accompany the carer's action or expression, it can lead to an inappropriate response from the person with Down's syndrome who is unable to read visual cues; yet verbal interaction in care homes often lasts for just a few seconds and takes place mostly in noisy communal areas [32].

Michael, like many others with Down's syndrome may always have had difficulty in clarity of speech often needing time to answer questions or formulate responses [33]. This will be no less of an issue now that he has dementia. Similarly, there are reports of self-talk among young people with Down's syndrome [34]. This can also be seen in older adults with Down's syndrome and may be a lifelong adaptive coping strategy. A carer who has no experience of working with people who have Down's syndrome may see this as an indication of pathology rather than a symptom of dementia or specific to the learning disability. This emphasizes the importance of knowing the past history of a person and all of their current and previous communication methods, which will be helped by asking the questions suggested in this framework.

Conclusion

Traditionally, specialist services for people with Down's syndrome and other learning disabilities have been developed with their own history, philosophy, staff, and practice approaches. It is only with the recent shift in demographics and a higher incidence of health problems such as dementia that the question of how to provide the best care for people ageing with Down's syndrome, who may live in a generic population, has arisen.

It seems apparent from the limited evidence available, and from practice examples, that placing someone with Down's syndrome in a care home for older people is not an effective care alternative. Yet, until there is more detailed and reliable evidence this is the only real option. This means that we need a better understanding of how to make this experience as supportive, caring, and effective as possible, with all the attendant complex staffing, service, and resource implications. If care homes are to remain a viable option for people with Down's syndrome, there needs to be a major change in approach and staff training, plus a greater understanding of learning disabilities. Despite strong opportunities for cross-sector learning between older people's and learning disability services, there is significant progress to be made before someone with a specific learning disability such as Down's syndrome can see a move to a care home as a positive choice for their continuing care.

Acknowledgement

The work looking at care homes in Scotland was funded by a studentship in the School of Health in Social Science, University of Edinburgh.

References

1. Bradley VJ, Knoll J (1990). *Shifting paradigms in services to people with developmental disabilities.* Cambridge, MA: Human Services Research Institute.
2. Heller T (1999). Emerging models, in Stanley SH, Germain W (eds) *Aging, rights and quality of life: prospects for older people with developmental disabilities*, pp. 149–166. Baltimore, MD: Paul H Brookes.
3. Moss S, Patel P (1992). Prevalence of mental illness in people with learning disability over 50 years of age, and the diagnostic importance of information from carers. *Irish J Psychol*, **14**, 26–35.
4. Department of Health (2001). *Valuing people: a new strategy for learning disability for the 21st century.* London: Department of Health.
5. Watchman K (2008). Changes in accommodation experienced by people with Down's syndrome and dementia in the first five years after diagnosis, *J Policy Pract Intellect Disabil*, **5**(1), 65–68.
6. Mason J, Scior K (2004). Diagnostic overshadowing amongst clinicians working with people with intellectual disability in the UK. *J Appl Res Intellect Disabil*, **17**(2), 85–90.
7. Bigby C (2008). Known well by no-one. Trends in the informal social networks of middle aged and older people with intellectual disability five years after moving to the community. *J Intellect Devl Disabil*, **33**(2), 148–157.

8. Mencap (2007). *Death by indifference.* London: Mencap.

9. Janicki MP, McCallion P, Dalton A (2000). Supporting people with dementia in community settings, in Janicki MP, Ansello EF (eds) *Community supports for aging adults with lifelong disabilities,* pp. 387–414. New York: Paul H Brooks.

10. Baird P, Sadovnik AD (1987). Life expectancy in Down syndrome. *J Pediatr,* **110**, 849–854.

11. Scottish Executive (2000). The same as you? A review of service for people with a learning disability. Edinburgh: The Stationery Office.

12. Tyrell J, Cosgrave M, McCarron M (2001). Dementia in people with Down's syndrome. *Int J Geriatr Psychiatry,* **16**, 1168–1174.

13. Prasher V, Krishna VHR (1993). Age-of-onset and duration of dementia in people with Down syndrome integration of 98 reported cases in the literature. *Int J Geriatr Psychiatry,* **8**, 915–922.

14. Lai F, Williams RS (1989). A prospective study of Alzheimer disease in Down syndrome. *Arch Neur,* **46**, 849–853.

15. Wilkinson H, Kerr D, Rae C, Cunningham C (2004). *Home for good? Preparing to support people with learning difficulties in residential settings when they develop dementia.* Brighton: Pavilion Publishing/ Joseph Rowntree Foundation.

16. Wilkinson H, Janicki MP (2002). The Edinburgh Principles with accompanying guidelines and recommendations. *J Intellect Disabil Res,* **46**(3), 279–284.

17. Forbat L, Wilkinson H (2008). Where should people with dementia live? Using the views of service users to inform models of care. *Br J Learn Disabil,* **36**(1), 6–12.

18. Department of Health (2001). *National service framework for older people.* London: Department of Health.

19. Watchman K (2007). Dementia and Down syndrome: the diagnosis and support needed. *Learn Disabil Pract,* **10**(2), 10–14.

20. McCarron M, Gill M, Lawlor B, Begley C (2002). Time spent caregiving for persons with the dual disability of Down's syndrome and Alzheimer's dementia. *J Learn Disabil,* **6**(3), 263–279.

21. Wilkinson H, Kerr D, Rae C (2003). Might it happen to me or not? What do people with learning disability understand about dementia? *J Dementia Care,* **11**(1), 27–32.

22. Hussein S, Manthorpe J (2007). Older people with learning disabilities: workforce issues *Int J Integr Care,* **13**(1), 17–23.

23. Thompson D, Wright S (2001). Misplaced and forgotten? *People with learning disabilities in residential services for older people.* London: The Foundation for People with Learning Disabilities.

24. Janicki MP, McCallion P, Dalton AJ (2002). Dementia-related care decision-making in group homes for persons with intellectual disabilities. *J Gerontol Soc Work,* **38**(1/2), 179–195.

25. Ford D, Stepney S (2003). Hospital discharge and citizenship rights of older people: will the UK become a test bed for Eastern Europe? *Eur J Soc Work,* **6**, 257–272.

26. Jönson H (2007). Is it racism? Scepticism and resistance towards ethnic minority care workers among older care recipients, *J Gerontol Soc Work,* **49**(4), 79–96.

27. Leslie P, Crawford H, Wilkinson H (2009). People with learning disability and dysphagia: a Cinderella population? *Dysphagia,* **24**(1), 103–104.

28. Goldsmith M (1998). *Hearing the voices of people with dementia.* London: Jessica Kingsley.

29. Cioffi J, Fleming A, Wilkes L, Sinfield M, Le Miere J (2007). The effect of environmental change on residents with dementia: the perceptions of relatives and staff. *Dementia,* **6**(2), 215–231.

30. Reilly S, Abendstern M, Hughes J, Challis D, Venables D, Pederson I (2006). Quality in long term care homes for people with dementia: an assessment of specialist provision. *Ageing Soc,* **26**, 649–668.

31. Wishart J (2007). Socio-cognitive understanding: a strength or weakness in Down syndrome, *J Intellect Disabil Res,* **51**(12), 996–1005.

32. Ward R, Vass A, Aggarwal N, Garfield C, Cybyk B (2008). A different story: exploring patterns of communication in residential dementia care. *Ageing Soc*, **28**, 629–651.

33. Kumin L (2006). Speech intelligibility and childhood verbal apraxia in children with Down syndrome. *Downs Syndr ResPract*, **10**(1) 10–22.

34. Glenn S, Cunningham C (2000). Parents reports of young people with Down syndrome talking out loud to themselves. *Ment Retard*, **38**, 498–505.

Chapter 10

Dementia care in developing countries

Sivaraman Shaji

Introduction

Demographic transition towards ageing is a global phenomenon and is one of humanity's greatest triumphs. Worldwide, the fastest rate of growth is in the age group of 60 years and above [1]. The percentage of elderly people is increasing overwhelmingly in the countries of Asia, Africa, and Latin America. For developing countries, population ageing has many serious connotations and challenges. The developed nations of the West 'became rich before they became old', but developing countries today are 'becoming old before they become rich'. In 2002, of the more than 600 million older persons (people aged over 60 years), almost 499 million were in developing countries. By 2025, of almost 1.2 billion people projected to be in this age group worldwide, about 840 million will be in developing countries. Half of the world's older persons will be in Asia [2].

The total population of the Asia-Pacific region in 2005, as estimated from United Nations data, is 3.58 billion. The population over 65 years is estimated as 238.9 million. The number of people with dementia will increase in the Asia-Pacific region from 13.7 million people in 2005 to 64.6 million by 2050 [3], out of a total population of 685.2 million. The population of elderly (aged over 60 years) in India in 1991 was about 55.3 million, comprising 6.6% of the total population. It reached 7.5% by 2001 and population projections predict a steady increase in the percentage of elderly people in the community [4]. As the economy and level of education improve, it is expected that there will be a significant increase in life expectancy in many of the Latin American countries. Population projections indicate that the life expectancy at birth in most of the Latin American countries will be 75 years and above by 2025 [5].

Prevalence of dementia in developing countries

Globally, demographic trends predict a steady increase in the number of people with age-related morbidities especially dementia. Though the pattern of age-related health problems has been well documented in the developed countries, there have been no reliable estimates of the particular problems in developing countries.

Epidemiological studies conducted in some of the developing countries has confirmed the presence of dementia as elsewhere in the world. A number of prevalence studies have been reported from various regions of India since the 1990s. Two epidemiological studies conducted in elderly people aged 60 years and above, one in the city of Chennai and another in the rural block of southern India, obtained prevalence rate of 27 per thousand and 37 per thousand, respectively [6,7]. Two prevalence studies conducted in Kerala (southern India), one from rural and the other from an urban community, reported prevalence rate of 44 per thousand and 33.6 per thousand in elderly people aged 65 years and above [4,8]. Studies conducted in northern parts of India reported lower prevalence rates [9,10]. Two studies from the 1980s, published in China reported very low prevalence rates for dementia. Prince and colleagues reviewed seven published prevalence surveys from the developing world and reported prevalence rates for dementia ranging from 13 to 53 per thousand for those aged 60 years and above and 17 to 52 per thousand for all those aged 65 years and over [11–15].

The age-adjusted prevalence of Alzheimer's disease (AD) reported from seven developing countries ranged from 0.6% to 1.8% [12]. It has been observed that there is regional variation in the relative proportion of AD compared with vascular dementia. The proportion of AD in studies from India ranged from 41% to 65% and the proportion of vascular dementia ranged from 22% to 58% [4, 6–8]. The studies from China, Taiwan and Japan have showed a significantly higher prevalence of vascular dementia compared with AD [16,17]. The reverse appears to hold in studies from Europe and North America which have reported AD to be more common [18,19].

Dementia as a public health problem

What are the challenges faced by developing countries when dementia is emerging as a major health problem for older people? There has been a paucity of research evidence from the developing world regarding various aspects of dementia. The 10/66-dementia research group has been formed to promote good quality, internationally comparable research into dementia in developing countries through active research collaborations. It is a network of over a hundred researchers mainly from developing countries like India, China, Africa, and Latin America. It is committed to encouraging better quality research in these regions where an estimated two third of all those with dementia live.

What is common about dementia in developing countries?

1. Dementia is a hidden problem and is underestimated

There are several possible reasons. Perhaps physicians do not diagnose dementia but use non-specific terms such as senility. Other postulates refer to the socio-economic realities and lack of awareness about dementia in the population studied. It is likely that there is a low survival rate after the onset of the disease. Poor access to technologically advanced health care may contribute to the death of patients resulting in lower estimates of the number of cases. Traditional attitudes towards older people can be a contributing factor in low survival. For example, family members will not inflict care and food onto older people who are bedridden and refuse to eat. It is also possible that there is a lower occurrence of underlying risk factors; or there are concomitant protective factors in the population studied that might account for the lower prevalence figures. There is some evidence that the occurrence of a specific gene, apolipoprotein E ε4, which is a known risk factor in AD, is lower in the Indian population than elsewhere. Additionally, gene-environment interactions have also been postulated as responsible factors for the lower number of cases in eastern countries [20,21].

2. Dementia is not thought of as a health condition

Most of the people consider dementia as an inevitable consequence of normal ageing not requiring any medical care; thus families do not seek help from the health care providers. In India, few people with dementia are seen by doctors [22]. In developing countries, not only are doctors more scarce, but also elderly people and their relatives may be less willing to consult them with problems such as failing memory, deteriorating speech or increasingly bizarre behaviour, either because mental illness is feared and stigmatized, or because doctors are perceived as having little or nothing to offer.

The primary care physicians are neither sensitive nor trained to detect the problems associated with dementia. A therapeutic nihilism exists regarding the care of people with dementia. Cultural responses to most illnesses differ. Dementia is no exception. In India, for example, cases of dementia involving anger and hot temper may be more easily recognized than those involving forgetfulness. In poor agricultural societies, older people may make few demands and dementia may not be noticed so quickly. People may not regard its consequences as seriously as they do in faster moving, more complex cultures. Different types of dementia may be responded to in different ways. In China, for instance, medical help may be sought after a stroke, but not in response to failing powers of memory [23].

3. Dementia is a stigmatized condition

In developing countries, there exists a tendency to perceive dementia as a psychiatric condition. Though it is a neurological illness with psychiatric manifestations, the negative feelings and attitudes directed towards mental illness are also seen directed towards dementia. So people tend to hide it once it occurs in the family. People often attribute it to abuse, neglect, and lack of love on the part of children towards their parents. Behavioural disturbances associated with dementia are often considered by others as intentional or deliberate on the part of people with dementia. These types of misinterpretations of the symptoms can be a source of family conflict or interpersonal problems. Some people tend to associate it with superstitious beliefs and attribute it to supernatural causes [24].

4. Traditional care is under strain

In many of the developing countries traditional family systems were beneficial in terms of care of older people. The traditional family system is crumbling in favour of nuclear families in many of the developing countries. The Chinese culture values caring for older people in the family and most of the families do so. The community is responsible for taking care of older people who have no family at all. However, because of the rapid social changes, a new way to take care of older people called community service has emerged. This implies that the family care model is changing in China [25].

In developing countries like India, the integrity of the traditional arrangements is increasingly threatened by the rapid socio-cultural and economic changes. It is widely believed that the extended family system acted as a safety net. A growing body of evidence suggests that this practice is increasingly compromised. Factors like fewer children born, increasing divorce, fewer two generational households, more middle-aged women returning to work, leave many elderly people isolated and alone [26].

These trends suggest there is growing pressure on care and a greater likelihood that many older people will be living without caregivers.

5. The problem of care burden is not acknowledged properly

Dementia exerts a disproportionate and multi-faceted impact on family and co-residents in most of the developing countries. There is a heavy reliance on family care. There is a widely held belief that the families are endowed with an inherent ability to cope with the stresses and strains of caregiving. This is far from reality, but the belief distracts people from the core problems and needs of caregivers. Studies conducted in these countries reveal that caregivers of people are strained owing to psychological, practical, and economic problems. The level of caregivers' strain was notably higher among caregivers of people with dementia in comparison with people living with depression. The economic strain was marked, and there was an increasing tendency to seek private medical care, which resulted in high health care costs [27].

6. Health care systems are not sensitive to the needs of patients with dementia

In many developing countries health care systems are oriented very much towards the priorities of maternal and child health and control of communicable diseases. Many of the community-based programmes are provided mainly for child and maternal health. The general health services are clinic-based. Often the condition is not identified at the primary care level; and, even if it is identified, the health care professionals are not properly trained to give practical advice or support to the caregivers. Caregivers' stress is neither assessed nor recognized and caregivers have no opportunities to discuss their difficulties. The number of specialist doctors, like psychiatrists, neurologists and physicians, is not adequate to meet the needs of the vast majority of people in the community. In general, people are not much worried about memory impairment or cognitive impairment [28–30]. People tend to seek medical help when the behavioural and psychological symptoms cross a certain threshold or when the disease becomes unmanageable.

Poverty is the greatest obstruction to the security of the aged in many developing countries. Many poor older people have little or no access to health services.

7. Lack of development of services

Services catering for the needs of patients with dementia are rare or non-existent in many developing countries. There has been little or no expectation of medical or nursing input and little available infrastructure of care beyond the family [31]. Psychogeriatric services have not yet evolved as a specialty. Adult psychiatrists and neurologists without any special training in the care of older people see most of the patients with dementia. The building up of multi-disciplinary teams, which is essential for any comprehensive dementia care programme, is conspicuous by its absence.

Developing dementia care services in the community – an Indian experience

India is the second most populous country in the world. It is the number of elderly people in India that is formidable rather than the percentage. Most of the people with dementia live with family members in the community. So community-based rehabilitation programmes are best suited for India.

Alzheimer's and Related Disorders Society of India (ARDSI) was formed in 1992 and became instrumental in starting dementia care programmes in India. It is a registered, national, non-profit, voluntary organization, dedicated to the care of, and support for people with dementia, as well as to training and research. It aims to improve the quality of life of people with dementia as well as the caregivers through support services, awareness campaigns, and a variety of other programs. ARDSI has 14 chapters spread across the country with its headquarters in Kerala. Through this network, it implements a number of services, which include: daycare, homecare, memory clinics, respite centres, and training programmes. One of its important objectives is to empower people in the community to cope with challenges caused by dementia.

The activities of ARDSI started with an epidemiological survey of dementia in a rural community. The training programme for the community geriatric health workers started simultaneously to provide care for identified patients.

Training of community geriatric health workers

The main objective of the training programme was to prepare people to take care of older people in various settings. Eligibility to the programme required that the applicant was an adult with a pass in matriculation. The duration of the course was 10 months. A multi-disciplinary team provided practical and theoretical training to the candidates. Community geriatric health workers were instrumental in providing care for older people in the community. They are entrusted with the following responsibilities:

1 Identification, referral, and follow up of cases in the community

2 Liaison between mental health professionals and family members

3 Providing care to the geriatric person in the community and other settings

4 Helping the family members in caregiving by providing educational inputs and emotional support

5 Transferring skills, attitudes, and knowledge to the caregivers to encourage better care

6 Facilitating the use of services from various agencies and the formation of self-help groups

7 Acting to ensure continuous and co-ordinated service for older people.

Urban community dementia care services (UCDS)

UCDS was a project for developing community-based comprehensive health care services for people with dementia. The centre provided health care to about 5000 elderly people. It was a joint venture of ARDSI and HelpAge India. The 3-year project started in1996. The main objectives of the project were:

1 To identify people with dementia

2 To provide services such as domiciliary care, day care, medical, and psychiatric services to people with dementia

3 To train community geriatric health workers

4 To organize support groups and to disseminate information about dementia

5 To encourage research.

A multi-disciplinary team worked in coordination to fulfil the objective of the project. The clinical team consisted of a medical officer, a psychiatrist (part-time), a clinical psychologist, a nurse, social workers and community geriatric health workers. The administrative staff included a project officer, accountant, and driver.

Six hundred elderly people received domiciliary care services during the years 1996–99 of which 102 people had a diagnosis of dementia. The health workers identified the cases through a community survey. They are trained to administer simple screening tools to pick up potential cases of dementia. All the suspected cases were subjected to clinical evaluation by the psychiatrists in their homes to confirm the diagnosis. An individualized care plan was formulated. The health workers carried out liaison work between the family and the experts. People from all socioeconomic classes availed themselves of the services. There was an increased demand from lower middle class and lower class households. Of the total patients, 72% had the diagnosis of Alzheimer's disease.

Forty-six people used the daycare service during this period. The diagnoses were: Alzheimer's disease 69%; vascular dementia 14%; mixed dementia 2%; mild cognitive impairment 6%; unspecified dementia 6%. Of the total number of patients, 47% belonged to upper middle class or upper class households. An evaluation study conducted revealed that the service was helpful to the majority of the caregivers (84%). The reasons for relief obtained through domiciliary care included: (1) receiving correct information to increase knowledge about dementia; (2) getting information about how to manage distressing symptoms; (3) helping to remove negative feelings towards those with dementia; and (4) providing respite to the caregivers and help through medical and nursing interventions [32].

Caregiver meetings were organized at least once a month. The meetings were usually conducted in patients' houses or local institutions. The carers who were in need of individual attention were referred to the counselling service of UCDS. The geriatric health workers training programme of the UCDS lasted for 12 months.

Raising awareness about dementia was an important objective of this project. The centre provided updated information about dementia. The 24-hour helpline provided easy access to the service and provided guidance and direction, when required.

Homecare by trained volunteers from the community

The volunteers from the community who had an aptitude to provide care were selected and trained to provide care to the people with dementia. Most of the volunteers belonged to a women's self-help group (Kudumbashre). They were given basic training regarding various aspects of dementia including psychosocial management. Their main duty was to help the patients and family members through simple interventions.

10/66 Caregiver intervention programme

The 10/66-dementia research group developed and tested a model for community-based rehabilitation of people with dementia. They have begun an ambitious but practical programme designed to complement local care with improved knowledge [33–35]. The integrated child development scheme (ICDS) is a part of a national health programme established by the government of India. Local, educated women are recruited as health workers after formal training in community-based maternal and child health care. The idea was that these health workers could be utilized for the care of older people in the community. The Thrissur Center (Kerala, India) of the 10/66 group developed an informant-based strategy to identify people with dementia residing in the community. The case identification method had been validated and proved to be both useful and cost-effective [36]. The 10/66 group developed a model for intervention to educate and train caregivers to manage people with dementia in the community better. Any intervention needs to consider the following facts: first, there should be some mechanism for the identification of cases in the community; secondly, the intervention needs to be capable of being delivered in the home setting using existing resources; thirdly, in developing the intervention, consideration must be given to the resource available to deliver it; finally, the content and level of intervention must be tailored to suit the cultural context.

Institutionalization and daycare services

The practice of institutionalization is comparatively less in developing countries. The most important reason for institutionalization is the inability of family members to cope with the behavioural and psychological symptoms of dementia [37]. Other reasons for institutionalization include absence of an informal caregiver, sickness, or disability in the primary caregiver, family problems, or interpersonal conflict. Most of the people in developing countries cannot afford institutionalization, as it is not cost-effective. Daycare services are also rare in many developing countries. The first daycare centre for people with dementia started in Cochin, India, in 1996. A study of the pattern of uptake of daycare services revealed that there are many barriers to the utilization of services. These include lack of awareness about the usefulness of the services, stigmatization, lack of consensus between family members regarding the use of services, and limitations related to the provision of services which prevent them from accommodating people with disorganized behaviours and various physical disabilities.

Minimum actions required for the care of people with dementia

An action plan was presented at the 20th international conference of Alzheimer's Disease International in 2004 in Japan (The Kyoto declaration). The 10 overall recommendations of this declaration are relevant to developing countries and appear below.

1. Provide treatment in primary care

There is a need to recognize dementia care as a component of primary health care and include the recognition and treatment on dementia in training curricula for all health professionals. There is also a need to develop locally relevant materials for training.

2. Make appropriate treatments available

Most of the anti-dementia drugs are not easily available or affordable for people in developing countries. The availability of essential drugs should be ensured in all health care settings. Basic education and training interventions for the caregivers need to be developed and evaluated.

3. Give the care in the community

Establish the principle that people with dementia are best assessed and treated in there own homes. Develop and promote standard needs assessments for use in primary and secondary care. Development of multi-disciplinary community health care teams is an essential pre-requisite for the development of services.

4. Educate the public

The most important impediment related to any intervention in dementia is the lack of awareness. Promoting public campaigns against stigma and discrimination and supporting governmental and non-governmental organizations to educate the public can be the initial step in raising awareness. The mass media have a great role in fostering positive attitudes. These campaigns may be helpful as a way to encourage early intervention and treatment.

5. Involve communities, families, and consumers

Promoting the formation of self-help groups may foster advocacy initiatives. It is essential to ensure representation of communities, families, and consumers in policymaking, service development, and implementation.

6. Establish national policies, programmes, and legislation

National policies, programmes, and legislation should be based on current knowledge and understanding of dementia. Dementia care programmes and policies should be formulated with existing social realities in mind. For example, people with dementia should be included in disability benefit schemes, caregivers in compensatory benefit schemes, and health and social care budgets established for older people.

7. Develop human resources

Psychogeriatric services are rare or non-existent in most of the developing world. Doctors, nurses, and other primary health care workers should be given training in old-age psychology and geriatric medicine. Developing training and resource centres and creating a network of national training centres for physicians, psychiatrists, psychologists, nurses, and social workers may be a great step forward.

8. Link with other sectors

An inter-sectoral approach to initiating community, school, and work place dementia awareness programmes and encouraging the activities of non-governmental organizations in this field is essential.

9. Monitor community health

Dementia as a topic must be included in basic health information systems. Surveying high-risk population groups and surveillance for early dementia in the community should be the part of this programme.

10. Support more research

There is a paucity of research in mental health in general and dementia in particular in developing countries. Conducting studies in primary health care settings on the prevalence, course and outcome of dementia and linking research to qualitative improvement in dementia care services must be kept as an important goal.

Conclusion

Dementia is emerging as an important public health problem in many of the developing countries, but its consequences are not properly acknowledged. There exist many factors that contribute to this insensitivity. These include a low level of awareness; culture bound beliefs regarding ageing and care of the aged and stigmatization. The services related to the care of people with dementia are rare or absent. There is a need to develop services of different types. Community based care is most suited to developing countries, as it is cost-effective and culturally acceptable. It is important to link dementia care with the existing health care delivery system. More research inputs, training of health personnel, awareness raising, and advocacy are needed. Combined, co-ordinated, and targeted efforts at various levels are required to prepare and support communities to cope with the challenges caused by the increasing population of elderly people with dementia.

References

1. WHO (2002). Active aging-a policy framework. Non-communicable Disease and Health promotion Department, Aging and life course, WHO, Geneva.
2. Awin N (2006). The role of government in health and aging—experiences of Malaysia, in Indira Jaiprakash (ed). *Aging with health and dignity*, pp. 1–12. Bangalore, India: Bangalore University.
3. Alzheimer's and Related Disorders Society of India (2006). *Dementia in the Asia Pacific region: the epidemic is here-executive summary of a report*, Kunnamkulam-680 5034: ARDSI.
4. Shaji S, Promodu K, Abraham T, Roy J, Varghese A. (1996). An epidemiological study of dementia in a rural community in Kerala, India. *Br J Psychiatry*, **168**, 745–749.
5. Mangone CA, Bueno A, A. Allegri R, *et al.* (2000), Behavioral and psychological symptoms of dementia in Latin America. *Int Psychogeriatr*, **12**(1), 415–418.
6. Raj Kumar S, Kumar S (1996). Prevalence of dementia in the community—a rural–urban comparison from Madras, India. *Aust J Ageing*, **15**, 9–13.
7. Rajkumar S, Kumar S, Thara R (1997). Prevalence of dementia in rural setting—a report from India. *Int J Geriatr Psychiatry*, **12**, 702–707.
8. Shaji S, Bose S, Varghese A (2005). The prevalence of dementia in urban population in Kerala, India. *Br J Psychiatry*, **186**, 136–140.
9. Chandra V, Ganguli M, Pandav R, Johnston J, Belle S, Dekosky ST (1998). Prevalence of Alzheimer's Disease and other dementias in rural India: The Indo–US Study. *Neurology*, **51**, 1000–1008.

10. Vas CJ, Pinto C, Panikker D, *et al.* (2001). Prevalence of dementia in an urban Indian population. *Int Psychogeriatr*, **13**, 439–450.

11. Prince M (2000). Dementia in developing countries: a preliminary consensus statement from the 10/66 dementia research group. *Int J Geriatr Psychiatry*, **15**, 14–20.

12. Prince M (2000). Methodological issues for population based research into dementia in developing countries. *Int J Geriatr Psychiatry*, **15**, 21–30.

13. Phanthumchinda K, Jitapunkul S, Sitthi Amorn, C, *et al.* (1991). Prevalence of dementia in an urban slum population in Thailand: validity of screening methods. *Int J Geriatr Psychiatry*, **6**, 639–646.

14. Li G, Shen YC, Chen C H, *et al.* (1989). An epidemiological survey of age related dementia in an urban area of Bejing. *Acta Psychiatr Scand*, **79**, 557–563.

15. Zhang MY, Katzman R, Salmon D, *et al.* (1990). The prevalence of dementia and Alzheimer's disease in Shanghai, China: impact of age, gender and education. *Ann Neurol*, **27**, 428–437.

16. Shibayama H, Kasahara Y, Kobayashi H (1986). Prevalence of dementia in a Japanese elderly population. *Acta Psychiatr Scand*, **74**, 144–151.

17. Hasegawa K, Homma A, Imai Y (1986). An epidemiological study of age related dementia in the community. *Int J Geriatr Psychiatry*, **1**, 45–55.

18. Jorm, A., F., Korten, A,E., Henderson, S,A.,(1987).The prevalence of dementia: a qualitative integration of the literature. *Acta Psychiatr Scand*, **76**, 465–479.

19. Jorm AF (1991). Cross national comparisons of the occurrence of Alzheimer's and vascular dementias. *Eur Arch Psychiatry Clin Neurosci*, **240**, 218–222.

20. Vas CJ, Rajkumar S, Tanyakitpisal P, Chandra V (2001). *Alzheimer's disease: the brain killer.* New Delhi, India: WHO, Regional Office for South East Asia.

21. Prince MJ (1997). The need for research on dementia in developing countries. *Trop Med Health*, **2**, 993–1000.

22. Patel V, Prince M (2001). Aging and mental health in a developing country: who cares? Qualitative studies from Goa. *India Psychol Med*, **31**, 29–38.

23. Alzheimer's Disease International (1999). Caring for the people with dementia around the world, *Fact sheet 5*, London, UK.

24. Shaji S (2007). Dementia-An Indian perspective of rehabilitation, Book of Abstracts, *13th National Conference of Alzheimer's and Related Disorders Society of India*, Chennai.

25. Xie X (1997). *Creating an integrated caring environment for the elderly, Central Union for the welfare of the aged*, Helsinki: Finnish Federation for the Social welfare and Health.

26. Shaji KS, Smitha K, Lal KP, Prince MJ (2003). Caregivers of patients with Alzheimer's Disease: a qualitative study from the Indian 10/66 Dementia research Network. *Int J Geriatr Psychiatry*, **18**, 1–6.

27. Dias A, Samuel R, Patel V, Prince M, Parameswaran R, Krishna-moorthy ES (2004). The Impact associated with caring for a person with dementia-a report from the 10/66 dementia research group, Indian network. *Int J Geriatr Psychiatry*, **19**, 182–184.

28. Cohen CI (2000). Racial differences in neuropsychiatric symptoms among dementia patients: a comparison of African Americans and Whites. *Int Psychgeriatr*, **12**(1), 395–402.

29. Liu HC (1994). Assessing cognitive abilities and dementia in a predominantly illiterate population of older individuals in Kinmen. *Psychol Med*, **24**, 763–770.

30. Chandra V (1994). Studies of epidemiology of dementia, comparison between developed and developing countries. *Aging Clin Exp Res*, **6**, 307–321.

31. Jolley D (2005) Dementia and dementia care: an International perspective, in Kar N, Jolley D, Misra B (eds). *Handbook of dementia*, pp. 306–322. Hyderabad, India: Paras Medical Publishers.

32. Sunny C (1999). *An evaluation of the urban community Dementia Services Center, Kochi*, Kalamasserry, Kochi, Kerala: The research Institute, Rajagiri College of Social Sciences.

33. Huang H, Shyu YL, Chen M, Chen S, Lin L (2003). A pilot study on a home based training programme for improving caregiver self efficacy and decreasing the behavioral problems of elders with dementia in Taiwan. *Int J Geriatr Psychiatry*, **18**, 337–345.

34. Prince M, Graham N, Brodatti H (2004). Alzheimer's Disease International's 10/66 Dementia Research Group: one model for action in developing countries. *Int J Geriatr Psychiatry*, **19**, 178–181.

35. The 10/66 Dementia Research Group (2004). Care arrangements for people with dementia in developing countries. *Int Psychogeriatr*, **19**, 170–177.

36. Shaji KS, Arun Kishore NR, Praveen MJ (2002). Revealing a hidden problem. An evaluation of a community dementia case finding program from the Indian 10/66 Dementia research Network. *Int J Geriatr Psychiatry*, **17**(3), 222–225.

37. Eke E, Ertan T (2000). Behavioral and psychological symptoms of Dementia in eastern and south Eastern Europe and the MiddleEast. *Int Psychogeriatr*, **12**(1), 409–413.

Chapter 11

Ingredients and issues in supportive care for people with dementia: summarizing from models of care

Julian C. Hughes, Mari Lloyd-Williams, and Greg A. Sachs

Introduction

In the chapters so far, we have seen different types of dementia from a variety of perspectives. The intention has been to reveal the models or frameworks that underpin different services. A word of caution is required. Our aim is to characterize a model of supportive care, but not to arrive at some sort of exact pathway of care for all people with dementia. In other words, although we hope to say what might constitute supportive care for people with dementia in a general way, individuals in individual contexts will need different ingredients of care at different times. We shall return to this theme in our final chapter. The importance of this point reflects an underlying point about person-centred care, which must be – at one and the same time – both ethical and practical. Supportive care in dementia must be person-centred and, as such, it must be individual.

In this chapter, our aims are more limited. We shall highlight some of the points that the authors of the preceding chapters have made. We shall summarize the issues that emerge. We shall derive from what has already been said the ingredients of a supportive care dementia service. We shall then look forward to the chapters that follow as they discuss the potential elements of supportive care.

Issues for supportive dementia care

The issues that emerge from the different models of care already considered show large degrees of overlap. Nonetheless, they are also quite various and are summarized in Box 11.1. This is split into different spheres (biological, psychological, social, spiritual, and ethical), but it has to be said immediately that these are not clear-cut divisions, as if our psychological and social aspects can be neatly divided. So, for example, we have placed the maintenance of well being as a psychological issue; but we have also listed regard to overall quality of life as a spiritual matter. The relationship between well-being and quality of life is conceptually complex. All we wish to acknowledge is that there is a state of psychological contentment that might be summed up by the phrase 'well-being'; and spirituality is also rightly concerned with issues connected with overall quality of life. Similarly, carer burden is both a psychological and a social issue; and the promotion of meaningful activities might have cognitive effects that could be detected biologically or might more simply help to guard against some of the effects of increasing physical frailty. It should also be said that the number of items occurring under a particular heading in Box 11.1 does not reflect its importance. Thus, although little emerged to flesh out the notion of spiritual care, spirituality is a notion that has emerged strongly in several of the chapters above.

Box 11.1 Issues for supportive dementia care derived from different models of care

Biological

Understanding underlying biology,
e.g. chemical and neuropathology
Genetic influences
Other biological risk factors
(e.g. cardiovascular, trauma, and alcohol)
Early diagnosis and importance of
diagnostic competence
Treatment appropriate to condition,
symptoms, and time
Recognition of brain frailty and consequent
susceptibility to confusion
Vulnerability to adverse effects of drugs;
Management of specific symptoms
(e.g. pain, dysphagia, constipation,
and contractures)
Nutritional issues
Mobility issues, including falls
Maintaining function

Psychological

Genetic counselling
Sympathetic, emotional support to person
with dementia and carers
Support of cognitive skills
Encouraging enjoyment
Understanding carer burden and need for
carer support
Therapeutic relationships
Comfort
Maintenance of well-being
Strategies for everyday living

Social

Environmental risk factors
Impact on family and family dynamics
Meaningful activities (e.g. music, dance,
and art)
Community support (e.g. home care, day
care, and respite care)
Stigma and need for education
Financial issues
Legal issues, including wills
Accommodation issues
Importance of communication
Safety
Individual care packages
Encouraging healthy lifestyles

Spiritual

Acknowledging and supporting spirituality
Regard to overall quality of life
Promoting dignity

Ethical

Personhood and person-centred care
Moral support
Advance care planning
Maintaining autonomy

In Chapter 2, Jolley has provided us with a useful overview of the dementias. One thing to emerge from this is the undoubted biological complexity of these conditions. It is clear from this account that dementia is rightly regarded as a specialized field. The number of issues to emerge is too large to recount in detail, but it is noteworthy that these span from the possibility of prevention, for example of vascular dementia or of dementia caused by trauma, to the need for appropriate psychosocial environments, as well as to the importance of spirituality.

Spirituality is a theme that emerges in the writings of Wallace in describing her own experience of dementia in Chapter 3. But we also find here a plea for continuity of care. Wallace is keen to emphasize the need for person-centred care and for practical advice and flexible support for carers. The need for flexibility is certainly something discussed by Pointon at various points in her description, in Chapter 4, of her journey with her husband from the time of his diagnosis to the time of his death. Like Wallace, she also commends the idea of a 'Dementia Adviser', which has emerged in the UK in the National Dementia Strategy. The continuity of care that might be assured by having such a person 'journeying alongside us', to use Pointon's phrase (see page 27), is a further theme that echoes the experience of Wallace. These first hand accounts provide powerful messages concerning the type of care people really want; as shown similarly in the account by Cooper in Chapter 6, which emphasizes the need for personalized care with an awareness of the person's history. This might be summed up in part by Pointon's memorable description of how essential it is that supportive care should provide 'time to attend' (page 32 above).

The PEACE programme, described in Chapter 5 by Shega and Sachs, makes clear some fundamentally important aspects of care for people with dementia. Amongst other things, community care must be coordinated; it must be patient and family-centred; and it must (unavoidably) be interdisciplinary. This point emerges in several of the other descriptions of services. For instance, in Chapter 7 in connection with Huntington's disease (HD), Bilney and Morris offer this definition of supportive care: 'an inter-professional approach to the management of the physical, cognitive, and emotional aspects of HD, providing assistance for the person with HD and their family throughout the disease' (see page 55 above). Again, there are several themes contained in this quote, such as the need to support the person and the family *throughout* the course of the disease, but it is worth highlighting the notion of *inter*-disciplinarity. This is more than just the stipulation that we need multi-disciplinary teams. The disciplines need to be inter-digitating, working hand in hand as it were. There must be no gaps. This is what really underpins the possibility of the *integrated* care pathways that Barber and Cooper mention in Chapter 6.

But to return to the PEACE programme, one of the other very important things to be demonstrated was that this approach can work and can produce measurable successes. It also incorporated a palliative approach to care and advocated the use of advance care planning. It is very likely that part of the success of the programme depended on the commitment and qualities of the individuals concerned. This should not be underestimated, even though the next iteration of PEACE will be attempting to use protocols to try to make assessments and interventions uniform and coordinated as efforts are made to serve larger numbers of patients across multiple practices. In the review of the younger persons team recorded by Barber and Cooper it is interesting that 'therapeutic relationships' were regarded so highly by those responding to the survey in connection with the team's work. This has obviously been of considerable importance to Wallace and Pointon, too, in their experiences of dementia.

A further feature of importance to emerge in the discussion of HD is, of course, the difficult mixture of mental and physical symptoms. But, as all of the other chapters attest, this is a feature of dementia across the board. The exact manifestations of mental and physical frailty differ in the different conditions at different times, but it is for this reason that the support that is required must be specialized. As Box 11.1 shows, there is a host of difficult physical factors to be considered. But these are different at different times within the course of any particular dementia and different in different types of dementia. Meanwhile, Box 11.1 demonstrates a raft of complicated social factors to be negotiated. Hence, the need for inter-professional teams, as Bilney and Morris suggest.

The complexities are exemplified in HIV-associated dementia (HAD) (described by Cohen and Schwartz in Chapter 8). In addition to the stigma of dementia, there is the stigma of HIV and AIDS. Similar to the case of HD (but equally true in dementia associated with Parkinson's disease or in the case of conditions such as progressive supranuclear palsy or Creutzfeldt-Jakob disease), in HAD there are not only the physical effects that come with the progression of any dementia, but also the devastating physical effects that are a primary manifestation of the disease. But perhaps most striking in the case of HAD is the possibility of prevention and treatment, for instance with the use of combination antiretroviral therapy (CART). Here is a case where cure and care potentially come together, where the dichotomy disappears. But here, too, is an area where there then emerge tremendous social and ethical tensions over the availability of treatment. The complexity of supportive care is evident.

A basic requirement of care is that people should be looked after in appropriate settings, but what might be appropriate has to be considered and, as Wilkinson and Watchman make plain in Chapter 9, this is an issue that has to be decided with considerable care. The issue of communication is vital in learning disabilities, but becomes increasingly important in all types of dementia. The issue for supportive care becomes partly a technical one to do with how to communicate effectively, but also an ethical one to do with providing person-centred care, which stresses the individuality and unique standing of people with dementia, who can otherwise be the victims of more or less overt stigma.

One weapon to combat stigma is education. In the developing world, as Shaji describes in Chapter 10, education is a crucial issue. But the themes, even if presenting with a different level of complexity in a multiplicity of social contexts, remain strikingly similar to those seen in the literature from more developed nations. People still require good diagnosis; there is still a need for support for families to decrease the burden of care; there is still a requirement for professionals from a variety of backgrounds to work in a co-ordinated manner to provide community care. Shaji also stresses the importance of good quality research. His emphasis on the need for access to technologically advanced health care makes the point that people in developing countries remain less fortunate because of the disparities in terms of economic wealth. Issues of dignity and quality of life depend in part on there being a basic level of health care provision. And he is surely right to draw attention to the public health implications globally of our increased and increasing longevity.

The issues raised, therefore, by this review of different experiences or provision of healthcare are many and various. Nevertheless, even from what has been said so far, the ingredients of a supportive care dementia service start to emerge.

Ingredients of supportive dementia care

As well as raising issues, the preceding chapters have also highlighted what the ingredients of a supportive care dementia service might be and these are summarized in Box 11.2.

Some of the ingredients in Box 11.2 seem almost mundane: of course good care (of whatever sort) should include coordinated, integrated, interdisciplinary, comprehensive care that is also flexible and able to provide holistic support: practical, emotional, moral, and spiritual. This sounds like motherhood and apple pie – a lovely idea but perhaps hopelessly optimistic and, perhaps, not completely achievable. And yet it is what people with dementia and their carers would want and it is what any of us would want for ourselves and for those close to us. These ingredients do not in themselves raise any questions. The only question is to do with practicalities and how this pattern of care might be achieved. Although we can gesture in the direction of an answer, for instance by (at least) commending (but then only provisionally) the idea of a Dementia Adviser, the details would need to be worked out locally, which may mean by individual services, or may involve national guidelines and incentives.

Of more interest is the idea that people must have the right sort of experience and skill at the right moment. The point here is crucial for supportive care from the time of diagnosis until death and beyond. Having the requisite knowledge concerning the use of antibiotics, for instance, is not enough. Instead, what is required is a matter of clinical judgement, because the use of antibiotics

Box 11.2 Ingredients of a supportive care dementia service derived from different models of dementia care

Coordination and integration (of health and social care)

Continuity of care with timely follow-up

Interdisciplinary care

Flexible support

Comprehensive care

Palliative care

Proper training and support to provide knowledgeable and experienced professionals equipped to deal with the various manifestations of various types of dementia in various contexts at various different stages of the particular condition

A mixture of practical, emotional, moral, and spiritual support

Ability to provide support recognizing how needs change over time

Community support

Liaison services to hospital and other institutional settings

Research and audit/quality improvement

when a person has mild dementia is different to the use of antibiotics when the person has very severe dementia. Attention to nutrition will be different at different stages of the disease. Even the provision of community support will need to be handled in an individual way depending on the exact circumstances for the particular person and where he or she is on his or her unique trajectory of dementia. Similarly, care in a nursing home will differ compared to care in the person's own home. Hence, one of the ingredients of supportive care must be the application of judgements that will be different, not just between people, but also within the course of the illness for a single individual. The supportive care framework should tend to encourage the broader view: a view of the illness over time during which priorities will change.

The place of palliative care within this framework needs further consideration. As we discussed in Chapter 1, the palliative care model provides a useful way to approach dementia. But we also saw some difficulties in its use. Supportive care seems to add something: the framework brings in, not only the potential of prevention and active treatment (doing away with the cure *versus* care dichotomy), but also the whole palliative care focus. The point to see is that palliative care, whilst not providing an overall framework, nevertheless is pervasive. All of the attitudes of palliative care, from the time of diagnosis, seem pertinent and important.

Community support is another important ingredient of a supportive care model. This notion carries a good deal of weight, because resting on it is the whole idea that people should be allowed to live the lives that they would wish and, furthermore, they should be encouraged to think of themselves as people who can *live with* dementia. Dementia should not preclude meaningful engagement and activities. Hence, there is a requirement that community support should be sufficient to allow people to pursue their own ends in a manner that is free and enhancing. This support should be person-centred, which includes the idea that it should be tailored to the individual. It should be palliative too, in the sense that it should emphasize quality of life and living up until the moment of death. The ingredients of a supportive care dementia service should have as its overall aim the preservation of the person's selfhood, where this is understood in a broad manner.

Looking forward

Having identified some of the issues and ingredients of supportive care in dementia, the chapters that follow are intended to outline the elements of supportive care. We shall move from medical approaches, which include looking at particular types of service, to psychological interventions, and to social support. Issues of spirituality, which include support for grieving, the importance of communication, and issues about maintaining the self, lead on to discussion of person-centredness and broadly ethical considerations, including discussion of advance care planning from the perspectives of Europe and America. Finally, before our concluding chapter, we discuss dying, both at home and in institutional care, and consider how the person and his or her family might be supported through the final stages of dementia.

Chapter 12

Pharmacological management of neuropsychiatric symptoms in people with dementia

Clive Ballard and Dag Aarsland

Introduction

Worldwide, there are almost 25 million people with dementia, the majority of whom have Alzheimer's disease (AD) [1]. It is a devastating illness resulting in a progressive decline in cognition and function, which causes immense distress to patients, their carers, and their families, and has an enormous impact on society. The treatment of neuropsychiatric symptoms in these individuals is one of the main therapeutic challenges, with more than 90% of people experiencing at least one of these symptoms over the course of the illness [2,3]. There are 3 main neuropsychiatric syndromes: agitation, psychosis, and mood disorders [2,4]. Agitation includes symptoms of aggression, irritability, restlessness, and pacing, usually associated with distress or anxiety. Aggression and non-aggressive agitation occur in 20% of the people with AD in contact with clinical services [2,5] or living in the community [6]. Frequencies are higher (40–60%) in care facilities [7].

The most frequent psychotic symptoms are visual hallucinations, auditory hallucinations, and delusions, which are present in 25% of the people with dementia in clinical settings [2,5]. The typical psychotic symptoms characteristic of schizophrenia almost never occur in people with dementia, and in contrast to functional psychoses, the psychotic symptoms are much less complex. Visual or second-person auditory hallucinations of people or animals, and simple persecutory delusions such as believing that possessions have been stolen are typical [2]. In a recent community study, 18% of the people with AD experienced delusions and 14% experienced hallucinations [6]. Mood symptoms, including depression, anxiety, and apathy, are frequent and important in people with dementia, with clinically significant depression occurring in 20% of the people with AD [2,5].

Neuropsychiatric symptoms are frequently distressing for patients [8], are stressful for caregivers [9,10] and are often a precipitant of nursing home care [11]. These symptoms are therefore frequent and important, and the clinical management of neuropsychiatric symptoms is a high priority for clinicians treating patients with dementia.

Overview of the current chapter

In the current chapter, we will summarize the evidence of benefits and harms related to antipsychotic drugs in people with AD, and review pharmacological approaches for the management of neuropsychiatric symptoms in these patients. Where the evidence is incomplete, we will offer our interpretation to help guide clinical decision-making. The current chapter focusses heavily on treatment issues in AD, predominantly because of the very limited evidence base related to the treatment of other dementias. Non-pharmacological approaches are likely to be equally applicable across all dementias (although this has not been established in clinical trials), but there are specific risks associate with antipsychotic medication in vascular dementia (VaD) [12] and dementia with Lewy bodies (DLB) [13] which highlight the priority of developing evidence based pharmacological approaches for the treatment of neuropsychiatric symptoms in these patient groups.

Antipsychotics for the treatment of neuropsychiatric symptoms in AD

Clinical Benefits

Typical antipsychotics

There have been 11 randomized, placebo-controlled trials of typical antipsychotics for the treatment of behavioural and psychiatric symptoms of dementia (BPSD), mostly involving small sample sizes, over periods between 4 and 12 weeks [14–17]. Using the convention of defining a good outcome as a 30% improvement on standardized behavioural rating scales, a significant but modest advantage of antipsychotics over placebo (59% versus 41%) has been reported, in the context of a high placebo response [14]. The most comprehensive evidence pertains to haloperidol, in which four randomized controlled trials (RCTs) have been completed, indicating a significant improvement in symptoms of aggression compared to placebo, but no significant improvement in other symptoms of agitation, and more modest improvements in psychotic symtpoms [18]. There is very little clinical trial evidence pertaining to other typical antipsychotics for the treatment of agitation, aggression, or psychosis.

Atypical antipsychotics

During the early 1990s, atypical antipsychotics such as risperidone, olanzapine, and quetiapine were introduced for the treatment of schizophrenia, and by the mid 1990s were in frequent clinical use as an 'off-license' treatment for agitation, aggression, and other BPSD. Since 1995, 18 placebo-controlled trials have examined the efficacy of atypical antipsychotics in people with AD, mainly over treatment periods of 6–12 weeks [12,19], although most are not fully in the public domain. Compared to placebo, risperidone is associated with a significant overall improvement of behavioral symptoms (combining all doses and studies), for total neuropsychiatric symptoms scores and aggression (preferential response at 2 mg per day), with a more modest benefit for psychosis (only at 1 mg per day) and no evidence of treatment benefits for non-aggressive agitation [12,19]. In addition, the only study focussing specifically on risperidone for the treatment of clinically significant psychosis in people with AD did not identify any significant benefits [20]. The studies of olanzapine [12,19] reported improvement in a combined score for agitation/aggression (at 5–10 mg/day) compared to placebo with an effect size intermediary between risperidone and haloperidol, but there was no significant improvement in psychosis in olanzpine-treated patients compared to those receiving placebo. Two trials with aripiprazole also indicate significant improvements in aggression [19]. The only published study with quetiapine did not indicate significant benefit in the treatment of agitation [21], but the number of unpublished studies precludes a meaningful meta-analysis. The beneficial effects of therapy are much more limited over longer treatment periods of 6–12 months [21–23].

The impact of atypical antipsychotic treatment on neuropsychiatric symptoms from a meta-analysis of 12 week RCTs of risperidone is summarized in Table 12.1. The Table focusses on

Table 12.1 Efficacy of risperidone for neuropsychiatric symptoms over 12 weeks of treatment (based on Ballard and Howard [12])

	Target symptom	Outcome measure	Mean difference from placebo
Risperidone 1 mg	Psychosis	BEHAV-AD	MD −0.79, 95%CI −1.31 to −0.27, $p = 0.03$
Risperidone 1 mg	Aggression	BEHAV-AD	MD −0.84, 95%CI −1.28 to −0.40, $p = 0.0002$
Risperidone 2 mg	Aggression	BEHAV-AD	MD −1.50, 95%CI −2.05 to −0.95, $p < 0.0001$

risperidone as there have been a larger number of trials conducted, and it is the only atypical antipsychotic for which all the trials are fully in the public domain.

Adverse effects of antipsychotic prescribing in people with Alzheimer's disease

The adverse effects of typical antipsychotics in patients with AD include parkinsonism, dystonia, tardive dyskinesia, and QTc prolongation on the electrocardiogram (ECG) [19,24,25]. QTc effects have been associated with several previously widely prescribed agents including thioridazine and droperidol [25]. Haloperidol, the most widely studied typical antipsychotic, has been evaluated in 4 placebo-controlled trials [18], which show a doubling in emergent extrapyramidal symptoms. Similarly, meta-anlaysis of placebo-controlled trials with risperidone also indicate that patients receiving risperidone were twice as likely to experience extra-pyramidal symptoms as those receiving placebo [12]. Data regarding extra-pyramidal symptoms have not been reported fully in trials evaluating other neuroleptics in people with dementia. Compared to placebo-treated patients, the meta-analysis also identified a significant increase in somnolence in both risperidone and olanzapine-treated patients [12], and an increase in peripheral oedema and fever amongst people treated with risperidone [12]. We do not interpret these data as indicating that risperidone has any greater side effects than other atypical antipsychotics, merely that the reporting of adverse events was more comprehensive in these trials.

Combining data from the placebo-controlled trials, risperidone is associated with a three-fold increased risk of serious cerebrovascular adverse events (including stroke), compared to placebo [12,19]. Summary data supplied by Eli Lilly and Company Ltd suggest a similar increase in the incidence of cerebrovascular adverse events in the placebo-controlled trials of olanzapine in AD (olanzapine 1.3% versus placebo 0.4%). In contrast, a large retrospective study of older people in Canada using healthcare databases did not identify an excess of strokes in people treated with typical or atypical neuroleptics [26], although this study did not specifically focus on people with dementia. The balance of evidence supports the conclusion that there is an increased risk of cerebrovascular adverse events in people with dementia treated with risperidone or olanzapine. However, it is unclear whether this is a class or drug-specific effect. Far less clinical trial information is available for other atypical antipsychotics. In the absence of clear clinical trial data for other drugs, there needs to be a high level of caution regarding the likelihood of an increased risk of adverse cerebrovascular events.

There is very little evidence about the potential impact of typical antipsychotics on stroke risk. A large retrospective Canadian study indicated a similar stroke incidence in people with dementia prescribed typical or atypical antipsychotics [27], but the absence of an 'untreated' comparison group makes the results difficult to interpret. It is unclear from the data presented whether patients with VaD, concurrent cerebrovascular disease, or amyloid angiopathy are at higher risk of these events.

In 2005, the Food and Drug Administration (FDA) [28] published a warning pertaining to a significant increase in mortality risk for people with AD treated with atypical neuroleptics, compared to individuals receiving placebo in RCTs. The FDA analysis was based on pooled data from 17 placebo-controlled trials of atypical neuroleptics, but data from individual trials were not provided. Hence, it is unclear whether the risk differs between individual drugs. Schneider and colleagues [29] have reviewed the evidence from 15 of these trials, confirming a significant increase in mortality (OR 1.54; 95%CI 1.06–2.23; $P = 0.02$), but finding no difference between specific agents. Mortality risk is even higher with typical neuroleptics, [30] and becomes increasingly pronounced with prolonged prescribing [31].

In a cohort study, McShane *et al.* [32] reported that neuroleptic-treated patients experienced twice the rate of cognitive decline as those not receiving these drugs. A more recent placebo-controlled trial with the atypical neuroleptic quetiapine also indicates an accelerated rate of cognitive decline, with quetiapine-treated patients experiencing a considerably greater decline than placebo-treated patients over 2 weeks [22]. A meta-analysis of mini-mental state examination (MMSE) change over 12 weeks in the placebo-controlled trials of atypical antipsychotics confirmed a significant increase in the rate of cognitive decline [20].

The evidence from meta-analyses pertaining to the adverse effects of antipsychotics in 12 week RCTs of risperidone in AD are shown in Table 12.2. The Table again focuses on risperidone as there have been a larger number of trials conducted, and it is the only atypical antipsychotic for which all the trials are fully in the public domain. In addition, the adverse event reporting was more comprehensive in these publications.

Summary of the evidence pertaining to antipsychotics in AD

Until 2000, thioridazine, promazine, and haloperidol were all widely used in the clinic, but prescribing practice has substantially changed following cardiac safety concerns related to thioridazine. Despite the increasing safety concerns, there have however been only very modest changes in the overall prescription rates, although atypical antipsychotics are now more widely prescribed than typical agents in most countries. The modest benefits of short-term therapy and the very limited evidence of ongoing treatment benefits need to be balanced against the adverse events. Reflecting this, best practice guidelines now highlight that the prescription of antipsychotics for AD patients should be restricted to people with severe symptoms causing risk or extreme distress that have not responded to other measures, and that treatment should only be continued beyond

Table 12.2 Adverse events associated with risperidone in 12 week RCTs in AD (based on Ballard and Howard (12))

	Adverse outcome	Odds ratio
Risperidone	Stroke/cerebral vascular event	3–4
Atypical antipsychotics	Mortality	1.5–1.8
Atypical antipsychotics	Accelerated cognitive decline	1.5–4
Risperidone (1–2 mg)	Ankle oedema	2.4–3.3
Risperidone (1–2 mg)	Chest infections	2.9
Risperidone (1–2 mg)	Extra-pyramidal symptoms	1.8–3.4
Risperidone (1–2 mg)	Sedation	2.4–4.5
Atypical antipsychotics	Falls	Unresolved

12 weeks in exceptional circumstances. Within this context, the remainder of the chapter focusses on best practice principles, non-pharmacological approaches and other potential pharmacological treatments for the treatment of neuropsychiatric symptoms in people with dementia.

General principles for the assessment and treatment of neuropsychiatric symptoms

Before any specific treatments are considered, a broad clinical assessment is very important. Physical health problems such as infection, pain, or dehydration are common, and often precipitate neuropsychiatric symptoms. Pain can be difficult to assess in people with dementia and is often under-diagnosed (see Chapter 14 for further discussion of pain). Urinary tract infections and chest infections are a frequent trigger for neuropsychiatric symptoms, but dental infections are also common and often not recognized. Treatment of concurrent physical health problems will frequently result in resolution of behavioural and psychiatric symptoms without recourse to any specific therapies. Visual and auditory impairment can also precipitate BPSD, and should be treated when possible. This may be as simple as changing glasses or a hearing aid, or encouraging them to be worn regularly. These principles are outlined in more detail by Lyketsos and colleagues [33].

It is also important to consider the severity and consequences of any behavioural or psychiatric symptoms. For example, many symptoms may occur very intermittently, only during specific situations or may not result in distress or risk to the individual or others. Symptoms which are not frequent or do not result in distress or risk may not require any specific therapy, or may be preferentially treated with a less invasive approach such as the various psychological approaches outlined in Chapter 17. Neuropsychiatric symptoms fluctuate greatly in severity and often resolve or improve spontaneously over 4–6 weeks. For mild-moderate symptoms, a period of monitoring by asking relatives or care staff to keep a diary of symptoms can often give valuable insights and can help avoid precipitous treatment for a symptom which may resolve spontaneously.

People with dementia are also often highly responsive to the environment they find themselves in. In general terms, the environment should be safe and familiar and unnecessary changes should be resisted. Safety is particularly important to allow a carer to leave a disturbed patient for a little while without worrying. An occupational therapy assessment of a home environment can be particularly useful to identify potential dangers and to instigate specific measures, such as locking away dangerous tools or kitchen implements. Wandering can be made safe by restricting a person to a specific area, but this entails constant attention to the need to balance personal autonomy against the management of the behaviour.

Pharmacological treatments

Given the serious adverse events associated with the use of antipsychotics in people with dementia, there is a strong imperative to develop better and safer pharmacological treatments. In current clinical practice, the key question is whether other available licensed compounds can provide useful pharmacological alternatives to atypical antipsychotics, and when the use of these drugs should be considered. The subsequent sections will review the evidence for the best candidate compounds and then suggest some recommendations for the use of these treatments in the clinic.

Cholinesterase inhibitors

There has been relatively little focus on whether cholinesterase inhibitors (ChEIs) have a potential role in the treatment of neuropsychiatric symptoms in AD or other dementias. A meta-analysis demonstrated a small but significant overall advantage of ChEIs compared to placebo over

24–26 weeks with regard to the overall treatment of neuropsychiatirc symptoms in AD [34]. Additional support for the benefits of ChEIs on neuropsychiatric symptoms comes from a randomized withdrawal study, in which cessation of donepezil in AD patients was associated with a significant worsening of the total Neuropsychiatric Inventory (NPI) score within 6 weeks [35]. However, there was no short-term benefit for treatment of clinically significant agitation with donepezil over 12 weeks in a large RCT, [36] suggesting that ChEIs do not appear to be useful in the management of acute agitation. ChEIs appear to have their greatest effects on depression/dysphoria, apathy/indifference, and anxiety [37] and may improve psychotic symptoms such as visual hallucination in people with DLB and related dementias [38]. They are probably not an effective treatment for clinically significant agitation, aggression, or psychosis in AD, at least over a 3-month period.

Memantine

Individual studies, meta- and pooled analyses indicate that memantine confers benefit in the treatment of irritability/lability, agitation/aggression, and to a lesser degree psychosis over 3–6 months, in patients with AD [39,40,41], and a Cochrane meta-analysis suggested that memantine conferred a modest but significant benefit in the treatment of neuropsychiatric symptoms in patients with VaD [41]. Whilst this evidence is very encouraging with respect to memantine, there are no RCTs specifically involving patients with clinically significant agitation or aggression. Prospective RCTs in people with AD who have clinically significant agitation are needed to support these findings. Ongoing RCTs in Canada and in the UK will hopefully clarify the role of memantine in the treatment of agitation/aggression in AD and VaD.

Antidepressants

The use of antidepressants to treat depression and other neuropsychiatric symptoms in AD dates back almost three decades, but despite this the literature remains limited. Several tricyclic antidepressants have been examined in clinical trials for the treatment of depression in people with AD, with limited evidence of benefit [42,43], perhaps in part because of the detrimental impact of side effects. Studies with selective serotonin reuptake inhibitors (SSRIs) have indicated better tolerability and generally a more favourable response to treatment (see [44] for an evidence based review), with the best study conducted so far indicating a good treatment response with sertraline [45]. Although widely used in clinical practice, there are no studies of the newer classes of antidepressants such as selective noradrenergic reuptake inhibitors (SNRIs). It should also be noted that clinical trials often exclude more severely depressed patients, which probably reduces the apparent treatment benefit in these studies. It should also be emphasized that the limited evidence from clinical trials should not be used as a reason to withhold anti-depressant treatment from a patient with AD who is severely depressed. Larger multi-site trials focussing on the treatment of depression in patients with AD are currently underway in the UK and US, and should hopefully address many of the currently unresolved issues.

The choice of anti-depressant drug is important because patients with dementia are often frail and may be expected to be more susceptible to side effects. Falls, possibly due to orthostatic hypotension (a fall in blood pressure on rising) and increased confusion in particular, are a problem with the tricyclic anti-depressants. Safety considerations and the current evidence base both favour SSRIs. For people residing in care homes or nursing homes, attention to care plans to increase social interaction and pleasant activities may be extremely effective for milder depression. In the absence of any specific evidence relating to the treatment of depression in VaD or DLB, the same treatment approaches as recommended for AD are probably the best guide for clinical practice.

Several other RCTs have examined the efficacy of sertraline, citalopram, and trazodone in the treatment of agitation in AD. In one of the RCTs, sertraline was generally well tolerated but did not appear to affect overall neuropsychiatric symptoms [46]. A *post hoc* analysis, however, examining patients with moderate or more severe agitation, suggested efficacy for sertraline compared to placebo in this sub-group [46]. In a second, smaller, 17-day trial of psychiatric in-patients with more severe neuropsychiatric symptoms, Pollock and colleagues [47] reported that citalopram was superior to placebo, with greatest efficacy for agitation/aggression, an effect not seen with perphenazine. In a later study, the same group found citalopram to be comparable in efficacy to risperidone, differentiated by its significant effect on agitation symptoms and superior tolerability, in the treatment of moderate to severe neuropsychiatric symptoms [48]. Despite initially encouraging results from open label and cross-over trials, double-blind comparisons of trazodone to placebo have failed to confirm any benefit in the treatment of neuropsychiatric symptoms [18, 49].

Anticonvulsants

With regard to anticonvulsants, there are some encouraging results for carbamazepine. A number of case series and small cross over trials provide preliminary evidence of possible efficacy for the treatment of agitation in AD (reviewed in [50,51]). There are only two small parallel group RCTs, both conducted over a 6-week period [52,53] both suggesting good tolerability, and with reasonable preliminary evidence of benefit on measures of agitation and global rating. A subsequent case-register study of subjects ≥ 65 years of age also suggested that carbamazepine confers less mortality risk than anti-psychotics [54]. Valproate studies have not shown treatment benefits for neuropsychiatric symptoms (reviewed in [51]). Data for other anticonvulsants is preliminary, and largely based upon small case series of patients receiving open-label treatment.

The evidence from these pharmacological approaches is summarized in Table 12.3.

Pimavanserin

Pimavanserin is a newly developed 5-HT2A agonist, with pre-clinical evidence of benefit in a rodent model of AD psychosis [55] and good tolerability in phase I and phase II trials in man.

Table 12.3 Non-antipsychotic pharmacological therapies for neuropsychiatric symptoms in AD

Sodium valproate for agitation/aggression	Low doses ineffective, higher doses poor tolerability
Carbamazepine for agitation/aggression	Two small and short duration RCTs focusing on agitation/aggression, both with positive outcomes. Needs formal meta-analysis and longer trials
Trazodone for agitation	Insufficient evidence to recommend as a treatment
Citalopram for agitation	Several promising comparative treatment RCTs, needs a formal meta-analysis and a placebo-controlled trial
Memantine for agitation and psychosis	Meta-analysis suggests significant benefit for 'behaviour' (2.76 points on neuropsychiatric inventory (NPI)) and promising post hoc pooled analysis. Meta-analysis also suggests benefit in treatment of neuropsychiatric symptoms in VaD. Needs prospective studies
Cholinesterase inhibitors for agitation	Ineffective over 12 weeks. Meta-analyses and pooled analyses suggest 1.5–2 point advantage on total NPI over 6 months, but main benefits in reducing emergence of neuropsychiatric symptoms and improving mood
Sertraline for depression	Best evidence for the pharmacological treatment of depression in AD is for sertraline, with good effect size in the best RCT so far conducted

In addition, the double-blind randomized controlled phase II trial for the treatment of psychosis in Parkinson's disease suggested improvement in psychotic symptoms [56] and a phase II trial for the treatment of psychosis in AD will commence shortly. The potential impact on other neuropsychiatric symptoms has not been examined. Although still at a relatively early stage of development, the initial studies are very encouraging.

In patients with moderate to severe AD, in whom memantine is indicated for the treatment of dementia, this is probably also the preferred treatment for agitation and has the advantage of an excellent safety profile. Otherwise, the main role of these pharmacological treatments is either in individuals who have not responded to other interventions, as a treatment for relapse of agitation or aggression after discontinuation of an atypical antipsychotic, or as a tool to enable the withdrawal of atypical antipsychotics if this cannot be safely achieved with non-pharmacological interventions.

Conclusions

There are limitations to our understanding of the biological basis of agitation and aggression (as well as other behavioral features) associated with AD, and the efficacy and safety of available drug treatments is controversial. Nevertheless, clinicians are required to treat patients on a case-by-case basis, using their best judgement. Careful identification of target symptoms and their consequences, initial trials of non-pharmacological approaches, and use of the least harmful medication for the shortest period of time, should be the guiding principles in the current management of neuropsychiatric symptoms in AD and other dementias.

References

1. Prince M (2004). Epidemiology of dementia. *Psychiatry*, **3**, 11–13.
2. Ballard C, Ayre G, Gray A (1999). Psychotic symptoms and behavioural disturbances in dementia: a review. *Revue Neurologique*, **155**, 44–52.
3. Steinberg M, Shao H, Zandi P, *et al.* (2008). Point and 5-year period prevalence of neuropsychiatric symptoms in dementia: the Cache County Study. *Int J Geriatr Psychiatry*, **23**, 170–177.
4. Aalten P, de Vugt ME, Lousberg R *et al.* (2003). Behavioral problems in dementia: a factor analysis of the neuropsychiatric inventory. *Dement Geriatr Cogn Disord*, **15**, 99–105.
5. Burns A, Jacoby R, Levy R (1990). Psychiatric phenomena in Alzheimer's disease. IV: disorders of behaviour. *Bri J Psych*, **157**, 86–94.
6. Lyketsos CG, Steinberg M, Tschanz JT *et al.* (2000). Mental and behavioral disturbances in dementia: findings from the Cache County Study on Memory in Aging. *Am J Psych*, **157**, 708–714.
7. Margallo-Lana M. Swann A, O'Brien J *et al.* (2001). Prevalence and pharmacological management of behavioural and psychological symptoms amongst dementia sufferers living in care environments. *Int J Geriatric Psych*, **16**, 39–44.
8. Gilley DW, Whalen ME, Wilson RS, Bennett DA (1991). Hallucinations and associated factors in Alzheimer's disease. *J Neuropsych Clin Neurosci*, **3**, 371–376.
9. Rabins PW, Mace NL, Lucas MJ (1982). The impact of dementia on the family. *JAMA*, **248**, 333–335.
10. Ballard CG, Eastwood C, Gahir M, Wilcock G (1996). A follow up study of depression in the carers of dementia sufferers. *BMJ*, **312**, 947.
11. Steele C, Rovner B, Chase GA, Folstein M (1990). Psychiatric symptoms and nursing home placement of patients with Alzheimer's disease. *Am J Psych*, **147**, 1049–1051.
12. Ballard C, Howard R (2006). Neuroleptic drugs in dementia: benefits and harm. *Nat Rev Neurosci*, **7**, 492–500.

13. McKeith I, Fairbairn A, Perry R, Thompson P, Perry E (1992). Neuroleptic sensitivity in patients with senile dementia of Lewy body type. *BMJ*, **305**, 673–674.

14. Schneider LS, Pollock VE, Lyness SA *et al.* (1990). A metaanalysis of controlled trials of neuroleptic treatment in dementia. *J Am Geriatr Soc*, **38**, 553–563.

15. Finkel SI, Lyons JS, Anderson RL, *et al.* (1995). A randomized, placebo-controlled trial of thiothixene in agitated, demented nursing home patients. *Int J Geriatr Psychiatry*, **10**, 129–136.

16. De Deyn PP, Rabheru K, Rasmussen A, *et al.* (1999). A randomized trial of risperidone, placebo, and haloperidol for behavioral symptoms of dementia. *Neurology*, **53**, 946–955.

17. Teri L, Logsdon RG, Peskind E, *et al.* (2000). Treatment of agitation in AD: a randomized, placebo-controlled clinical trial. *Neurology*, **55**, 1271–1278.

18. Lonergan E, Luxenberg J, Colford J, Birks J (2005). Haloperidol for agitation in dementia. *Cochrane Database Syst Rev*, **4**, CD002852.

19. Schneider LS, Dagerman K, Insel PS, (2006). Efficacy and adverse effects of atypical antipsychotics for dementia: meta-analysis of randomized, placebo-controlled trials. *Am J Geriatr Psych*, **14**, 191–210.

20. Mintzer J, Greenspan A, Caers I, *et al.* (2006). Risperidone in the treatment of psychosis of Alzheimer disease: results from a prospective clinical trial. *Am J Geriatr Psych*, **14**, 280–291.

21. Ballard C, Margallo-Lana M, Juszczak E *et al.* (2005). Quetiapine and rivastigmine and cognitive decline in Alzheimer's disease: randomised double blind placebo controlled trial. *BMJ*, **330**, 874.

22. Tune LE, Steele C, Cooper T *et al.* (1991). Neuroleptic drugs in the management of behavioral symptoms of Alzheimer's disease. *Psychiatr Clin North Am*, **14**, 353–373.

23. Schneider LS, Tariot PN, Dagerman KS *et al.* (2006). CATIE-AD Study Group. Effectiveness of atypical antipsychotic drugs in patients with Alzheimer's disease. *New Engl J Med*, **355**, 1525–1538.

24. Ballard C, Margallo Lana M, Theodoulou M *et al.* (2008). A randomised blinded placebo controlled in dementia patients continuing to take or discontinued from treatment with neuroleptics (the DART-AD trial). *PLoS Med*, **5**, e76.

25. Reilly JG, Ayis SA, Ferrier IN, Jones SJ, Thomas SH (2000). QTc-interval abnormalities and psychotropic drug therapy in psychiatric patients. *Lancet*, **355**, 1048–1052.

26. Gill SS, Rochon PA, Herrmann N *et al.* (2005). Atypical antipsychotic drugs and risk of ischaemic stroke: population based retrospective cohort study. *BMJ*, **330**, 445.

27. Herrmann N, Mamdani M, Lanctot KL (2004). Atypical antipsychotics and risk of cerebrovascular accidents. *Am. J. Psych*, **161**, 1113–1115.

28. Food and Drug Administration (FDA) (2005). Deaths with antipsychotics in elderly patients with behavioral disturbances. US Food and Drug Administration, FDA Public Health Advisory, Centre for Drug Evaluation and Research.

29. Schneider LS, Dagerman KS, Insel P (2005). Risk of death with atypical antipsychotic drug treatment for dementia: meta-analysis of randomized placebo-controlled trials. *JAMA*, **294**, 1934–1943.

30. Wang PS, Schneeweiss S, Avorn J *et al.* (2005). Risk of death in elderly users of conventional vs. atypical antipsychotic medications. *N Engl J Med*, **353**, 2335–2341.

31. Ballard C, Hanney ML, Theodoulou M *et al.* (2009). The dementia antipsychotic withdrawal trial (DART-AD): long-term follow-up of a randomised placebo-controlled trial. *Lancet Neurol*, **8**, 151–157.

32. McShane R, Keene J, Gedling K, Fairburn C, Jacoby R, Hope T (1997). Do neuroleptic drugs hasten cognitive decline in dementia? Prospective study with necropsy follow up. *BMJ*, **314**, 266–270.

33. Lyketsos CG, Colenda CC, Beck C *et al.* (2006). Position statement of the American Association for Geriatric Psychiatry regarding principles of care for patients with dementia due to Alzheimer disease. *Am J Geriatr Psychiatry*, **14**, 561–572.

34. Trinh NH, Hoblyn J, Mohanty S, Yaffe K. (2003) Efficacy of cholinesterase inhibitors in the treatment of neuropsychiatric symptoms and functional impairment in Alzheimer disease: a meta-analysis. *JAMA*, **289**, 210–216.

35. Holmes C, Wilkinson D, Dean C et al. (2004). The efficacy of donepezil in the treatment of neuropsychiatric symptoms in Alzheimer disease. *Neurology*, **63**, 214–219.

36. Howard RJ, Juszczak E, Ballard CG et al. (2007). CALM-AD Trial Group. Donepezil for the treatment of agitation in Alzheimer's disease. *New Eng J Med*, **357**, 1382–1392.

37. Gauthier S, Feldman H, Hecker J et al. (2002). Efficacy of donepezil on behavioral symptoms in patients with moderate to severe Alzheimer's disease. *Int Psychogeriatr*, **14**, 389–404.

38. McKeith I, Del Ser T, Spano P et al. (2000). Efficacy of rivastigmine in dementia with Lewy bodies: a randomised, double-blind, placebo-controlled international study. *Lancet*, **356**, 2031–2036.

39. Gauthier S, Loft H, Cummings J et al. (2008). Improvement in behavioural symptoms in patients with moderate to severe Alzheimer's disease by memantine: a pooled data analysis. *Int J Geriatr Psychiatry*, **23**, 537–545.

40. Wilcock GK, Ballard CG, Cooper JA et al. (2008). Memantine for agitation/aggression and psychosis in moderately severe to severe Alzheimer's disease: a pooled analysis of 3 studies. *J Clin Psychiatry*, **69**, 341–348.

41. McShane R, Areosa Sastre A, Minakaran N (2006). Memantine for dementia. *Cochrane Database Syst Rev*, **2**, CD003154.

42. Reifler BV, Teri L, Raskind M et al. (1989). Double-blind trial of imipramine in Alzheimer's disease patients with and without depression. *Am J Psychiatry*, **146**, 45–49.

43. Petracca G, Teson A, Chemerinski E, Leguarda R, Starstein SE (1996). A double-blind placebo-controlled study of clomipramine in depressed patients with Alzheimer's disease. *J Neuropsychiatry Clin Neurosci*, **8**, 270–275.

44. Bains J, Birks JS, Dening TD (2002). Antidepressants for treating depression in dementia. Cochrane Dementia and Cognitive Improvement Group. *Cochrane Database Syst Rev*, **4**, CD003944.

45. Lyketsos CG, Delcampo L, Steinberg M et al. (2003). Treating depression in Alzheimer disease: efficacy and safety of sertraline therapy, and the benefits of depression reduction: the DIADS. *Arch Gen Psychiatry*, **60**, 737–746.

46. Finkel SI, Mintzer JE, Dysken M, Krishnan KR, Burt T, McRae T (2004). A randomized, placebo-controlled study of the efficacy and safety of sertraline in the treatment of the behavioral manifestations of Alzheimer's disease in outpatients treated with donepezil. *Int J Geriatr Psychiatry*, **19**, 9–18.

47. Pollock BG, Mulsant BH, Rosen J et al (2002). Comparison of citalopram, perphenazine, and placebo for the acute treatment of psychosis and behavioral disturbances in hospitalized, demented patients. *Am J Psychiatry*, **159**, 460–465.

48. Pollock BG, Mulsant BH, Rosen J et al. (2007). A double-blind comparison of citalopram and risperidone for the treatment of behavioral and psychotic symptoms associated with dementia. *Am J Geriatric Psych*, **15**, 942–952.

49. Sultzer DL, Gray KF, Gunay I, Berisford MA, Mahler ME (1997). A double-blind comparison of trazodone and haloperidol for treatment of agitation in patients with dementia. *Am J Geriatr Psychiatry*, **5**, 60–69.

50. Tariot PN, Loy R, Ryan JM, Porsteinsson A, Ismail S (2002). Mood stabilizers in Alzheimer's disease: symptomatic and neuroprotective rationales. *Adv Drug Deliv Rev*, **54**, 1567–1577.

51. Konovalov S, Muralee S, Tampi RR (2008). Anticonvulsants for the treatment of behavioral and psychological symptoms of dementia: a literature review. *Int Psychogeriatr*, **20**, 293–308.

52. Tariot PN, Erb R, Podgorski CA et al. (1998). Efficacy and tolerability of carbamazepine for agitation and aggression in dementia. *Am J Psychiatry*, **155**, 54–61.

53. Olin, J.T., Fox LS, Pawluczyk S, Taggart NA, Schneider LS (2001). A pilot randomized trial of carbamazepine for behavioral symptoms in treatment-resistant outpatients with Alzheimer disease. *Am J Geriatr Psychiatry*, **9**, 400–405.

54. Hollis J, Grayson D, Forrester L, Brodaty H, Touyz S, Cumming R (2007). Antipsychotic medication dispensing and risk of death in veterans and war widows 65 years and older. *Am J Geriatric Psych*, **15**, 932–941.

55. McFarland K, Gorman SA, Price DL, Johnson RW, Bonhaus DW (2008). Antipsychotic like activity of pimavanserin, a 5-HT2A inverse agonist, in putative animal models of Alzheimer's disease and psychosis. Poster presented at American Academy of Neurology annual conference, April 2008.
56. Revell S, Friedman JH, Mills R, Williams H, Johnson AD, Bahr D (2008). A double-blind placebo controlled, dose escalation trial of pimavanserin in Parkinson's disease and psychosis. Poster presented at American Academy of Neurology annual conference, April 2008.

Chapter 13

Hospital admissions in dementia

Elizabeth L. Sampson

Hospital admissions

How common is dementia in the acute hospital?

Older people currently use approximately 40% of the health-care resources in the United Kingdom and occupy two-thirds of hospital beds [1]. The frailty and age of patients in the acute hospital reflects and amplifies the prevalence of dementia found in the community. Less than half of those with dementia ever receive a correct diagnosis and when they do, this is often at a time of crisis, e.g. during an emergency hospital admission [2]. Even after admission, detection rates remain low at between 37–46% [3,4]. Prevalence estimates for dementia (ICD-10 or DSM-IV) for acute medical in-patients, over the age of 65 years, range from 9.1–50.4% on acute general hospital wards [5,6] and from 63.0–79.8% on specialized geriatric and elderly care wards [7,8]. Patients with hip fractures have a reported prevalence of cognitive impairment of 31 –88% [9].

Why are people with dementia admitted to the acute hospital?

The commonest underlying causes of hospital admission in people with dementia are aspiration pneumonia, cystitis or urinary tract infection, syncope and collapse, septicaemia, and hip fracture [10]. In patients from nursing homes with Alzheimer's disease, 15% of the admissions are due to pneumonia, 11% for gastroenteritis, and 7% for kidney or other urinary tract infections [11]. These three diagnoses are 'Ambulatory Care Sensitive Conditions'—conditions for which hospitalizations are thought to be avoidable or manageable with prompt access to medical care, and could have been prevented or treated in the community. Interestingly, they are markers of the quality of health service provision. These findings may reflect the problems that people with dementia have in accessing community health care [12].

Clinical characteristics of people with dementia admitted to the acute hospital

People with dementia have complex medical, social, and psychological needs and these may be exacerbated by physical illness and adverse interactions between the health care system, the patient, and their family or caregivers. They are a vulnerable and frail population who differ significantly from those without dementia.

People with dementia on acute medical wards are significantly older by 5–9 years [13,14], more likely to be female [15,16], have lower levels of educational attainment [4,16], are more impaired in activities of daily living [7,17], and are more likely to be admitted from nursing homes [16,17]. Unfortunately there is lack of data on the important comorbidities of depression and delirium [9]. There is a higher prevalence of depression amongst acute hospital in-patients with dementia compared to those who are not cognitively impaired [4]. It is, therefore, likely that these distressing conditions are under-recognized and under-treated in this group of patients.

In people with dementia who have undergone acute hospital admission, the number and severity of co-morbid illnesses have been found to be marginally increased [16] or lower than cognitively intact controls [17]. However, post mortem studies suggest that serious physical illnesses are often not detected in these patients prior to their death [18,19]. Factors contributing to underdiagnosis include poorer access to screening programmes and delayed diagnosis, particularly for cancers [20], the difficulties that people with dementia have in reporting physical symptoms, and the (sometimes appropriate) reluctance of clinicians to 'over-investigate'.

People with dementia are more acutely physiologically unwell when they are admitted to hospital and this worsens with the severity of cognitive impairment (Sampson *et al.*) [21]. This may be caused by delayed presentation or the higher prevalence of pneumonia and sepsis. They have poorer nutritional status on admission, with lower body mass index [17,22,23], cholesterol, and albumin levels [22]. They are more dehydrated [14,24] with greater electrolyte disturbance [24], and more likely to present with lymphocytosis [22].

The experience of people with dementia who are admitted to the acute hospital

The acute hospital is a challenging environment for frail older people with dementia and complex needs. The emphasis on high throughput, moving patients rapidly from the accident emergency department, often to a medical assessment unit and then onto a 'base ward' may increase the risk of disorientation and mis-communication for patients unable to advocate for themselves. Concerns have been raised regarding the ability of acute hospital staff to diagnose and provide person-centred care effectively for people with dementia [25].

People with dementia are at higher risk of iatrogenic harm through polypharmacy [17], and have higher complication rates [26]. The functional impairment associated with dementia increases the amount of nursing time required to assist each person per day by up to 3 hours [27]. Despite the high mortality experienced by patients with dementia who are admitted to the acute hospital, they receive as many burdensome and painful investigations and procedures (e.g. arterial blood gas sampling) [28] and are more likely to be physically restrained than patients who are cognitively intact [29]. This suggests that clinicians fail to adopt a palliative or supportive approach to patient care, possibly because people with advanced dementia are not perceived to be suffering from a 'terminal illness'. Other vital components of good end-of-life and person-centred care are also neglected with little acknowledgement of spiritual needs, withdrawal of inappropriate medications, or referral to hospital palliative care teams [28]. Significantly more dementia patients experience pain in the last 6 months of life compared to those with cancer (75% versus 60%) [30], but pain control is often inadequate. In a study of patients with fractured neck of femur, cognitively impaired patients were prescribed a third as much analgesia as cognitively intact controls [31].

The impact of dementia on outcomes in the acute hospital

Dementia is an independent predictor of functional decline in acute hospital in-patients [32]. This loss of ability is thought to occur in two stages: an initial decline secondary to the acute physical illness, just prior to acute admission; and a subsequent failure to improve or maintain function after hospitalization [16]. Decline occurs in both basic and more complex 'instrumental' activities of daily living and in mobility which is less cognitively demanding [16]. The causes of functional decline are complex but include the effects of bed rest and limited mobility. Functional decline significantly increases the need for nursing or residential home care after admission [4,17].

The majority of studies have found that dementia or pre-existing cognitive impairment significantly increases the length of hospital admission by 4 days [14,33] to more than 23 days [13,26].

This is often secondary to 'delayed discharge' of patients who need to be transferred to residential or nursing homes [7,26]. Dementia mediates the increase in length of hospital stay via a range of factors such as iatrogenic harm and the development of inter-current infections. This consequently increases the costs of hospitalization and promotes further functional decline and loss of autonomy.

Amongst acute medical in-patients, dementia has a marked and independent effect on short and longer term mortality. Dementia significantly increases the risk of death during the index admission. Fields et al. [26] found that 17% of the people with dementia died during acute hospital admission compared to 5% of those who were cognitively intact. Mortality is independently associated with the severity of the cognitive impairment [21]: 7.5% of those scoring 24–30 on the MMSE died during index admission compared to 10% of those scoring 16–23 and 24% of those scoring 0–15. The adjusted hazard ratio for mortality risk for mild dementia was 1.34 (95%CI 0.60–3.15) and for moderate/severe dementia was 2.6 (95%CI 1.28–5.39). Both of these studies comprised people admitted with a range of underlying admission diagnoses. A similar effect has been demonstrated in-patients with dementia and pneumonia. Six month mortality was 53% compared to 13% of those who were cognitively intact (adjusted hazard ratio 4.6, 95%CI 1.8–11.8) [34]. Dementia also significantly and independently increases the risk of death after hip fracture: 6 month mortality risk is 2.57 (1.65–04.01) compared to those without dementia [35]. In advanced dementia, this effect is more marked. The 6-month mortality in patients with severe impairment was 55% whilst only 13% of those who were cognitively intact died (adjusted hazard ratio 5.8, 95% CI 1.7–20.4) [29]. This may be caused by increased general frailty or a higher risk of post-operative adverse events and iatrogenic harm.

Improving acute hospital care for people with dementia

Kitwood defined personhood as 'a standing or status that is bestowed upon one human being by others in the context of particular social relationships and institutional arrangements' [36]. The deterioration seen in dementia may not be caused wholly by the disease but by how the person is treated; this results in the subsequent loss of personhood. Personhood is, therefore, directly threatened by the environment, treatment, staff attitudes, and processes that occur within the acute hospital. There is much evidence that the quality of care that people with dementia receive is poor [2], but a range of simple interventions may improve this situation. These will be dealt with in the following sections, first focussing on specific interventions that fit the model of supportive care and secondly looking at more holistic approaches.

Avoiding acute hospital admission: the role of advance care planning

People with dementia are often admitted to the acute hospital for reasons that are deemed to be 'inappropriate', including breakdown in the social care package and the inability of family caregivers to continue coping. The emergency transfer of patients from residential and nursing home, the majority of whom will have dementia, has been highlighted as an area of particular concern – over 50% of these are thought to be avoidable [37]. Often this is due to poor support from out-of-hours health services, lack of training amongst care home staff and concerns about the medico-legal consequences of *not* transferring someone to hospital. A number of initiatives and mechanisms can be implemented to address these issues, from those determined by the person with early dementia for themselves, to systemic changes in health and social care systems.

Advance care planning (see Chapters 28 and 29) is a key method of avoiding repeated acute hospital admissions and allows a more 'holistic' assessment of the person with dementia that may, in some cases, be able to take into account their previously expressed wishes. A number of tools and modes of advance care planning, are available and are appropriate at different stages.

Ideally, advance care planning should begin at the earliest stages of dementia, when a person still has the competence and capacity to make decisions. The *Mental Capacity Act 2005* gives competent adults in England and Wales the legal right to refuse treatment (i.e. artificial feeding and nutrition, cardiopulmonary resuscitation) through the writing of an 'advance decision'. People can also make an 'advance statement', which reflects their general beliefs and personal values, about the sort of care they would like to receive in the future. For example, they can express the wish to die at home and not in hospital. Further discussion of the *Mental Capacity Act* and dying at home can be found in Chapter 30 in this volume.

Lasting Powers of Attorney were also introduced in the *Mental Capacity Act* and enable the appointment of an attorney to make proxy decisions when the person with dementia no longer has the capacity to do so. A 'Personal Welfare' Lasting Power of Attorney allows the attorney to give or refuse consent to medical treatment, if this has been expressed in the document. Similar frameworks are available in other countries to facilitate advance care decisions. For example, the 'Let Me Decide' programme from Australia has led to a significant decrease in the transfer of nursing home residents to acute hospital with no changes in overall mortality [38]. The emergency admission of a person with dementia to the acute hospital can be used as an opportunity to engage with carers to consider advance care planning [39].

The United Kingdom '*Gold Standards Framework*' (GSF) identifies patients requiring palliative or supportive care towards the end of life, assessing their needs, symptoms, and preferences and planning care around these, in particular supporting patients to live and die where they choose. Although not developed specifically for patients with dementia, the GSF was developed for care homes and enhances communication between GPs and other specialists, particularly out of hours, and supports the training of care home staff in end of life care. Tailored individual care plans are developed for residents. This has been shown to reduce acute hospital admissions and hospital deaths [40].

Increasing specialist medical support to nursing homes and 'Hospital at Home Schemes' for residents with acute medical illness can decrease the risk of delirium, show no significant negative impact on mortality, have significant cost savings, and – most importantly – are associated with high levels of patient and carer satisfaction [41,42].

Once a person with dementia has been admitted to the acute hospital, consideration of individual needs and a number of simple measures can significantly improve quality of care.

Feeding and nutrition

Malnutrition occurs in up to 60% of the older people who are admitted to the acute hospital [43]. This increases mortality and morbidity and significantly impairs quality of life: the enjoyment of food is a basic pleasure and social activity that even people in the advanced stages of dementia can experience. Factors contributing to difficulties with eating include the loss of ability to recognize food, problems coordinating the use of cutlery secondary to apraxia, and loss of the physiological drivers of appetite and satiety. People can develop physical difficulties with the act of swallowing (dysphagia), or aspirate. Difficulties related to the environment of the acute hospital ward include not taking account of an individual's likes and dislikes, lack of appropriately trained staff to assist with feeding, unappetizing presentation of food or simple factors such as placing food trays out of reach. A speech and language therapist or dietician can assist with formulating individualized care plans to facilitate swallowing (i.e. by thickening food) and supplement intake. Other simple interventions advocated in the United Kingdom include the 'red tray' system, where those needing help with eating are identified on admission and their meal placed on a red tray to signal the need for help. Protected mealtimes, where non-urgent activity such as ward and drug rounds are restricted, so that patients can eat their meals without being interrupted and ward staff have time to assist, can be very effective. The decision to place a feeding tube is often complex, emotive, and is made hurriedly in the stressful environment of the acute medical ward. There is little evidence to suggest that this improves quality of life or decreases adverse outcomes such as aspiration pneumonia or malnutrition [44]. It also deprives people with advanced dementia of the opportunity for interacting with others, denies them the basic enjoyment of the taste of food, reduces dignity and autonomy, and makes personal care even more 'instrumental' and task-oriented.

Orientation and communication

Communication is an essential component of continuity of care and this is impaired when people with dementia are unable to remember information or express their needs to staff. Given that dementia is widely under-recognized in this setting, even simple steps such as relatives drawing attention to the fact that a person has dementia, can improve care and ensure appropriate treatment decisions are made. Leaving a notepad by the bed so that reminders and messages can be written down for the patient or leaving familiar objects by the bedside can reduce anxiety. Simple measures such as making sure the person has the correct glasses and that these are clean, or that hearing aid batteries are not flat, will improve orientation [45]. Photographs by the patient's bed can enhance person-centred care by providing hospital staff with talking points and placing the person with dementia in a wider social context. Reality orientation therapy techniques have a useful role on acute wards [46]; some hospital wards do not have large, easily seen clocks and little access to windows or natural daylight. The date and the name of ward can be provided on whiteboards and 'incontinence' decreased by signposting toilets.

Achieving adequate pain control

Pain is under-recognized and under-treated in people with dementia and the complex reasons for this are covered in the next chapter. Often behaviours that are interpreted as 'difficult to manage' on the acute ward, such as agitation or crying out, are secondary to under-treated pain. Pain management can be improved by contacting relatives or carers of the person with dementia who may be aware of individual responses to pain (e.g. social withdrawal or grimacing) and by good nursing care to avoid pressure sores. Simple interventions with regular analgesia such as paracetamol can be extremely effective [47].

Care at the end of life

Many patients with dementia who are admitted to the acute hospital will die there. The evidence base on how care may be improved is somewhat limited [48] and mainly focusses on specific interventions such as 'fever management policies', or pain control rather than on a 'holistic' approach to palliative care as defined by the World Health Organization:

> The active, total care of patients whose disease is not responsive to curative treatment. Control of pain, of other symptoms, and of psychological, social and spiritual problems is paramount. The goal of palliative care is achievement of the best quality of life for patients and their families. [49]

Much of the person-centred approach to dementia care is concordant with this definition throughout the whole disease trajectory, and this area is a key example of how advance care planning from the earliest stages of dementia to the end of life is part of the spectrum of supportive care.

Ahronheim et al. [50] conducted a randomized control trial of an intervention where patients received assessment and care plan recommendations from a palliative care team with the goal of enhancing patient comfort in an acute hospital. The intervention did not decrease rates of re-admission to hospital, average length of stay or mortality but there was a significant increase in written palliative care plans and patients received fewer intravenous drugs. The authors highlighted the 'unique barriers' to providing good end of life care, including prognostic uncertainty, and suggested that care planning may be more effective when done outside the busy acute hospital environment.

Another approach has been that of the 'Dementia Special Care Unit' (DSCU). Volicer *et al.* [51] compared this approach to traditional long term care settings and found that the DSCU, which provided a palliative care approach focussing on 'maintenance of patient's comfort rather than maximal survival', led to less discomfort, fewer antibiotic prescriptions, intravenous drugs, and decreased transfers to the acute hospital. Mortality in the DSCU was higher, but costs significantly lower (see also Professor Volicer's discussion in this volume in Chapter 31).

The Liverpool Care Pathway was originally developed to improve care in hospital for cancer patients during the last 48 hours of life [52]. It has been modified for use in people dying with other diagnoses such as renal disease and heart failure and different settings including hospices and nursing homes. The pathway has three phases: initial assessment of the patient, ongoing assessment, and care after death. As well as attending to medical needs, such as the discontinuation of inappropriate interventions and medications and the provision of comfort measures (e.g. mouth care), the pathway enhances person-centred care by assessing the patient's insight into their situation, their psychological and spiritual needs, and those of their family. Implementation of the pathway involves training staff, rigorous evaluation of the quality of care, and audit of variance from the pathway. The pathway is credited with bringing significant improvements to care of the dying. There are, however, a number of issues pertinent to people with dementia that may challenge implementation for these patients. Prognostic uncertainty in dementia is a key concern and hospital staff may not perceive dementia to be a 'terminal' disease; the pathway is only of use if it is recognized that a patient is moving into the 'dying phase'. Concerns have been raised that in dementia 'dying' can take many years [53], however, the pathway is flexible and it is entirely appropriate that patients are sometimes moved from the pathway back to more 'active' management should their clinical condition improve. Certainly, a future adaptation and evaluation of the pathway for use in people with dementia would significantly enhance quality of care.

'Holistic' approaches

Many of the above interventions focus on specific clinical needs such as feeding or on particular stages of dementia, e.g. end of life care. Good person-centred care requires a more holistic approach and number of 'multicomponent' interventions and pathways have been developed that may improve the quality and outcomes of care for older people with dementia in the acute hospital.

The Palliative Excellence in Alzheimer Care Effort (PEACE) Programme

This American-based programme (see Chapter 5) was set up to improve end of life care for people with dementia but takes a long term disease management model, integrating 'palliative care into ongoing comprehensive primary care of persons with dementia over the disease course, from initial diagnosis to death'[54]. The patient-centred principles of the programme include advance care planning, education on the disease process, improved care co-ordination and family support. This is implemented by clinical nurse specialists who coordinate care between families, physicians, and other health and social care professionals. This approach is relevant to the acute hospital as those involved in the programme were more likely to die in hospice or a place of their choosing, less likely to die in the acute hospital, and their carers were more satisfied with the quality of care received [55].

The Hospital Elder Life Programme (HELP)

This programme, also developed in America, takes a structured and supportive approach to the care of the older person admitted to the acute hospital. Its principle aim is to reduce the incidence of delirium but it has also decreased the risk of cognitive and functional decline, the number of in-hospital adverse events, and rates of re-admission. The HELP programme provides a pragmatic system 'to actually do what everyone knows 'should be done' in the care of older persons' [56]. As well as targeting biological parameters such as hydration, the programme uses trained hospital staff and volunteers to ensure that patients receive daily visitors to provide them with conversation and emotional support, therapeutic activities involving socialization and cognitive stimulation, maintenance of mobility and, importantly, companionship during meals. This programme is well-validated and evaluated and has been shown to reduce delirium, functional decline, and discharges to nursing homes significantly [56].

Care Services Improvement Partnership (CSIP) 'Dementia in acute care settings' programme

This is a practice development guideline to improve acute nursing care for people at all stages of dementia, developed after extensive qualitative focus groups with acute hospital nurses [57]. Preliminary work found that dementia was defined as a 'thing' that impacted on the behaviour of the patient. This behaviour was then interpreted as 'non-directed', 'without purpose', 'irrational', and 'without meaning'. The guideline contains publicity materials for the ward, an educational tool and the key component, an 'information gathering' sheet which involves the structured collection of personalized and individual information regarding the person with dementia. The headings used include the person with dementia's preferred methods of communication, the best times to communicate, practical ways that constraints can be minimized, non-verbal ways in which the person expresses unhappiness or withdrawal of cooperation, and interactions that the person enjoys and which can elicit a positive response. The tool helps nursing staff to develop a reciprocal relationship with people with dementia, it 'legitimizes' time not spent on nursing tasks and promotes conversation and human interaction and, thus, the 'person-centeredness' of care. It has been successfully piloted in the UK National Health Service but not extensively validated.

Dementia care mapping in the acute hospital

Dementia care mapping was originally designed as a tool to assess the quality of care that people with dementia receive, from their own perspective. It is based on the work of Kitwood [36] and the philosophy of person-centred care and aims to promote a holistic approach (as discussed in more detail in Chapter 25). A trained observer assesses people with dementia continuously over representative time periods (usually around 6 hours). They make detailed notes, both qualitative and quantitative, on the care received. Activities are detailed and quantified under structured headings including 'Personal Detractors' – short episodes of care that may lead to loss of self-esteem in the person with dementia. These may include incidents leading to increased institutionalization, disempowerment, and exclusion. More general judgements are also made including measures of 'ill being/well-being'.

The data is analysed and interpreted and can then be used to improve care. The technique is well established and validated and has been used in a variety of settings including mental health wards for older people and nursing homes.

Kitwood has defined the psychological needs of people with dementia as comfort, occupation, inclusion, identity, and attachment. It is easy to see how these needs are not currently well met on the acute hospital ward: identity and attachments are lost through rapid transfers from one ward to another, comfort and occupation can be difficult to provide with high staff turnover and lack of training in dementia care. Kitwood's principles may offer a useful template to uphold patient dignity in these circumstances. Preliminary work [58] suggests that Dementia Care Mapping is feasible and useful on the acute hospital ward and development of this work may bring future benefits in terms of person-centred care and dignity.

Conclusions

Given the problems faced by people with dementia who are admitted to the acute hospital, it is understandable how they may be 'lost' in this system, how they experience adverse events and outcomes, and how it is difficult to provide good quality holistic care. It would be unfortunate, however, if this led to therapeutic nihilism on the part of health care professionals. The number of difficulties and challenges described actually open up many points at which the quality of care and a more person-centred and supportive approach could be adopted. What is notable is that none of the changes required is 'high tech' or expensive, indeed many may be cost-neutral and just involve basic communication and respect for the autonomy of the patient. Improvements will occur when acute hospital staff are adequately trained and supported, people with dementia are encouraged to plan decisions early in their illness, and their carers feel empowered to demand the high quality care that people with dementia deserve.

References

1. Department of Health (2001). *National service framework for older people*. London: Department of Health.
2. Bourne J (2007). *Improving services and support for people with dementia*. London: National Audit Office.
3. Harwood DM, Hope T, Jacoby R (1997). Cognitive impairment in medical inpatients. II: Do physicians miss cognitive impairment? *Age Ageing*, **26**(1), 37–39.
4. Joray S, Wietlisbach V, Bula CJ (2004). Cognitive impairment in elderly medical inpatients: detection and associated six-month outcomes. *Am J Geriatr Psychiatry*, **12**(6), 639–647.
5. Hickey A, Clinch D, Groarke EP (1997). Prevalence of cognitive impairment in the hospitalized elderly. *Int J Geriatr Psychiatry*, **12**(1), 27–33.
6. Feldman E, Mayou R, Hawton K, Ardern M, Smith EB (1987). Psychiatric disorder in medical in-patients. *Q J Med*, **63**(241), 405–412.
7. Torian L, Davidson E, Fulop G, Sell L, Fillit H (1992). The effect of dementia on acute care in a geriatric medical unit. *Int Psychogeriatr*, **4**(2), 231–239.
8. Adamis D, Treloar A, Martin FC, Macdonald AJ (2006). Recovery and outcome of delirium in elderly medical inpatients. *Arch Gerontol Geriatr*, **43**(2), 289–298.
9. Holmes JD, House AO (2000). Psychiatric illness in hip fracture. *Age Ageing*, **29**(6), 537–546.
10. Zhao Y, Kuo TC, Weir S, Kramer MS, Ash AS (2008). Healthcare costs and utilization for medicare beneficiaries with Alzheimer's. *BMC Health Serv Res*, **8**, 108.
11. Carter MW, Porell FW (2005). Vulnerable populations at risk of potentially avoidable hospitalizations: the case of nursing home residents with Alzheimer's disease. *Am J Alzheimers Dis Other Demen*, **20**(6), 349–358.

12. Nelson T, Livingston G, Knapp M, Manela M, Kitchen G, Katona C (2002). Slicing the health service cake: the Islington study. *Age Ageing*, **31**(6), 445–450.

13. Erkinjuntti T, Wikstrom J, Palo J, Autio L (1986). Dementia among medical inpatients. Evaluation of 2000 consecutive admissions. *Arch Intern Med*, **146**(10), 1923–1926.

14. Lyketsos CG, Sheppard JM, Rabins PV (2000). Dementia in elderly persons in a general hospital. *Am J Psychiatry*, **157**(5), 704–707.

15. Kolbeinsson H, Jonsson A (1993). Delirium and dementia in acute medical admissions of elderly patients in Iceland. *Acta Psychiatr Scand*, **87**(2), 123–127.

16. Sands LP, Yaffe K, Covinsky K *et al.* (2003). Cognitive screening predicts magnitude of functional recovery from admission to 3 months after discharge in hospitalized elders. *J Gerontol A Biol Sci Med Sci*, **58**(1), 37–45.

17. Zekry D, Herrmann FR, Grandjean R *et al.* (2008). Demented versus non-demented very old inpatients: the same comorbidities but poorer functional and nutritional status. *Age Ageing*, **37**(1), 83–89.

18. Kammoun S, Gold G, Bouras C *et al.* (2000). Immediate causes of death of demented and non-demented elderly. *Acta Neurol Scand Suppl*, **102**(176), 96–99.

19. Fu C, Chute DJ, Farag ES, Garakian J, Cummings JL, Vinters HV (2004). Comorbidity in dementia: an autopsy study. *Arch Pathol Lab Med*, **128**(1), 32–38.

20. Gupta SK, Lamont EB (2004). Patterns of presentation, diagnosis, and treatment in older patients with colon cancer and comorbid dementia. *J Am Geriatr Soc*, **52**(10), 1681–1687.

21. Sampson EL, Blanchard MR, Jones L, Tookman A, King M (2009). Dementia in the acute hospital: prospective cohort study of prevalence and mortality. *Br J Psychiatry*, **195**, 61–66.

22. Cattin L, Bordin P, Fonda M, *et al.* (1997). Factors associated with cognitive impairment among older Italian inpatients. Gruppo Italiano di Farmacovigilanza nell'Anziano (G.I.F.A.). *J Am Geriatr Soc*, **45**(11), 1324–1330.

23. Pedone C, Ercolani S, Catani M, *et al.* (2005). Elderly patients with cognitive impairment have a high risk for functional decline during hospitalization: The GIFA Study. *J Gerontol A Biol Sci Med Sci*, **60**(12), 1576–1580.

24. Seymour DG, Henschke PJ, Cape RD, Campbell AJ (1980). Acute confusional states and dementia in the elderly: the role of dehydration/volume depletion, physical illness and age. *Age Ageing*, **9**(3), 137–1346.

25. Morris J, Beaumont D, Oliver D (2006). Decent health care for older people. *BMJ*, **332**(7551), 1166–1168.

26. Fields SD, MacKenzie CR, Charlson ME, Sax FL (1986). Cognitive impairment: can it predict the course of hospitalized patients? *J Am Geriatr Soc*, **34**(8), 579–585.

27. Erkinjuntti T, Autio L, Wikstrom J (1988). Dementia in medical wards. *J Clin Epidemiol*, **41**(2), 123–126.

28. Sampson EL, Gould V, Lee D, Blanchard MR (2006). Differences in care received by patients with and without dementia who died during acute hospital admission: a retrospective case note study. *Age Ageing*, **35**(2), 187–189.

29. Morrison RS, Siu AL (2000). Survival in end-stage dementia following acute illness. *JAMA*, **284**(1), 47–52.

30. McCarthy M, Addington-Hall J, Altmann D (1997). The experience of dying with dementia: a retrospective study. *Int J Geriatr Psychiatry*, **12**(3), 404–409.

31. Morrison RS, Siu AL (2000). A comparison of pain and its treatment in advanced dementia and cognitively intact patients with hip fracture. *J Pain Symptom Manage*, **19**(4), 240–248.

32. Covinsky KE, Palmer RM, Fortinsky RH *et al.* (2003). Loss of independence in activities of daily living in older adults hospitalized with medical illnesses: increased vulnerability with age. *J Am Geriatr Soc*, **51**(4), 451–458.

33. Fulop G, Strain JJ, Fahs MC, Schmeidler J, Snyder S (1998). A prospective study of the impact of psychiatric comorbidity on length of hospital stays of elderly medical-surgical inpatients. *Psychosomatics*, **39**(3), 273–280.

34. Reisberg B, Ferris SH, de Leon MJ, Crook T (1982). The Global Deterioration Scale for assessment of primary degenerative dementia. *Am J Psychiatry*, **139**(9), 1136–1139.

35. Holmes J, House A (2000). Psychiatric illness predicts poor outcome after surgery for hip fracture: a prospective cohort study. *Psychol Med*, **30**(4), 921–929.

36. Kitwood T (1997). The experience of dementia. *Aging Ments Health*, **1**(1), 13–22.

37. Saliba D, Kington R, Buchanan J *et al.* (2000). Appropriateness of the decision to transfer nursing facility residents to the hospital. *J Am Geriatr Soc,* **48**(2), 154–163.

38. Caplan GA, Meller A, Squires B, Chan S, Willett W (2006). Advance care planning and hospital in the nursing home. *Age Ageing*, **35**(6), 581–585.

39. Sampson EL, Thune-Boyle I, Kukkastenvehmas R *et al.* (2008). Palliative care in advanced dementia; A mixed methods approach for the development of a complex intervention. *BMC Palliat Care*, **7**, 8.

40. NHS End of Life Care Programme. *The gold standards framework*. Available at: http://www. goldstandardsframework.nhs.uk/ (accessed 10 November 2008).

41. Caplan GA, Ward JA, Brennan NJ, Coconis J, Board N, Brown A (1999). Hospital in the home: a randomised controlled trial. *Med J Aust*, **170**(4), 156–160.

42. Board N, Brennan N, Caplan GA (2000). A randomised controlled trial of the costs of hospital as compared with hospital in the home for acute medical patients. *Aust N Z J Public Health*, **24**(3), 305–311.

43. Naber TH, Schermer T, de BA, Nusteling K *et al.* (1997). Prevalence of malnutrition in nonsurgical hospitalized patients and its association with disease complications. *Am J Clin Nutr*, **66**(5), 1232–1239.

44. Finucane TE, Christmas C, Travis K (1999). Tube feeding in patients with advanced dementia: a review of the evidence. *JAMA*, **282**(14), 1365–1370.

45. Alzheimer's Society. *Care on the hospital ward*. Available at: http://www.alzheimers.org.uk/ factsheet/477 (accessed 10 November 2008).

46. O'Connell B, Gardner A, Takase M *et al.* (2007). Clinical usefulness and feasibility of using Reality Orientation with patients who have dementia in acute care settings. *Int J Nurs Pract*, **13**(3), 182–192.

47. Lloyd-Williams M, Payne S (2002). Can multidisciplinary guidelines improve the palliation of symptoms in the terminal phase of dementia? *Int J Palliat Nurs*, **8**(8), 370–375.

48. Sampson EL, Ritchie CW, Lai R, Raven PW, Blanchard MR (2005). A systematic review of the scientific evidence for the efficacy of a palliative care approach in advanced dementia. *Int Psychogeriatr*, **17**(1), 31–40.

49. World Health Organisation. (1990). *Cancer Pain Relief and Palliative Care.* Technical Report Series No. 804. WHO: Geneva.

50. Ahronheim JC, Morrison RS, Morris J, Baskin S, Meier DE (2000). Palliative care in advanced dementia: a randomized controlled trial and descriptive analysis. *J Palliat Med*, **3**(3), 265–273.

51. Volicer L, Collard A, Hurley A, Bishop C, Kern D, Karon S (1994). Impact of special care unit for patients with advanced Alzheimer's disease on patients' discomfort and costs. *J Am Geriatr Soc*, **42**(6), 597–603.

52. Ellershaw J (2007). Care of the dying: what a difference an LCP makes! *Palliat Med*, **21**(5), 365–368.

53. Treloar AJ (2008). Continuous deep sedation: Dutch research reflects problems with the Liverpool care pathway. *BMJ*, **336**(7650), 905.

54. Shega JW, Levin A, Hougham GW, *et al.* (2003). Palliative excellence in Alzheimer care efforts (PEACE): a program description. *J Palliat Med*, **6**(2), 315–320.

55. Shega JW, Hougham GW, Stocking CB, Cox-Hayley D, Sachs GA (2008). Patients dying with dementia: experience at the end of life and impact of hospice care. *J Pain Symptom Manage*, **35**(5), 499–507.

56. Inouye SK (2004). A practical program for preventing delirium in hospitalized elderly patients. *Cleve Clin J Med*, **71**(11), 890–896.

57. Care Services Improvement Partnership. *Dementia in acute care settings. A resource for caring for people with dementia on medical and surgical wards.* Available at: http://www.changeagentteam.org.uk/index. cfm?pid=250 (accessed 10 November 2008).

58. Woolley RJ, Young JB, Green JR, Brooker DJ (2008). The feasibility of care mapping to improve care for physically ill older people in hospital. *Age Ageing*, 37(4), 390–395.

Chapter 14

Distress and pain in dementia

Alice Jordan and Mari Lloyd-Williams

Introduction

The loss of cognitive and communication abilities that are seen as dementia advances creates great difficulties in assessing distress [1]. There may be a variety of causes of distress, i.e. depression, agitation, and isolation, as well as pain. Clearly, if distress and pain are not managed adequately, this will impact on the person's quality of life. Initially in this chapter, the issues regarding pain prevalence and assessment will be discussed, followed by consideration of how distress might be assessed and managed.

Evidence regarding pain prevalence

It has long been appreciated that pain is often under-recognized and under-treated in elderly people. Ferrell et al. [2]. carried out a pilot epidemiology study of 92 nursing home residents with an average Mini Mental State Examination (MMSE) of 20.7. Using semi-structured interviews, medical records review and two pain instruments (Pain Experience Measure and the McGill Present Pain Intensity Scale) they demonstrated that sixty-five subjects (71%) indicated the presence of pain at least some of the time, 47% reporting intermittent pain, and 24% constant pain. Only 15% of those with pain had received any analgesic medication in the previous 24 hours. Other authors have also demonstrated the under-recognition and under-treatment of pain in elderly patients [3–6], with the prevalence of pain in this group recognized as being between 49 and 83% [7]. Although it may be possible to extrapolate data from studies carried out in general elderly populations, there is a relative lack of evidence surrounding pain in those with cognitive impairment. This is more marked with those with severe dementia as this group is invariably excluded from studies into pain in those with cognitive impairment [8].

There are some published studies regarding pain prevalence in those with moderate cognitive impairment. Further work carried out by Ferrell et al. involved nursing home residents with a mean MMSE of 12.1 [9]. Participants were interviewed about their pain, medical notes and charts were reviewed, and the subjects were shown five scales to rate the intensity of their pain. In this study, 62% of the participants complained of pain, however, 17% were unable to complete any of the scales presented. Although this study does involve those with more marked cognitive impairment, 70 subjects were excluded from the initial sample as they were essentially mute and unresponsive and no meaningful information could be obtained from the patient interview. Presumably many in this group were severely demented and again information regarding their pain experience is not provided.

Further work carried out by Shega et al. of geriatric outpatients involved a sample of patients with a mean MMSE of 16.6 who were interviewed regarding the levels of pain [10]. From those interviewed, 32% reported experiencing pain at that time. Although this study provides information regarding levels of pain in those with moderate cognitive impairment, those unable to attend an outpatient clinic or who were unable to communicate were excluded. Work carried out by Schuler *et al.* investigating the psychometric properties of the German PAINAD tool involved a sample of 99 nursing home residents with a mean MMSE of 12.9 [11]. They asked nursing staff to judge whether the participants were in pain during an observation period whilst the pain tool was also completed. The nursing staff concluded that 39% of the sample was in pain. Additional information regarding symptoms (including pain) experienced in the terminal stages of dementia is provided by a case note audit carried out by Lloyd-Williams [12]. It was demonstrated that in the 17 case notes reviewed, pain was one of the most common symptoms recorded, however, the management of the identified pain was variable. Further work demonstrated that using multi-disciplinary guidelines regarding symptom control improved the management of pain in those dying with dementia [13].

These studies provide some information regarding how common pain might be as dementia progresses; but does dementia itself alter pain perception? Although age-related changes in pain perception are probably not clinically significant [14], there is evidence suggesting that there is an alteration in the perception of pain due to the effects of the dementing process on the brain. Case reports have been published of patients with Alzheimer's disease who had experienced physical trauma of various kinds and yet did not exhibit normal pain behaviour nor give verbal reports of pain commensurate with the tissue damage they had incurred [15]. By requesting reports via the Alzheimer Disease Society newsletter, additional reports of patients failing to exhibit a normal pain experience in response to acute accidents, infections, acute surgical conditions, and chronic conditions have been published. It has been suggested, therefore, that there may be a sub-set of Alzheimer's patients who do not experience pain as might be expected. By relating the neuropathological changes seen in dementia to the pathways of the constructs involved in the pain experience, it is possible to demonstrate that the medial pain system may be affected in Alzheimer's disease [16]. Recent work carried out by Cole *et al.* has challenged some of the evidence surrounding pain perception in Alzheimer's disease [17]. They used fMRI techniques to analyse responses to pain in patients with early Alzheimer's disease and demonstrated that activity in both medial and lateral pathways was preserved.

In vascular dementia, infarcts can occur at many locations and hence could influence both the lateral and medial pain systems. These infarcts could alternatively provoke or ameliorate the suffering associated with pain [18]. Disruption of connections within the cortex and between cortex and sub-cortex by white matter lesions seen in vascular dementia can cause increased pain, termed central post-stroke pain. Hence it is possible that those suffering from vascular dementia suffer from an increase in pain. There are relatively few studies examining what effect this might have clinically for those with vascular dementia [19,20].

The assessment of pain in dementia

Several different approaches have been employed to assess pain in those with cognitive problems. As it has been demonstrated that self-reporting of pain by elderly patients with cognitive impairment will correlate with known physical pathology [21], obtaining self report, where possible, will provide valid information for pain assessment. The American Geriatrics Society Panel on Persistent Pain in Older Adults has therefore recommended that for older adults with mild to moderate dementia, the practitioner should attempt to assess pain by directly querying the patient [14]. They recommend considering the use of a multidimensional pain instrument in this group and highlight the importance of allowing adequate time, observing for changes in behaviour and framing questions in the present tense owing to potential difficulties with recall.

Pain assessment tools such as Visual Analogue Scales, Verbal Rating Scales, and Pain Faces Scales have been used in a variety of studies in elderly patients with varying levels of cognitive impairment [9,22–24]. Some of these studies excluded those who were severely demented [24] or found that many scales could not be completed with worsening cognitive ability [9]. Other studies have demonstrated that at least one of the scales could be completed, but this differed from person to person, making it difficult to recommend one scale for all [22]. Similar conclusions were reached by Stolee *et al.* in their systematic review of pain assessment tools for use in older persons with cognitive impairment [25]. They reviewed 30 self-report instruments and found completion in those with cognitive impairment varied between 20% and 100%. The higher completion of the self-report tools was found for those with mild to moderate cognitive impairments. These studies and reviews demonstrate that although some patients with dementia are able to complete certain self-report scales, this can vary tremendously. The validity and reliability of these scales for assessing pain in severe dementia has not been conclusively demonstrated. It would, therefore, seem logical to use a different method to assess pain than scales reliant on self-report in this group of patients. Behavioural assessment tools offer an alternative approach and have consequently been evaluated in this population.

The use of pain behaviour assessment tools in severe dementia

The use of such tools forms part of a framework of techniques to assess pain alongside self-report, a search for potential causes of pain, surrogate reporting, and analgesic trial [26]. The American Geriatrics Society recommended assessing pain in those with severe dementia by direct observation for pain behaviours [14]. This forms the first step of their algorithm for assessing pain, followed by meeting comfort needs, looking for underlying causes and considering an empirical trial of analgesia.

The idea of using observed behaviour for assessing pain is not new. Behavioural tools and observational procedures have been identified in the literature as methods of assessing pain in various populations from neonates to older adults. Such tools have a wide array of behaviours that can indicate pain including those related to posture, facial expressions and change in functional ability. Although such tools could be used in patients with dementia, this assumes that the signs that are normally indicative of pain in a general population are also representative of pain in elderly patients with dementia. Recent work by Horgas *et al.* [27] compared pain behaviours observed using the Pain Behaviour Measure in older adults who self-reported pain. They demonstrated no significant difference in pain behaviours between cognitively intact older adults and older adults with mild to moderate dementia. Concerns have been raised, however, that less obvious or atypical behavioural presentations may be observed in some people with dementia, behaviours that may not appear on pain tools used in those with cognitive impairment [28]. As a result, numerous tools to be used specifically in those with dementia have been developed over the past 15 years. Two assumptions underlie the development of such tools: first, that discomfort can be observed although it may not be verbally expressed; secondly, that those with dementia cannot voluntarily control their expressions or demeanour. Thus, observed behaviours can be considered external markers of internal states [29].

Challenges associated with using behavioural pain assessment tools

Although it is clear that behavioural tools are a sensible approach in identify pain in those with severe dementia, there are multiple pitfalls to this approach. There is no evidence for any behaviour that solely indicates pain [30], which could lead to an over-diagnosis of pain when the behaviour is due to a different cause. Pain behaviours are not unique from those that might indicate other problems such as boredom or depression [31]. The uniqueness of individuals and their disease means that a behaviour indicating pain in one patient may indicate contentment in another. Hence, there is a danger that important cues are overlooked or misinterpreted. The behaviours seen can be complex and difficult to capture adequately by behavioural tools not tailored to that individual [32]. Having behaviours on a scale that the person would not ever display runs the risk of their pain behaviours not scoring highly on a scale and, therefore, not being taken as seriously. Hence, any scoring system attached to a behavioural scale is merely a representation of the number of behaviours seen, not an intensity rating [33].

Behavioural scales may also measure a different aspect of the pain experience to self-report [34], which may explain only moderate correlations demonstrated between self-report and behavioural pain assessment scales [35]. As some responses to chronic pain can be decreased activity, rather than an increase in certain types of behaviour, this may not be adequately identified on a uni-directional pain behaviour measure [36]. Finally, the tools rely on the abilities of nursing staff to identify and interpret the behaviour correctly, which may be difficult because of constraints on time or desensitization [32].

Despite these potential problems, the concerns raised regarding the under-recognition and under-treatment of pain in this population have increased the drive to develop suitable assessment tools to identify pain [37]. Without the promotion of pain assessment tools, it is possible that many behaviours, caused by pain, may simply be ascribed to that person's dementia. One review of 10 assessment tools concluded, however, that currently there is no standardized tool that may be recommended for broad adoption in clinical practice [38]. Another review of 12 papers concluded that none of the scales was convincingly the most appropriate scale for assessing pain in elderly people with dementia [39]. A further review published recently was again unable to recommend one tool for use across population and settings [36]. Although these reviews are critical of aspects of current assessment tools, all have emphasized that the use of behavioural tools in this population form an important part of assessing pain [38,39]. Indeed, around 25% of nursing homes in a recent study were using a pain assessment tool to assess the pain of their residents [40]. With the lack of conclusive evidence recommending one specific tool, it may be appropriate for practitioners to decide which tool might be most suited for their use, utilizing knowledge regarding the current evidence base. The website updated by Herr *et al.* [41]. is useful in providing such information. It is worth emphasizing that there are limitations with any assessment tool, as discussed previously, and the use of behavioural tools should form only part of the assessment of pain.

Understanding how best to use such tools, as well as appreciating their limitations, is vital in developing strategies for assessing and managing pain in severe dementia. Recent work carried out in nursing homes has suggested that, although the acute causes of pain are often readily identified by staff (potentially caused by more obvious behavioural changes), the worsening of chronic painful conditions may go unnoticed [42]. There may be a role, therefore, for the regular use of assessment tools in those with severe dementia, however, further work is required to establish how this might be carried out.

The management of pain in dementia

Once pain has been identified, evaluating the underlying cause is important as this will govern its management. If the underlying cause can be treated, then this should be done where possible. As many patients with dementia are elderly, it is worth highlighting that they are particularly susceptible to drug side effects, and adverse drug reactions occur more frequently than in younger patients. The alterations in pharmacokinetics and pharmacodymamics seen in the elderly lead to varying oral bioavailability, differing drug distribution, changes in metabolic clearance and differing end organ responses to drugs [43]. These issues can lead to an increased frequency of constipation, confusion, and orthostatic hypotension owing to drug treatments [44]. Hence a sensible approach when prescribing analgesia is to start with the lowest anticipated effective dose, monitor frequently on the basis of expected absorption and known pharmacokinetics of the agent and then titrate the dose on the basis of likely steady state blood levels and clinically demonstrated effects [14]. Using drugs with a short half life may be useful initially as the elderly are particularly susceptible to drug accumulation. Using a combination of pharmacological and non-pharmacological techniques often results in more effective pain control and less reliance on medications that have major side effects in elderly patients [45]. There may also be issues surrounding the administration of oral medication as a significant proportion of those with dementia will develop swallowing difficulties as the condition progresses [46].

The mechanisms underlying pain are often divided into the categories of nociceptive and neuropathic pain. Nociceptive pain results from direct stimulation of pain receptors and arises from inflammation, tissue injury or mechanical deformity. This type of pain often responds well to the analgesics that form the WHO analgesic ladder. Neuropathic pain results from injury to nerve fibres from compression, infiltration or degeneration of neurons. Although neuropathic pain may respond to the analgesics of the WHO ladder, it also responds to adjuvant agents, such as antidepressants or anticonvulsants. Some pain may have both nociceptive and neuropathic elements.

The principles governing analgesic use have been encapsulated in a series of slogans by the WHO [47]. Drugs should be given by mouth where possible, by the clock and by the ladder, using a three-step analgesic ladder. Prescribing drugs on an 'as required' basis partly requires the individuals to request medication. Many people with cognitive impairment are often unable to initiate a request for analgesia even if they can report pain when asked directly. This may therefore lead to under-treatment of pain in those with cognitive impairment [48]. The first step of the analgesic ladder is the prescription of non opioid drugs such as paracetamol and NSAIDs, followed by adding weak opioids as step 2 and then step 3 is the prescription of strong opioids with non opioids. Adjuvant analgesics (neuropathic agents, psychotropic medication) can be added at any step.

As mentioned previously non pharmacological management strategies are often very effective when used in combination with drug strategies [45]. Physical methods, such as heat (stimulating production of endogenous opioids) and cold (suppressing the release of products from tissue damage), can be effective. Massage has been shown not only to reduce pain scores [49], but also to reduce anxiety, agitation and other dysfunctional behaviour [50]. Transcutaneous electrical nerve stimulation (TENS) and acupuncture are thought to cause endogenous opioid release, however, it is debatable how well these approaches may be tolerated by those with severe dementia. It would seem sensible that as well as treating pain as it is recognized, efforts should be made to prevent painful conditions from occurring. Gentle exercise may help reduce immobility and inactivity that can worsen pain [14,45], as well as improving psychological wellbeing. The frequency of fractures in the elderly can be reduced by preventing falls occurring in the first place and by using hip protectors and treating osteoporosis [43]. In addition, preventing painful pressure ulcers from developing by the use of pressure relieving aids, frequent turning and maintaining adequate nutrition is also important [43].

Evaluating whether the management instituted to alleviate pain has been of benefit is an essential part of effective pain management. The same principles used in identifying pain in the first instance can be used to assess whether it has been alleviated, for example whether the behaviour thought to be caused by pain has resolved. If there are concerns that the management instituted has not been effective, it is important to consider whether the drug dose is effective for the level of pain, whether the appropriate drug is being given for the type of pain and whether the sole cause is pain, as there may be elements of anxiety or another cause all together.

The identification and management of distress in dementia

It has previously been highlighted that behavioural pain assessment tools, when used for people unable to communicate their needs, may identify behaviours owing to a variety of causes, not just pain. This has been identified by the creators of behaviour pain assessment tools [51], who have suggested that when using such tools, alternative causes for the behaviour observed need to be excluded. Recent work using the Doloplus-2, a behavioural assessment tool designed for cognitively impaired patients, has also suggested that the tool may identify discomfort related to grief, anxiety, and agitation rather than purely somatic pain [52].

A recent study used a behavioural pain assessment scale (PAINAD – Pain Assessment in Advanced Dementia scale) to observe a group of patients with severe dementia to assess whether the patients were in pain at three different times in their day [42]. Although half of the patients observed scored significantly on the PAINAD scale, only a third of those with significant scores were felt to be in pain. Those who were not felt to be in pain, but had displayed observable behaviour found on a pain scale, were felt to be distressed owing to a variety of causes. This included distress caused by not understanding the situation (leading to fear or frustration) or distress from environmental factors.

The importance of identifying and managing distress in patients with dementia is being increasingly recognized. Over 90% of those with dementia will experience 'behaviour disturbance' with symptoms such as aggression, delusions, wandering, and agitation [53]. These non-cognitive symptoms seen in dementia are often described under the umbrella term of behavioural and psychological symptoms of dementia (BPSD). Evidence suggests that these symptoms are important determinants of patients' distress, quality of life, carer burden and outcome in dementia [54]. The symptoms are also important in leading to prescriptions of psychotropic drugs and nursing home placement [53,55]. Multiple factors cause these symptoms, including the underlying brain disease, host factors and the environment. Thorough investigation of all the contributing dimensions is required in order to plan logical intervention [56], with treatment designed to address the underlying cause where possible [57].

It has been suggested that rather than attempting to identify a specific cause of distress such as pain, identifying global distress is the only possible starting point in those with severe communication difficulties [30]. The use of the carer's knowledge of the person has been highlighted as a method of identifying when distress is occurring. Once it has been established that the person is distressed; then the cause of the distress should be sought. The use of an 'ABC' approach to evaluate such behaviour has been suggested, with the antecedents, the behaviour itself, and the consequences of the behaviour being identified to understand the cause of the behaviour observed. Clearly pain may be one potential cause of distressed behaviour. It is worth highlighting, however, that an important (and at times unappreciated) consequence of pain in those with dementia is fear. The memory of the social context and beliefs that would have modified the experience of pain may be lost, causing those with cognitive impairment to be excessively frightened by pain episodes [58]. Therefore, any behaviour identified may have several underlying causes; some may be more amenable to treatment than others. The importance of evaluating and alleviating behaviours of distress, whether caused by pain or by other factors, is imperative to the care of those with severe dementia.

References

1. Robinson L, Hughes J, Daley S, Keady J, Ballard C, Volicer L (2005). End-of-life care and dementia. *Rev Clin Gerontol*, **15**(2), 135–148.

2. Ferrell BA, Ferrell BR, Osterweil D (1990). Pain in the nursing home. *J Am Geriatr Soc*, **38**(4), 409–414.

3. Won A, Lapane K, Gambassi G, Bernabei R, Mor V, Lipsitz LA (1999). Correlates and management of nonmalignant pain in the nursing home. SAGE Study Group. Systematic Assessment of Geriatric drug use via Epidemiology. *J Am Geriatr Soc*, **47**(8), 936–942.

4. Roy R, Thomas M (1986). A survey of chronic pain in an elderly population. *Can Fam Physician*, **32**, 513–516.

5. Cairncross E, Magee H, Askham J (2007). *A hidden problem: pain in older people. A qualitative study.* Oxford: Picker Institute Europe.

6. Bernabei R, Gambassi G, Lapane K *et al.* (1998). Management of pain in elderly patients with cancer. *J Am Med Assoc*, **279**(23), 1877–1882.

7. Fox PL, Raina P, Jadad AR (1999). Prevalence and treatment of pain in older adults in nursing homes and other long-term care institutions: a systematic review. *Can Med Assoc J*, **160**(3), 329–33.

8. Huffman JC, Kunik ME (2000). Assessment and understanding of pain in patients with dementia. *Gerontologist*, **40**(5), 574–581.

9. Ferrell BA, Ferrell BR, Rivera L (1995). Pain in cognitively impaired nursing home patients. *J Pain Symptom Manage*, **10**(8), 591–598.

10. Shega JW, Hougham GW Stocking CB, Cox-Hayley D, Sachs GA (2004). Pain in community-dwelling persons with dementia: frequency, intensity, and congruence between patient and caregiver report. *J Pain Symptom Manage*, **28**(6), 585–592.

11. Schuler MS, Becker S, Kaspar R, Nikolaus T, Kruse A, Basler HD (2007). Psychometric properties of the German pain assessment in advanced aementia scale (PAINAD-G) in nursing home residents. *J Am Med Dir Assoc*, **8**, 388–395.

12. Lloyd-Williams M (1996). An audit of palliative care in dementia. *Eur J Cancer Care*, **5**, 53–55.

13. Lloyd-Williams M, Payne S (2002). Can multidisciplinary guidelines improve the palliation of symptoms in the terminal phase of dementia? *Int J Palliat Nurs*, **8**(8), 370–375

14. Ferrell BA, Casarett D, Epplin J, Fine P, Gloth M, Herr K *et al.* (2002). The management of persistent pain in older persons (AGS panel on persistent pain in older persons). *J Am Geriatr Soc*, **50**, S205–S224.

15. Fisher-Morris M, Gellatly A (1997). The experience and expression of pain in Alzheimer patients. *Age Ageing*, **26**(6), 497–500.

16. Scherder EJ, Sergeant JA, Swaab DF (2003). Pain processing in dementia and its relation to neuropathology. *Lancet Neurol*, **2**(11), 677–686.

17. Cole LJ, Farrell MJ, Duff EP, Barber JB, Egan GF Gibson SJ (2006). Pain sensitivity and fMRI pain related brain activity in Alzheimer's disease. *Brain*, **129**, 2957–2965.

18. Farrell, MJ, Katz B, Helme RD (1996). The impact of dementia on the pain experience. *Pain*, **67**(1), 7–15.

19. Scherder EJ, Sergeant JA, Swaab DF (2003). Pain assessment in patients with possible vascular dementia. *Psychiatry*, **66**(2), 133–145.

20. Achterberg WP, Scherder E, Pot AM, Ribbe MW (2007). Cardiovascular risk factors in cognitively impaired nursing home patients: A relationship with pain? *Eur J Pain*, **11**, 707–710.

21. Parmelee PA, Smith B, Katz IR (1993). Pain complaints and cognitive status among elderly institution residents. *J Am Geriatr Soc*, **41**(5), 517–522.

22. Jones KR, Fink R, Hutt E *et al.* (2005), Measuring pain intensity in nursing home residents. *J Pain Symptom Manage*, **30**(6), 519–527.

23. Closs SJ, Barr B, Briggs M, Cash K, Seers K (2004). A comparison of five pain assessment scales for nursing home residents with varying degrees of cognitive impairment. *J Pain Symptom Manage*, **27**(3), 196–205.

24. Chibnall, JT, Tait RC (2001). Pain assessment in cognitively impaired and unimpaired older adults: a comparison of four scales. *Pain*, **92**(1–2), 173–186.

25. Stolee P, Hillier LM, Esbaugh E, Bol N, McKellar L, Gauthier N (2005). Instruments for the assessment of pain in older persons with cognitive impairment. *J Am Geriatr Soc*, **53**(2), 319–326.

26. Herr K, Coyne PJ, Key T *et al.* (2006). Pain assessment in the nonverbal patient: position statement with clinical practice recommendations. *Pain Manag Nurs*, **7**(2), 44–52.

27. Horgas AL, Elliott AF, Marsiske M (2009). Pain assessment in dementia: relationship between self-report and behavioural observation. *J Am Geriatr Soc*, **57** (1), 126–132

28. Scherder E, Oosterman J, Swaab D *et al.* (2005). Recent developments in pain in dementia. *Br Med J*, **330**(7489), 461–464.

29. Hurley AC, Volicer B, Hanrahan PA, Houde S, Volicer L (1992). Assessment of discomfort in advanced Alzheimer patients. *Res Nurs Health*, **15**(5), 369–377.

30. Regnard C, Reynolds J, Watson B, Matthews D, Gibson L, Clarke C (2007). Understanding distress in people with severe communication difficulties: developing and assessing the disability distress assessment tool (DisDAT). *J Intellect Disabil Res*, **51**(4), 277–292.

31. Snow AL, Shuster JL (2006). Assessment and treatment of persistent pain in persons with cognitive and communicative impairment. *J Clin Psychol*, **62**(11), 1379–1387.

32. Davies E, Male M, Reimer V, Turner M (2004). Pain assessment and cognitive impairment: part 2. *Nurs Stand*, **19**(13), 33–40.

33. Pasero C, McCaffery M (2005). No self report means no pain intensity rating. *Am J Nurs*, **105**(10), 50–53.

34. Monina E, Falzetti G, Firetto V, Mariani L, Caputi CA (2006). Behavioural evaluation in patients affected by chronic pain: a preliminary study. *J Am Geriatr Soc*, **7**, 395–402.

35. Pautex S, Michon A, Guedira M *et al.* (2006). Pain in severe dementia: self-assessment or observational scales? *J Am Geriatr Soc*, **54**, 1040–1045.

36. Hadjistavropoulos T, Herr K, Turk DC *et al.* (2007). An interdisciplinary expert consensus statement on assessment of pain in older persons. *Clin J Pain*, **23**(1), S1–43.

37. Zwakhalen SMG, Hamers JPH, Berger MPF (2006). The psychometric quality and clinical usefulness of three pain assessment tools for elderly people with dementia. *Pain*, **126**, 210–220.

38. Herr K, Bjoro K, Decker S (2006). Tools for assessment of pain in nonverbal older adults with dementia: a state-of-the-science review. *J Pain Symptom Manage*, **31**(2), 170–192.

39. Zwakhalen, SM, Hamers JPH, Abu-Saad HH, Berger MPF (2006). Pain in elderly people with severe dementia: a systematic review of behavioural pain assessment tools. *BMC Geriatr*, **6**(3) (27 January).

40. Allcock N, McGarry J, Elkan R (2002). Management of pain in older people within the nursing home: a preliminary study. *Health Soc Care Community*, **10**(6), 464–471.

41. Herr K, Bursch H, Black B. *State of the art review of the tools for assessment of pain in nonverbal older adults*. Available at: http://prc.coh.org/PainNOA/OV.pdf (accessed 24 February 2009).

42. Jordan AI (2008). *The assessment of good practice in pain management in severe dementia* (MD Thesis). Newcastle-upon-Tyne, UK: Newcastle University.

43. Grimley-Evans J, Williams TF, Beattie BL, Michel JP, Wilcock GK (2000). *Oxford textbook of geriatric medicine*, 2nd edn. Oxford: Oxford University Press.

44. Stein WM (2001). Pain in the nursing home. *Clin Geriatr Med*, **17**(3), 575–594.

45. Ferrell BA (1995). Pain evaluation and management in the nursing home. *Ann Intern Med*, **123**(9), 681–687.

46. Feinberg MJ, Ekberg O, Segall L, Tully J (1992). Deglutination in elderly patients with dementia: findings of videofluorographic evaluation and impact on staging and management. *Radiology*, **183**, 811–814.

47. WHO (1990). Cancer pain relief and palliative care. Geneva: World Health Organization.

48. Miller L, Nelson L, Mezey M (2005). Comfort and pain relief in dementia: awakening a new beneficence. *J Gerontol Nurs*, **26**(9), 33–40.

49. Sansone P, Schmitt L (2000). Providing tender touch massage to elderly nursing home residents: a demonstration project. *Geriatr Nurs*, **21**(6), 303–308.

50. Ballard CG, O'Brien JT, Reichelt K, Perry EK (2002). Aromatherapy as a safe and effective treatment for the management of agitation in severe dementia: the results of a double blind placebo controlled trial. *J Clin Psychiatry*, **63**(7), 553–558.

51. Warden V, Hurley AC, Volicer L (2003). Development and psychometric evaluation of the pain assessment in advanced dementia (PAINAD) scale. *J Am Med Dir Assoc*, **4**(1), 9–15.

52. Hølen JC, Saltveldt I, Fayers PM, Hjermstad MJ, Loge JH, Kaasa S (2007). Doloplus-2, a valid tool for behavioural pain assessment? *BMC Geriatr*, **7**(29) (19 December).

53. Ballard C, O' Brien J (1999). Treating behavioural and psychological signs in Alzheimer's disease. *Br Med J*, **319**, 138–139.

54. Banerjee S, Smith SC, Lamping DL *et al.* (2005). Quality of life in dementia: more than just cognition. An analysis of associations with quality of life in dementia. *J Neurol Neurosurg Psychiatry*, **77**, 146–148.

55. Michel JP, Gold G (2001). Behavioural symptoms in Alzheimer's disease: validity of targets and present treatments. *Age Ageing*, **30**, 105–106.

56. McKeith I, Cummings J (2005). Behavioural changes and psychological symptoms in dementia disorders. *Lancet Neurol*, **4**, 735–742.

57. Class AC, Schneider L, Farlow M (1997). Optimal management of behavioural disorders associated with dementia. *Drugs Aging*, **10**(2), 95–106.

58. Weiner DK, Hanlon JT (2001). Pain in nursing home residents. *Drugs Aging*, **18**(1), 13–29.

Chapter 15

The role of the family doctor in supportive care for people with dementia

Gillie E. Evans and Louise Robinson

The general practitioner (GP) is a doctor who provides personal, primary, and continuing medical care to individuals and families. . . . He will work in a team and delegate where necessary. His diagnosis will be composed in physical, psychological, and social terms. He will intervene educationally, preventatively, and therapeutically to promote his patients' health. [1]

Supportive care is the multi-disciplinary holistic care of patients and their families from the time around diagnosis, through treatments aimed at cure or prolonging life, and into the phase currently acknowledged as palliative care. It involves recognizing and caring for the side effects of active therapies as well as patients' comorbidities, psychological, social, and spiritual concerns. It also values the role of family carers and helps them in supporting the patient, as well as in attending to their special needs [2].

On reflection, the two definitions above, about the nature of general practice and the concept of supportive care, appear to be closely linked; similarities include a multi-disciplinary, holistic approach to patient care, with an emphasis on continuity of care from the point of diagnosis to a patient's death. The primary care team, and in particular, the role of the family doctor or GP, would seem to be pivotal in the co-ordination and delivery of supportive care for people with dementia. In theory, the GP should possess an in-depth knowledge of the person with dementia, their immediate family, and community support networks and be able to assess their physical, psychological, and social needs, as well as the needs of their main carers. The aim of this chapter is to reflect upon the role of the family doctor in the provision of supportive care for people with dementia, to examine existing evidence concerning the delivery of such care, and to consider how they might improve upon this. So let's start with the detection, diagnosis, and disclosure of a diagnosis of dementia.

Making a diagnosis of dementia

Evidence has shown that it can take up to 4 years from initial presentation of suspicious symptoms to a person with dementia receiving confirmation of their diagnosis, but on average the process takes between 18–30 months [3]. In the United Kingdom, a recent report considered this delay to be unacceptable and called for greater public awareness of the illness with improved training at both undergraduate and postgraduate levels to minimize such diagnostic delays [4]. Although in some cases delays may be caused by a reluctance of the patient and family to accept symptoms and acknowledge difficulties, or to different cultural beliefs around normal ageing, primary and community care professionals need to be more aware and refer for an expert opinion from their old age psychiatry colleagues sooner rather than later [5].

Currently, international consensus is that earlier diagnosis allows patients and their families more time to adjust both emotionally, socially, and practically to living with dementia, even though they may find the initial process of disclosure distressing [6]. Also, people in the earlier stages of dementia are more able to discuss their management preferences and wishes for future care allowing a more person-centred approach.

Assessment of cognitive function

Simple cognitive tests are available for use in the community to make an initial assessment of a person's cognitive function. Currently, routine screening for dementia is not considered clinically or cost-effective [5]. The most commonly used cognitive assessment tool is the Mini-Mental State Examination (MMSE) [7]. The General Practitioner Assessment of Cognition (GPCOG) [8], and two other cognitive screening tests, the Mini-Cog Assessment Instrument and the Memory Impairment Screen, have been found to be as clinically and psychometrically robust and more appropriate for use in primary care than the MMSE [9].

Diagnosis of dementia

However, cognitive assessment tests alone are not sufficient to diagnose dementia; a detailed history and examination by the GP is required. This should include exploration of the patient's symptoms and their ideas and concerns, and a comprehensive assessment of the patient's social functioning via their family carers. The GP should perform routine blood tests (full blood count, biochemistry, glucose, thyroid function, vitamin B_{12}, and liver function), and perhaps a chest x-ray and ECG if indicated, before referring the patient for a specialist, secondary care assessment. This should preferably be by an old age psychiatrist [5], who can confirm the diagnosis via detailed mental state examination and possibly neuroimaging. Memory clinics are increasingly being established to provide specialist centres for such an assessment. Evaluation of a specialist memory clinic service has revealed high patient satisfaction, an estimated increase in the number of new patients seen of around 60%, and a two-fold increase in successful engagement with ethnic minority patients [10].

In the UK, recent NICE guidelines for health and social care professionals on dementia provide a clear pathway for the detection and referral of people with a suspected dementia [5]. Notwithstanding such clarity, a recent UK report on dementia highlighted the poor performance in this area [4], with the reported time to diagnosis in the UK twice that of some other European countries and a deteriorating confidence in the ability of GPs to diagnose dementia. Research in the UK has revealed that family doctors appear to carry out a 'watchful waiting process' on people presenting with suspicious symptoms, rather than referring them at an early stage [3]. This is probably accounted for by: a tendency to assume such cognitive changes are merely caused by 'old age', limited access in some areas of the country to specialist mental health services [11], and restrictions on the prescribing of anti-dementia drugs (acetylcholinesterase inhibitors) in the UK in the early stages of the illness [12]. However, following a judicial review in 2007, this NICE guidance has been amended and the prescribing of such drugs is not solely dependent on MMSE scores now, but on a more holistic assessment of the person's functioning.

Studies have already confirmed that evidence-based practice protocols can enhance detection rates in primary care [13]; research however needs to be translated into practice and not left on an academic journal shelf! The addition of a short cognitive assessment tool (e.g. the GPCOG) into routine care of those at greater risk of developing dementia, such as those with high blood pressure and heart disease, may help.

Disclosing a diagnosis of dementia

However, another important area of concern is our apparent difficulty with saying the 'D word' openly. A systematic review, focussed on the process, found that the disclosure of the diagnosis was rated by GPs as one of the five most difficult areas in dementia management; they were less likely to use the correct terminology than psychiatrists; and carers were more likely to be told the diagnosis than patients [14]. Although disclosure has been reported as having negative consequences for people with dementia, including effects on their self esteem and anxiety about the future, reported benefits include an 'end to uncertainty', with subsequent easing of relationship tensions, confirmation of suspicions, access to support, and better understanding of the situation [14].

In the UK, a National Dementia Strategy for England has been developed in consultation with 'relevant stakeholders'[15]. This should begin to address the need for a major national awareness programme and a long awaited change in service provision. Finally, as healthcare professionals, we need to overcome our own personal demons and be able to say the word 'Dementia' openly and sensitively to patients without whispering behind their backs to their relatives!

At this early stage in the illness, GPs could signpost to patients and their families the sorts of information and sources of practical and emotional support provided by key voluntary organizations such as the Alzheimer's Society, who can play a crucial role in helping people to live with dementia.

Supportive care: ensuring care is both patient and carer centred

The concept of person-centred care has been widely promoted in dementia care [16] (see also Chapter 25 in this volume) and has become integrated into health and social care policy in some countries. Evidence-based guidance on dementia care also advocates this approach for people with dementia and their carers [5]. Patient-centred care, like supportive care, reflects a need to focus on the individual, not the illness, and adopt a broader more holistic approach. Despite achieving a theoretical consensus, practical guidance for healthcare professionals on how to deliver person-centred care for people with dementia is unfortunately limited. Another potential barrier to delivering person-centred care in dementia is that the majority of GP consultations with people with dementia also involve their carers, who have their own individual needs (i.e. triadic consultations).

Research has shown that in triadic consultations, older people tend to be less involved, and less assertive [17,18]. Carers themselves report that when they are present in medical consultations, people with dementia become increasingly marginalized and less involved in decision-making [18,19]. Although communication skills training is an essential component for doctors in the UK, there is a lack of compulsory training on dementia and older people's mental health in both the undergraduate medical and the nursing curricula. The importance of certain communication skills in consultations with people with dementia, such as appropriate pacing of questions and the use of non-verbal communication has been emphasized [5]; however, current UK postgraduate training in old age psychiatry does not include any formal skills training to address this requirement. More importantly, there is a lack of evidence-based training for health professionals on how to facilitate triadic consultations successfully, to ensure both patient and carer concerns are identified, and their individual needs met. Training for health and social care professionals in these areas is urgently needed to facilitate supportive care in dementia.

Supportive care in dementia through a collaborative care model

Key roles for the family doctor in caring for people with long-term conditions include acting as a gate-keeper to other services and as a care co-ordinator through liaison with other services. However, in the UK, there is consistent evidence that the overall standard of dementia care is in urgent need of improvement, with frequent failure to deliver services in a timely, integrated, and cost-effective manner [4]. A collaborative care model for dementia, based within primary care, has been recommended for people with dementia [5].

The collaborative care model comprises several core components: a care manager (or key worker) to provide information and co-ordinate care, the use of care pathways (evidence-based protocols) for common areas of dementia management, and timely access to specialist advice. The collaborative care model has already been shown to be effective in the management of other long-term conditions, such as diabetes and depression. Initial results from USA-based trials evaluating a collaborative care model reveal promising results in terms of both patient care and carer support [20]. This model of care would also appear to be favoured by people with dementia and their family supporters [4].

How would such a model work in practice? The care manager would need to be knowledgeable in dementia care, have experience of working in multi-disciplinary teams, and possess skills in information provision, practical advice, and psychological support. He or she would be based in the community either within a primary care team or a community mental health team, and would liaise regularly with the family doctor and secondary care specialists. The use of evidence-based care pathways for common areas of dementia care such as agitation and other behavioural and psychological symptoms, depression, incontinence, and carer support, would ensure a consistent approach to clinical and care management for all health and social professionals involved. Although significant amounts of research funding have been allocated to evaluating the effectiveness of drugs in treating dementia and the behavioural problems related to it, there have been limited studies exploring the effectiveness and acceptability of different models of service delivery for dementia care, such as the Admiral Nurse service (see Chapter 16) [21].

A community-based care manager focussing principally on the person with dementia would complement existing innovative services and would also, in theory, promote better integration of health and social care, facilitate more patient-centred care packages, and allow time for advance care planning which, although now part of the UK *End of Life Strategy* [22], is not yet integrated into clinical practice. Earlier discussion and documentation of the views of a person with dementia with regard to their preferred place of future care and their specific wishes on treatments and potential interventions should improve the quality of end-of-life care and may reduce unnecessary hospital admissions. Allowing time, in the privacy and comfort of a person's home, would encourage a broader, less clinically focused and, perhaps, more sensitive, and personal discussion.

As the dementia became more advanced, the care manager would also be pivotal in liaising with the family doctor, community palliative care teams, and Admiral Nurse team in ensuring a smooth transition into end-of-life care. However, the collaborative care model for dementia remains a theoretical concept, and confirmation of its effectiveness in a variety of health care settings is required. Until then, the role of the care manager in providing supportive care for people with dementia, from diagnosis to dying, usually falls to their family doctor, or their social worker.

Care homes

As dementia progresses, about a third of those people affected will eventually be admitted to a care home, either following a hospital admission or when the family and community support network can no longer meet their required level of care. This is often a time of anxiety and distress for all concerned requiring supportive counselling from the GP. Some people enter care homes within their own neighbourhood, but others move to a care home close to family members, which may be in a different part of the country. In so doing, they lose the continuity of care from the GP who may have looked after them for many years.

In 2002, it was estimated that about 62% of residents in UK care homes have dementia to some degree [23], but many will not have a formal diagnosis. Until recently, there was a positive disincentive to making a diagnosis of dementia for residents in homes without dementia care beds; but now, as long as care needs can be met, moving the resident is not inevitable. GPs need to assess cognitive difficulties arising amongst their care home patients and treat remediable causes such as hypothyroidism. The effects of depression, institutionalization, or lack of stimulation may mimic early dementia and must not be accepted as such without assessment, appropriate investigation, and treatment.

The GP care home visit is usually made in response to an acute problem. Initial discussion about the patient often takes place within earshot of other residents and visitors. The patient may need transfer by hoist from his or her place at the dining table to the nearest bedroom to be examined. For persons with dementia, this can be distressing as they struggle to understand what is happening. GPs recognize that they have not always offered a good standard of care under these circumstances, and some will admit that they do not enjoy looking after patients in care homes. This stance needs challenging not collusion. GPs have a pivotal role to play in changing from a reactive to a proactive approach to the complex needs of these patients.

Our experience has shown that some care homes have patients registered with as many as 17 practices, so staff may need to liaise with 60 different GPs. Rationalizing working practices to establish a committed GP practice per care home and a named GP taking personal responsibility for the patients has the potential to enable better holistic care for patients and improved relationships with care home staff. Practice-based commissioning and locally enhanced service agreements may be available to provide financial support to practices taking on responsibility for a named care home, but the managing authority (in the UK presently, the Primary Care Trust) will need to involve the majority of local GPs if it is to be successfully implemented.

A regular GP visit to a care home may require restructuring of the working day and consideration of a morning or afternoon session during traditional surgery hours. In response, the care home can reasonably be asked to provide a dedicated, fully briefed member of staff and a private room in which to discuss patients and see those who are up and about before others visiting their rooms. The provision of a dedicated phone line may allow secure remote access to the practice computer records via a laptop computer. Apart from acute emergencies, most problems can wait for the weekly visit or will have been anticipated in advance. Care structured in this way can be delivered by both part- and full-time GPs.

Advance care planning

The Gold Standards Framework (GSF) [24] is recognized as a valuable tool in proactive planning for patients with cancer. The underlying principles are as relevant for those with dementia. The regular meeting between GPs, district and Macmillan (i.e. palliative) nurses facilitates the sharing of up-to-date information. In the care home, the GP or care home manager can take the lead in co-ordinating a similar approach. Any resident who is deteriorating can be discussed and plans made to cover potential palliative care needs. Information can then be shared with other involved agencies including the Out-of-Hours service provider.

The advance care plan (see also Chapters 28 and 29) is part of this proactive approach and, in England and Wales, under the terms of the 2005 Mental Capacity Act [25], all those involved are required to create appropriate opportunities for people with dementia to participate in discussions and any decision-making process about their care, if able to do so. The Act also places a duty on health professionals to ensure that the views of anyone caring for a person or interested in his or her welfare must be taken into account and this gives legal recognition and status to families and carers, in contrast to the past.

The plan itself can be a simple document and GPs can take the lead in establishing its use in the community and in any care home for which they are responsible, in liaison with the staff. A single side of paper containing questions about the wishes of all those closely involved, with reference to aspects of care that they would or would not like to happen, their preferred place of care, and any special arrangements, will suffice. Ideally, it should be filled in soon after diagnosis or when a resident first arrives at a care home, but it is a dynamic document and taking advantage of lucid intervals, or a moment of quiet discussion, can allow it to be updated at any time. It provides an opportunity to talk about the progressive nature of dementia, to help all those involved to come to terms with this, and to let them know the primary care team and/or the care home staff can meet end-of-life care needs. Completing the plan occasionally reveals unrealistic expectations or disputes between family members that will need further discussion.

In March 2006, GSF guidance [26] was produced to help identify patients nearing the last 6–12 months of life and thus trigger better assessment and planning of care related to their needs. For patients with dementia it includes the 'surprise question' ('*Would you, as a health professional, be surprised if this patient died within the next year?*'), clinical indicators of dementia, and markers of physical decline. Within the community or in the care home setting, support for these patients can then be directed towards end-of-life care planning with the focus on comfort and dignity.

Medication

Reviews of medication form an extremely important aspect of the GP's role in the care of the person with dementia. From a quality perspective, the GP care home alignment proposal has the potential to improve prescribing by limiting the number of prescribers for each resident. After a period of adjustment to the care home, it is often possible to reduce the dose of anti-psychotic or sedative medication from that previously needed at home or in a hospital ward. Very frail patients can sometimes be seen to improve dramatically and regain a degree of communication, mobility, enjoyment of food, and response to family visits.

Supportive care of the person with dementia also involves a detailed review of medication for longstanding conditions. The dose of anti-hypertensive drugs can often be significantly reduced when the patient has lost weight in advanced dementia. Decisions need to be made about prescribing potentially toxic drugs such as digoxin, amiodarone and warfarin, and continuing acetylcholinesterase inhibitors, and drugs to reduce vascular risk factors. The ethical dilemmas raised by continuing or stopping such treatment will need to be addressed.

End-of-life care

The experience gained from looking after the patient described in Box 15.1 highlighted the difficulties inherent in providing good end-of-life care for people with dementia and led to the formation of a Palliative Care in Dementia Group in Peterborough, which could provide a model for other areas in the country. It is a multi-disciplinary group bringing together primary and secondary care, and based at the Sue Ryder Thorpe Hall Hospice. The Group has promoted sharing of expertise and supported the development of practical tools to improve end-of-life care for patients with dementia. The associated documentation has been adapted for ease of use in the daily life of a busy care home. The Group has also taken on an educational role in the local

Box 15.1 End-of-life care

One of my patients had advanced dementia and had lived in the local care home for 5 years. Over Christmas he developed a chest infection from which he was clearly not recovering and he appeared distressed and possibly in pain. My impression was that he was dying. After discussion with his family and the staff, it was clear that his best interests would be served by enabling him to stay in the care home, but he needed active management of his symptoms. Contact was made with the local Palliative Care Consultant who provided advice and support, despite the patient's non-cancer diagnosis. A syringe driver was set up and he died peacefully, with his family beside him, 36 hours later.

primary care and care home communities. Further details about the Group and generic versions of all the documents and associated protocols are available on line [27].

Increasingly, attention is being paid to the need to assess pain in people with dementia and the accepted position is that it is under-detected and under-treated. Scales have been developed for assessment of pain and distress in patients with cognitive impairment (see Chapter 14 in this volume). Family members, nursing and care staff can be empowered to recognize their contribution to the assessment of pain, agitation, and distress, by noting subtle changes in response and behaviour. The resulting palliative care requires active management of symptoms and not simply 'tender loving care'. GPs may need advice on prescribing for opiate naïve patients or those who are acutely agitated, and nurses in the care home setting may need syringe driver training.

Using an end-of-life care pathway provides a structured approach to care for the person with dementia in the last few days of life. However, identification of end-stage dementia is difficult, and any end-of-life pathway needs to accommodate that difficulty. Using the standard end-of-life care pathway template, but removing disorientation as a criterion, provides entry requirements appropriate to the assessment of the person with dementia (see discussion of the Liverpool Care Pathway on page 122 above). Awareness that removal from the pathway is an option is a further reassurance for the GP and team taking the decision that a patient is imminently dying. The pathway supports nursing and care staff in the community or the care home in the delivery of a high standard of end-of-life care, with recognition of the additional needs of relatives.

Emergency situations

In the care home, the GP can take the lead in educating and empowering staff to make decisions in an acute situation. The assessment of a person who has collapsed and lost consciousness needs to include consideration of the possible causes, the most appropriate immediate response, whether or not further medical help is needed, and to take into account best interests. The distress of a trip to hospital for a person with dementia should be avoided (see Box 15.2), unless there are exceptional circumstances such as a hip fracture.

Consideration also needs to have been given to the possibility of a resident having a cardiopulmonary arrest. In practical terms, GPs must consider the question of resuscitation for all their care home patients. The chance of a successful resuscitation outside hospital in patients who are physically frail and have dementia, is extremely low. The risk of harm, such as rib fractures or further brain damage, is significant. The potential for a very distressing, undignified death is high. This does not mean making a judgement on the quality of life of a person with dementia, but must take account of his or her views if known, and those of others most closely involved, as well

Box 15.2 Emergency decisions

During a weekly visit, there was a sudden flurry of activity and a patient was wheeled past, tipped back in a wheelchair, waxy-faced and unconscious. I followed slowly behind and by the time I reached his room he was lying on the bed. Although apparently unconscious, when asked how he was feeling, he opened his eyes and replied that he was 'floating'. There was a pause; he shut his eyes and lay still, very pale and barely breathing, but in no apparent distress. I left him with a member of staff and continued seeing other residents, finding his condition unchanged on review later on. I heard no more but when I visited a week later, he was up and dressed and responded to me with his usual brisk rebuff.

If I hadn't been there, staff admitted that someone would have dialled 999 even before he had reached his room. The ambulance crew would have had no choice but to scoop and run and he would have had a very distressing trip to hospital.

as consider the benefits and burdens of active resuscitation. Such decisions should be appropriately recorded and shared with any other health professionals involved in the patient's care.

The onset of acute confusion in a patient usually prompts a search for a remediable cause such as acute infection or constipation. For those with dementia, a sudden deterioration or change in behaviour needs to be approached initially in a similar manner and factors such as pain should also be considered. Persisting behavioural change, especially aggressive or noisy behaviour, may put the person, family members, or other care home residents and staff at risk, and the GP will be required to weigh up the needs of all those involved in deciding how to address the situation. Most 'challenging behaviour' represents a means of communication for the person with dementia (see Chapter 17 in this volume); trying to understand and address the person's needs is time-consuming but can be successful. In the care home, staff can adapt their approach at times of increased agitation or aggression, such as when attending to personal care needs. Techniques such as distraction or allowing wandering within a secure environment may be helpful. Dementia care mapping by staff trained in its use can provide invaluable insight into the pattern and nature of interaction between a particular resident and other residents and members of staff [28].

All these measures can be tried before considering prescribing, but at times the GP will need to consider medication if the situation remains too distressing, or risky for the patient and others (see Chapter 12). Knowing that the behavioural problems escalate at a certain time of the day may allow changes to the timing of existing medication to good effect. GPs may wish to take advice from the local mental health team for the elderly before prescribing, but often decisions have to be made in an acute and worsening situation. Using the lowest possible dose, reviewing frequently, and having responsibility for that patient in the longer term will help support any prescribing decision made.

In advanced dementia, physical problems, such as difficulty swallowing, may occur and assessment by a speech therapist (who will also have an important role in training and providing on-going support) may reveal that the patient has 'an unsafe swallow' and cannot be fed orally without risk of aspiration. The GP must take responsibility for the decisions that follow this assessment; it is important that GPs understand the risks and benefits of artificial feeding and can convey these to all those involved (for further discussion see Chapters 27 and 28). Relatives and care staff who are feeding a person under these circumstances may be very apprehensive and feel responsible when death eventually occurs and may require considerable support from the GP.

Conclusion

The GP has a pivotal role to play in providing good supportive care for the person with dementia from before diagnosis until death. There are substantial opportunities for tangible improvements in health and well-being at every stage. The challenge to GPs is to recognize those opportunities and use all the clinical skills at their disposal to address them fully. In so doing, GPs need to take a proactive approach to the care of people with dementia and to consider the ethical dimension of that approach. There is a need to improve identification and treatment of symptoms and provide active management of supportive and palliative care needs. GPs can take a leadership role and empower relatives, nurses, and carers so that they recognize the value of the contributions they can make to all aspects of care. Reviewing significant events can lead to positive changes, including improved communication, and reduced hospital admissions, especially close to death. Finally, GPs have the potential to ensure that people with dementia have a good death – secure, dignified, and peaceful – and thus provide families with a positive experience at the end of this devastating illness.

References

1. Royal College of General Practitioners. (1972). *The future general practitioner: learning and teaching.* London: RCGP.

2. Ahmedzai SH (2005). The nature of palliation and its contribution to supportive care, in Admedzai S, Muers M (eds). *Supportive care in respiratory disease,* pp. 3–38. Oxford: Oxford University Press.

3. Bamford C, Eccles M, Steen N, Robinson L (2007). Can primary care record review facilitate earlier diagnosis of dementia? *Fam Pract,* **24**, 108–116.

4. National Audit Office (2007). *Improving services and support for people with dementia.* London: The Stationery Office.

5. NICE/SCIE (2006). *Dementia: supporting people with dementia and their carers in health and social care.* London: National Institute for Clinical Excellence and Social Care Institute for Excellence (NICE/SCIE).

6. Waldemar G, Phung KTT, Burns A *et al.* (2007). Access to diagnostic evaluation and treatment for dementia in Europe. *Int J Geriatr Psychiatry,* **22**, 47–54.

7. Folstein MF, Folstein SE, McHugh PR (1975). Mini-mental state: a practical method for grading the cognitive state of patients for the clinician. *J Psychiatr Res,* **12**, 189–198.

8. Brodaty H, Pond D, Kemp NM *et al.* (2002). The GPCOG: a new screening test for dementia diagnosed for general practice. *JAGS,* **50**, 530–534.

9. Milne A, Culverwell R, Guss R, Tuppen J, Whelton R (2008). Screening for dementia in primary care: a review of the use, efficacy and quality of measures. *Int Psychogeriatrics,* **3**, 431–458.

10. Banerjee S, Willis R, Matthews D, Contell F, Chan J, Murray J (2007). Improving the quality of care for mild to moderate dementia: an evaluation of the Croydon memory service model. *Int J Geriatr Psychiatry,* **22**, 782–788.

11. Audit Commission (2002). *Forget me not.* London: Audit Commission.

12. National Institute for Health and Clinical Excellence (2006). *Donepezil, galantamine, rivastigmine (review) and memantine for the treatment of Alzheimer's disease (amended).* London: NICE.

13. Downs M, Turner S, Bryans M *et al.* (2006). Effectiveness of educational interventions in improving detection and management of dementia in primary care: a cluster randomised controlled study. *Br Med J,* **332**, 692–696.

14. Bamford C, Lamont S, Eccles M, Robinson L, May C, Bond J (2004). Disclosing a diagnosis of dementia: a systematic review. *Int J Geriatr Psychiatry,* **19**(2), 151–169.

15. Department of Health (2009). *Living well with dementia: a national strategy.* Available at: http://www.dh.gov.uk/en/SocialCare/Deliveringadultsocialcare/Olderpeople/NationalDementiaStrategy/index.htm (accessed 25 March 2009).

16. Kitwood T (1997). *Dementia reconsidered: the person comes first*. Buckingham: Open University Press.

17. Greene MG, Majerovitz SD, Adelman RD, Rizzo C (1994). The effects of the presence of a third person on the physician-older patient medical interview. *JAGS*, **42**, 413–419.

18. Beisecker AE, Chrisman SK, Wright LJ (1997). Perceptions of family caregivers of persons with Alzheimer's disease: communication with physicians. *Am J Alzheimers Dis*, March/April, 73–83.

19. Hirschman KB, Xie SX, Feudtner C, Karlawish HT (2004). How does an Alzheimer's disease patient's role in medical decision making change over time? *J Geriatr Psychiatry Neurol*, **17**, 55–60.

20. Callahan CM, Boustani MA, Unverzagt FW *et al.* (2006). Effectiveness of collaborative care for older adults with Alzheimer disease in primary care: a randomized controlled trial. *JAMA*, **295**(18), 2148–2157.

21. Woods R, Wills W, Higginson I, Hobbins J, Whitby M (2003). Support in the community for people with dementia and their carers: a comparative outcome study of specialist mental health service interventions. *Int J Geriatr Psychiatry*, **18**, 298–307.

22. Department of Health (2008). *End of life care strategy: promoting high quality care for all adults at the end of life*. London: Department of Health.

23. Matthews F, Dening T (2002). Prevalence of dementia in institutional care. *Lancet*, **360**(9328), 225–226.

24. Department of Health (2005). *Gold standards framework*. Available at: www.goldstandardsframework. nhs.uk (accessed 17 September 2008).

25. Department of Health (DoH) (2005). *The mental capacity act 2005*. Available at: http://www.opsi.gov. uk/acts/acts2005/ukpga_20050009_en_1 (accessed 25 March 2009).

26. Gold Standards Framework (2006). *Palliative care and the GMS contract prognostic indicator guidance*. Available at: http://www.goldstandardsframework.nhs.uk/content/gp_contract/QOF_Introduction_ Paper_1.pdf (accessed 25 March 2009).

27. Jenner Health Centre (2007). Available at: http://www.dementia.jennerhealthcentre.co.uk/ (accessed 25 March 2009).

28. Brooker D, Surr CA (2005). *Dementia care mapping: principles and practice*. Bradford: University of Bradford.

Chapter 16

Community mental health nursing and supportive care

John Keady and Philip Hardman

Introduction

Supportive care in mental health nursing is a new and previously untested concept. This chapter provides an overview of the role of the community mental health nurse (CMHN) in dementia care and uses the anchor points of the recovery model and the senses framework to develop supportive care within this professional context. A case study on the acceptance and adjustment to an early diagnosis of dementia is presented to 'flesh out' a supportive care philosophy. The chapter will conclude with the importance of education and a shared understanding on the meaning of supportive care if the approach is to become embedded within the rubric and lexicon of everyday CMHN practice.

CMHN practice in dementia: an overview

The Nursing and Midwifery Council (NMC) is the governing, accrediting, and registration body for all nursing practice in the United Kingdom (UK) and its report 'Standards for proficiency for pre-registration nurse education' [1] provides a definition of the role and practice boundaries of the mental health nurse; this definition is shown in Box 16.1. At present, mental health nurses comprise the largest professional group in mental health services in the UK with some 48,000 registered nurses (mental health) working in the National Health Service (NHS) [2]. Mental health nurses undertake a variety of roles in hospital, community, and residential services and the work of the CMHN is, therefore, just one of a number of potential options available upon qualification and in following a career pathway.

Within the NHS, the CMHN has a rich and varied history, one that stretches back to the late 1950s and formed part of the progressive first wave of services that decanted the Victorian asylums in favour of a more holistic, community-orientated approach to mental health care [3,4]. At that time, there were only a handful of psychiatric nurses undertaking this community role and their function was chiefly to 'provide psychological support for patients and relatives, supervise medication and deal with difficulties before they became entrenched' ([4], p. 11). This supportive and preventative function was undertaken with a broad population of 'patients' and included older people and those living with dementia [5]. This 'new' community orientated nursing role proved to be a popular and successful innovation and by 1966 Nolan [3] reported that in the UK, there were approximately 225 CMHNs 'employed by 42 psychiatric hospitals' (p. 13). The steady increase in the number of CMHNs continued over the next three decades with the fourth quinquennial national CMHN census of England and Wales reporting that the total number of CMHNs in these two countries had risen from 4000 in 1990 to nearly 7000 by 1996 [6] – the last time the census count was taken.

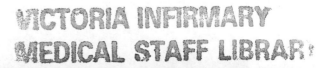

Box 16.1 Definition of mental health nursing

Mental health nurses care for people experiencing mental distress, which may have a variety of causative factors. The focus of mental health nursing is the establishment of a relationship with service users and carers to help bring about an understanding of how they might cope with their experience, thus maximising their potential for recovery. Mental health nurses use a well developed and evidence-based repertoire of interpersonal, psychosocial and other skills that are underpinned by an empathetic attitude towards the service user and the contexts within which their distress has arisen. Mental health difficulties can occur at any age and service users may be cared for in a variety of settings, including the community and their own homes. They may require care for an acute episode or ongoing support for an enduring illness. Mental health nurses work as part of multi-disciplinary and multi-agency teams that seek to involve service users and their carers in all aspects of their care and treatment.

Source: ([1], p. 24)

Community mental health nurses are usually based in primary or secondary care settings and operate as members of interdisciplinary and integrated Community Mental Health Teams (CMHTs), such as child and adolescent mental health services, forensic mental health services, adult mental health teams, community learning disability teams, drug and alcohol action teams, older people's mental health services, and so on. Recently, CMHNs have been described as the 'backbone' of specialist mental health services in the UK ([7], p. 185), thus underscoring their importance to the smooth running of mainstream service provision. For dementia care services specifically, CMHNs are usually located within older people's CMHTs and may carry either a dedicated dementia care caseload or a 'mixed' (organic-functional) one; such service configuration will usually depend upon historical practice and local team priorities. Community mental health nurses in dementia care may also take on other specialist community roles, for instance, as members of younger people with dementia teams [8,9], memory assessment and treatment services [10,11], and in providing dedicated support to carers of people with dementia, such as through the Admiral Nurse service ([12,13,14] and see Box 16.2).

Box 16.2 Role of the Admiral Nurse

All Admiral Nurses are Registered Nurses (Mental Health), most with previous experience of practising as a CMHN. The Admiral Nurse role originally commenced in the 1990s by the charity *for dementia* (formerly the Dementia Relief Trust) to address the needs of carers of people with dementia living in the community. There are, at present, over 60 Admiral Nurses working in the UK in areas such as London, the South East, the West Midlands, the North West of England, North Wales and North Lincolnshire. Admiral Nursing encompasses a variety of posts that enhance the core nursing role, including Admiral Nurse Consultant, Lecturer Practitioner and Research Practitioner. Many of the Admiral Nurse teams are located within NHS secondary mental health services and integrated health and social care trusts. However, each team works collaboratively with a range of local service providers including primary care, tertiary care, social care and voluntary and independent providers. This is a way of working that reflects the complex nature of dementia and the experiences of individuals and families.

Source: ([13], p. 345).

One of the earliest descriptions of the 'psychiatric nurse in the community nursing service' was provided by John Greene, chief male nurse at Moorhaven Hospital in Plymouth, UK. In his seminal paper outlining this 'new' role, Greene [5] argued that 'psychogeriatric' and 'partially confused' patients required a different approach to services than other client groups, and then went on to give a detailed (but dense) critique of what this specialist work looked like. Unpacking the role attributes from this critique, Keady and Adams ([15], p. 37) suggested that this early role description encompassed:

1 The value of experience in working with people having dementia and their families
2 A knowledge of dementia and its likely course
3 Attention to personal care needs
4 Information-sharing with families
5 Promotion of autonomy for people with dementia
6 Maintaining regular visits and contact
7 Establishing trust with both the person with dementia and their family
8 Service co-ordination.

Forty years on, the role of the CMHN in dementia care can still be seen in this initial summary. However, perhaps the greatest change over recent years is that contemporary CMHN practice in dementia care is predominantly conducted through a time-limited 'psychosocial intervention' (PSI) and reserved for those with the most complex and enduring needs [16,17,18]. This shift in practice philosophy has replaced the traditional, long-standing relationships of old where large caseload numbers and an absence of discharge criteria were the hallmarks of CMHN practice in dementia care [16,17]. Three recent studies are described below to help illuminate this practice shift.

Study 1

Esme Moniz-Cook and her colleagues [7] undertook an evaluation of training CMHNs in a systematic PSI to help family carers manage behavioural problems in their relatives with dementia. This PSI programme consisted of 3 components: problem-solving; stress-coping interventions; and functional behavioural analysis in dementia. One hundred and thirteen families received the PSI from 9 CMHNs and outcome measures were obtained at baseline 6, 12, and 18 months and compared with a 'usual practice' cohort comprising 20 CMHNs and their caseloads. The study demonstrated that problem behaviours reduced in the experimental group families, although a prolonged period of engagement was necessary to moderate carer mood. The paper also highlighted the need for dementia-specific practice arrangements (rather than a 'mixed' functional-organic caseload), training and sustained clinical supervision in the delivery of a successful PSI; a finding that has been reported previously [19].

Study 2

Cantley and Caswell [20] outlined the role of the CMHN in assertive outreach through the Intensive Community Treatment Team in Hull and East Riding Community Health NHS Trust, UK. Independently evaluated by *Dementia North*, the aims of the project were to: provide timely, realistic, and co-ordinated packages of care; maximize the individual's well being, independence, choice, and dignity; prevent admissions to hospital or care homes; facilitate a planned approach to necessary admissions as a means of ensuring the best possible outcome for people with dementia and their carers; and provide comprehensive packages of therapeutic interventions to enable people with dementia to return home from hospital sooner than would otherwise be possible. In this pilot study, the CMHN carried an average of 6 cases and focus was placed upon the immediacy of the referral criteria, such as: deterioration in the client's mental health and/or increasing cognitive impairment; aggressive or disruptive behaviour; evident risks; carer struggling to cope; poor compliance with medication; and the client resisting service input. The evaluation demonstrated that a 'high proportion' of problems were met by the team and that intervention was between 12 weeks (the ideal) to 18 weeks.

Study 3

In a retrospective case note study of a sample of 404 consecutive referrals over an 18-month period to a north of England memory clinic (175 patients were eventually diagnosed as having dementia), Page and his colleagues [21] demonstrated that initial home assessment by two specialist dementia care nurses offered a 'high level of accuracy in their diagnostic capabilities' (p. 32). The paper went on to report that the specialist nurses may require additional training and support in the identification of subtypes of dementia.

Attempting to further develop such 'new ways of working' [2], two recent national reviews of mental health nursing practice, one conducted in England by the Chief Nursing Officer (Christine Beasley) and entitled *'From values to action'* [22] and the other in Scotland conducted by their Chief Nursing Officer (Paul Martin) and entitled *'Rights, Relationships and Recovery'* [23], have proved highly influential. The mental health nursing review *'From values to action'* [22] outlined three values that are to be used to underpin mental health nursing clinical care, training, and relationships with service users, carers and families, these being (slightly abridged):

1 The recovery approach
2 The principle of equality
3 The need for evidence-based practice (p. 17).

The review [22] also linked 'recovery' to the adoption of a palliative care model to meet the needs of people with dementia, particularly those in its 'severe stages' (p. 26). Within the context of this chapter, therefore, it is the emphasis on the first of these values, the recovery approach, which has the most natural link with the values of supportive care as championed by this book. Accordingly, the main components of this approach are further considered in the next section.

The recovery approach

As stated in *'Rights, Relationships and Recovery'* [23], the recovery approach evolved out of service users' movements from around the world with several states in the United States of America committing their mental health service to a recovery ethos. The language of 'recovery' is therefore owned by, and is in the possession of, the service user movement. Box 16.3 outlines a widely agreed definition of 'recovery' [24].

Box 16.3 Definition of 'recovery'

'[Recovery is] a deeply personal, unique process of changing one's attitudes, values, feelings, goals, skills and roles. It is a way of living a satisfying, hopeful and contributing life, even with the limitations caused by illness. Recovery involves the development of new meaning and purpose in one's life as one grows beyond the catastrophic effects of mental illness'.

Source: ([24], p. 14).

Rights, Relationships and Recovery [23], however, went on to develop this description by suggesting that recovery is not simply based on the absence of symptoms (as Box 16.3 implies) but, instead, is more reflective of the journey of discovery taken by the service user within the context of their life story and experiences:

> '[Recovery] is based on hope, involvement, participation, inclusion, meaning, purpose, control, and self-management, and emphasizes the importance of peer support, meaningful activity, employment, maintaining social networks, and activities when distressed and having the chance to contribute, or give back, in some way'. ([23], p. 18)

Within the context of mental health nursing care, therefore, 'recovery' is a set of values about a person's right to build a meaningful life for him or herself and is centred around self-determination and self-management. Moreover, as Shepherd, Boardman and Slade [25] succinctly argue, 'hope' is the glue that links together both these belief structures and provides the bridge necessary for 'sustaining motivation and supporting expectations of an individually fulfilled life' (p. 1). Thus, within the recovery approach, it is not the 'treatment and [medical] cure' model that holds sway, rather it is the person's self-narrated perception of their quality of life – both actual and potential – and their hope(s) about how this could be achieved that becomes the transcending service goal and rationale for 'professional' intervention.

Reconfiguring mental health services to respond to this (individual) lived construction of hope, illness, and recovery is a significant challenge and requires recovery-orientated services and practices that act to rehabilitate the service user and create the conditions necessary for 'recovery' to occur. Such a reconfiguration of professional values and treatment goals also requires a number of relationship-building skills and collaborative values to be present in any inter-personal exchange between professional and service user, including openness, equality of relationship and reciprocity [26]. Developing these points a little further, *'From values to action'* [22] suggested that in mental health nursing practice the recovery approach should promote the values of:

1 Working in partnership with service users (and/or carers) to identify realistic life goals, which they are then enabled to achieve

2 Stressing the value of social inclusion

3 Stressing the need for professionals to be optimistic about the possibility of positive individual change (p. 17).

Whilst these partnership goals are to be applauded, one criticism that could be levelled against the present construction of the recovery approach and its wholesale adoption by the mental health nursing profession is that it is predominantly built from the narrative and experience of adults living with serious mental illness(es); the contribution of people with dementia to this dialogic is unknown at this time. Recently, Keady and his colleagues [27] have suggested that the adoption of a 'recovery' narrative within CMHN practice in dementia care has potential, but its use may give rise to a number of questions such as:

1 Is 'recovery' a narrative that is – or could be – owned by people with dementia and their families?

2 Is recovery an ethical term to use when working with people having progressive and enduring cognitive disability and whose diagnosis may lead to premature death?

3 What does recovery mean to dementia care nurses generally and to CMHNs in dementia care specifically?

After debating and reflecting upon these questions, the authors conclude that the 'recovery approach' has resonance, but it is best viewed as a dimension of supportive care in dementia and one that could act as a platform for evidence-based practice built from an individual – and/or family – construction of need and quality of life. It is the development of this conceptualization that forms the substance of the next section.

CMHN practice and supportive care in dementia

As CMHNs work with people having dementia from across the spectrum of the condition, i.e. from community screening to diagnosis to behaviour that challenges and on to palliative care and beyond to the support of bereaved carers, one approach that may help give a vision to supportive care in the CMHN field is to see supportive care underpinned by the senses framework and embedded within a recovery narrative. For some years now, the first author and his colleagues have been promoting a more 'inclusive' vision of gerontological and dementia care practice based on relationship-centred values and the senses framework [28,29,30]. The 'six senses' that comprise the senses framework [29] were developed in close collaboration with older people and both family and paid carers, and were developed using the notion that if people with chronic illness are to receive high quality care they need to experience:

1 A sense of security

2 A sense of belonging

3 A sense of continuity

4 A sense of purpose

5 A sense of fulfilment

6 A sense of significance.

These senses are not presented in a hierarchical order, rather they identify intrinsic human values and their use in practice is based upon the principles of transparency, negotiation and equality between all stakeholders; in this instance, the person with dementia, family carer(s) and the professional worker. All views are significant in the articulation of each of the senses and, as such, care planning and intervention is based upon a supportive care philosophy, i.e. 'done with' rather than 'done to'. This idea will be developed further through a short case study that is a composite of recent real-life cases within our own areas of clinical practice.

Case study

Alan is a 68-year-old married man from Cheshire who was recently diagnosed with Alzheimer's disease following attendance at a local memory assessment treatment and support service. Alan is married to Stella and he had worked as a secondary school teacher for most of his adult life; as such, he is a well known figure in the local community. For the last 2 months, however, Alan has had real difficulty in accepting and coming to terms with his diagnosis and he has expressed thoughts to his wife, children and general practitioner that he 'no longer wanted to carry on and face the future'. Alan was fearful of getting older with Alzheimer's disease as the information he had read on the internet about the condition said that he would eventually lose all his faculties and become dependent upon the people he loved for his future care and quality of life. He also read that the timing of his death could not be predicted and that his death may be painful and prolonged. Alan did not want any of this and said that he would rather be 'out of it now' than accept this as his future. Following referral to his CMHN for his low mood and suicidal ideation, attempts were made to support a recovery approach by instilling a sense of purpose in Alan's life.

Using the words of Alan and Stella, a snapshot of the assessment and supportive care planning process relating to the recovery of a sense of purpose is presented in Table 16.1.

Table 16.1 The supportive care approach

Presenting issue: recovering Alan and Stella's sense of purpose		
Sense	Alan's belief structure	Stella's belief structure
Purpose	'I feel afraid of the future and I don't want to be a burden to my family'	'I want to be there for Alan, but he just shuts me out all the time.
	'I love my wife and family and home but think they will be better off without me'	'He is my husband and the father of our children. We belong together but I am finding it hard'
	'My retirement and diagnosis has brought about major life transitions and adjustments in my life. I haven't coped well with them and feel useless around the house'	
	'I can't see a role for myself anymore. It's as if all the lights in my life have gone out'	
	'What can I achieve now I have Alzheimer's? Nothing'	
	'My wife and family are the most important things in my life – but just look at me now, what good am I to them?'	

CMHN: supportive care plan

Aim: recovering Alan and Stella's sense of purpose

Alan:

Primary actions

1 Start individual counselling and relationship building
2 Perform a daily risk assessment
3 Commence biographical work to locate networks and interests
4 Partnership working and daily visits
5 Undertake structured depression and quality of life measures

Medium-term goal

1 Introduce Alan to a diagnostic support group and positive living skills course
2 Potential for befriending involvement

Stella:

Primary actions

1 Involve Admiral Nurse in providing independent support
2 Undertake structured depression and quality of life measures

Medium term goal

1 Recover shared activities through the development/re-instigation of mutual interests

Other actions

1 Daily evaluation of supportive care plan
2 Keep CMHT and GP updated at weekly meeting forums
3 Bring case to weekly peer supervision meetings
4 Involve Alan and Stella's children in the supportive care plan

As can be seen, such a supportive care approach is time intensive as the CMHN puts into place a psychosocial approach that aims to recover a sense of purpose – and balance – in Alan and Stella's life. The CMHNs involvement is consistent with the relationship building foundations of the recovery approach and in engendering hope in (eventually) living positively with dementia, a cognitive shift necessary to pull Alan (and Stella) from the brink of despair. For the CMHN, therefore, enhancing the problem-solving coping capacity of both Alan and Stella, identifying (any) immediate emotional, physical, or practical risks that may impinge upon the quality of life (for one partner or both), opening avenues of communication between the couple, cognitively reframing negative thoughts into positive, adaptive ones and exposing the couple to other family and outside contacts becomes the evidence-base of CMHN practice. Such a professional role is cognisant with the recovery approach but operationalized through a supportive care philosophy and evidenced (in this instance) through the senses framework.

Discussion

To date, CMHNs in dementia care have been largely operating in a practice vacuum where descriptions of practice efficacy, rather than structured evaluations of care, have been 'the norm' [16,17]. As recent work has made clear, the absence of a guiding philosophy of care for CMHNs practising in dementia has largely left the profession vulnerable and their role open to professional and public uncertainty [17,31,32]. As this chapter has shown, the philosophical, practical, and conceptual development of supportive care could be the missing link that provides a context and meaning for CMHN practice in dementia. However, in order for this to occur, three conditions need to be met.

First, the vast majority of CMHNs working in the UK would need to 'buy into' the concept of supportive care and be prepared to define and apply a supportive care approach across the spectrum of the condition. Perhaps more importantly, people with dementia and their families would need to 'own' the language of supportive care and believe that this approach has real meaning to/ for their lives. Without this shared belief structure, the relational aspects of the senses framework and the modified use of the recovery approach, as illustrated in this chapter through Alan and Stella's case study, would have little meaning and utility.

Secondly, it would be necessary to introduce supportive care into the curriculum and training of all mental health nurses. At present, pre-registration mental health training equips a mental health nurse upon qualification to practise as a CMHN, including with people with dementia and their families. This could be a major hurdle as the content of mental health nurse training in dementia care varies considerably across the UK [33] and the NMC sets no minimum standards of exposure to dementia care work prior to qualification. This has led to an *ad hoc* and piecemeal exposure to dementia care education and the acquisition of practice-based knowledge that does not do anyone any favours, least of all people with dementia and their families.

Thirdly, and finally, mental health nurse leaders and policy makers would need to accommodate recovery as a dimension of supportive care, and not see the 'recovery approach' as the sole way forward for the mental health nursing profession. Combating this shift in attitudes would, again, be a challenging exercise but ultimately a necessary one, as the message of hope contained in contemporary definitions of recovery (see Box 16.3 for example) requires modification if it is to be 'owned' by people with dementia and their families. This is not meant to be a negative appraisal, only a sensitive and realistic one given the terminal and ultimately degenerative nature of cognitive and self-care abilities following a diagnosis of dementia.

If these three conditions could be met, the adoption of supportive care holds real promise for the advancement of CMHN practice in dementia care.

References

1. Nursing and Midwifery Council (2004). *Standards for proficiency for pre-registration nurse education*. London: Nursing and Midwifery Council.

2. Department of Health (2007). *Mental health: new ways of working for everyone. developing and sustaining a capable and flexible workforce. Progress report*. London: HMSO

3. Nolan P (2003). Voices from the past: the historical alignment of dementia care to nursing, in Keady J, Clarke CL, Adams T (eds) *Community mental health nursing and dementia care: practice perspectives*, pp. 3–16. Buckinghamshire: Open University Press/McGraw Hill Publications.

4. Nolan P (2003). The history of community mental health nursing, in Hannigan B, Coffey M (eds) *The handbook of community mental health nursing*, pp. 7–18. London London: Routledge.

5. Greene J (1968). The psychiatric nurse in the community nursing service. *Int J Nurs Stud*, **5**, 175–184.

6. White E (1999). The 4th quinquennial national community mental health nursing census of England and Wales. *Aust N Z J Ment Nurs*, **8**(3), 86–92.

7. Moniz-Cook E, Elston C, Gardiner E *et al.* (2008). Can training community mental health nurses to support family carers reduce behavioural problems in dementia? An exploratory pragmatic randomised controlled trial. *Int J Geriatr Psychiatry*, **23**, 185–191.

8. Williams O, Keady J, Nolan M (1995). Younger-onset Alzheimer's disease: learning from the experience of one spouse carer. *J Clin Nurs*, **4**, 31–36.

9. Beattie AM, Daker-White G, Gilliard J, Means R (2002). Younger people in dementia care: a review of service needs, service provision and models of good practice. *Aging Ment Health*, **6**(3), 205–212.

10. Page S (2007). Nurse prescribing and the CMHN: assuming new responsibilities: in dementia treatment, in Keady J, Clarke CL, Page S (eds) *Community mental health nursing and dementia care: practice perspectives*, pp. 125–141. Buckinghamshire: Open University Press/McGraw Hill Publications.

11. Keady J, Williams S, Hughes-Roberts J (2005). Emancipatory practice development through life-story work: changing care in a memory clinic in North Wales. *Pract Devel Health Care*, **4**(4), 203–212.

12. Woods RT, Wills W, Higginson IJ, Hobbins J, Whitby M (2003). Support in the community for people with dementia and their carers: a comparative outcome study of specialist mental health service interventions. *Int J Geriatr Psychiatry*, **18**(4), 298–307.

13. Keady J, Ashcroft-Simpson S, Halligan K, Williams S (2007). Admiral nursing and the family care of a parent with dementia: using autobiographical narrative as grounding for negotiated clinical practice and decision-making. *Scand J Caring Sci*, **21**, 345–353.

14. Soliman A (2003). Admiral nurses: a model of family assessment and intervention, in: Keady J, Clarke CL, Adams T (eds) *Community mental health nursing and dementia care: practice perspectives*, pp. 171–185. Buckinghamshire: Open University Press/McGraw Hill Publications.

15. Keady J, Adams T (2001). Community mental health nursing and dementia care. *J Dem Care*, **9**(1), 35–38.

16. Keady J, Clarke CL, Adams T (eds) (2003). *Community mental health nursing and dementia care: practice perspectives*. Buckinghamshire: Open University Press/McGraw Hill Publications.

17. Keady J, Clarke CL, Page S (eds) (2007). *Partnerships in community mental health nursing and dementia care: practice perspectives*. Buckinghamshire: Open University Press/McGraw Hill Publications.

18. Adams T (ed) (2007). *Dementia care nursing: promoting well-being in people with dementia and their families*. Basingstoke: Palgrave Macmillan.

19. Keady J, Woods B, Hahn S, Hill J (2004). Community mental health nursing and early intervention in dementia: developing practice through a single case history. *Int J Older People Nursing*, **13**(6b), 57–67.

20. Cantley C, Caswell P (2007). Assertive outreach and the CMHN: a role for the Future? in Keady J, Clarke CL, Page S (eds) *Community mental health nursing and dementia care: practice perspectives*, pp. 232–244. Buckinghamshire: Open University Press/McGraw Hill Publications.

21. Page S, Hope K, Bee P, Burns A (2008). Nurses making a diagnosis of dementia: a potential change in practice? *Int J Geriatr Psychiatry*, **23**, 27–33.

22. Department of Health (2006). *From values to action: the chief nursing officers review of mental health nursing*. London: HMSO.

23. Scottish Executive (2006). *Rights, relationships and recovery: the report of the national review of mental health nursing in Scotland*. Edinburgh: Scottish Executive.

24. Anthony WA (1993). Recovery from mental illness: the guiding vision of the mental health service in the 1990s. *Psychosoc Rehab J*, **16**, 11–23.

25. Shepherd G, Boardman J, Slade M (2008). *Making recovery a reality*. London: Sainsbury Centre for Mental Health.

26. Borg M, Kristiansen K (2004). Recovery-orientated professionals: helping relationships in mental health services. *J Ment Health*, **13**, 493–505.

27. Keady J, Clarke CL, Page S, Adams T (2007). Signposts to the future: some personal reflections and messages for CMHN practice, in Keady J, Clarke CL, Page S (eds) *Community mental health nursing and dementia care: practice perspectives*, pp. 327–332. Buckinghamshire: Open University Press/McGraw Hill Publications.

28. Nolan M, Davies S, Brown J, Keady J, Nolan J (2004). Beyond 'person-centred' care: a new vision for gerontological nursing. *Int J Older People Nursing*, **13**(3a), 45–53.

29. Nolan M, Brown J, Davies S, Nolan J, Keady J (2006). *The senses framework: improving care for older people through a relationship-centred approach*. GRIP Report Number 2, Sheffield: University of Sheffield.

30. Nolan M, Davies S, Ryan T, Keady J (2008). Relationship-centred care and the 'senses' framework. *J Dem Care*, **16**(1), 26–28.

31. Pickard S (1999). Coordinated care for older people with dementia. *J Interprof Care*, **13**(4), 345–354.

32. Pickard S, Glendenning C (2001). Caring for a relative with dementia: the perceptions of relatives and CPNs. *Qual Ageing: Pol, Pract Res*, **2**(4), 3–11.

33. Pulsford D, Hope K, Thompson R (2007). Higher education provision for professionals working with people with dementia: a scoping exercise. *Nurs Edu Today*, **27**(1), 5–13.

Chapter 17

From psychological interventions to a psychology of dementia

Graham Stokes

Introduction

The contribution of psychology to dementia has a history that goes back more than 40 years. In the beginning psychological approaches were 'symptom-specific' and mechanistic (e.g. reality oriented) regarding people with dementia as a homogeneous group with uniform needs and failings. In part, negativity prevailed because definitions of success were bedevilled by unrealistic expectations and conceptual muddle, and this absence of realism often arose because the question that was rarely addressed was at which point does the devastation of cognition render therapeutic success improbable or impossible, and conversely when is there greater prospect of therapeutic benefit?

Nowadays, psychological interventions are embedded within and tailored to the needs of a person with dementia. A person living with a progressive cognitive disability is struggling to learn, recall, reason, and communicate, yet remains a person nevertheless. No longer does anyone seriously argue that the erosion of cognitive function leaves a person 'nonhuman', to be regarded as a physical entity devoid of self and feeling. Instead we embrace a person with a psychology that is dimmed by dementia but not destroyed; a person with a unique life history that exerts influence over how they live in a world that is rendered more complex, mysterious and, if history is our guide, increasingly unsupportive.

A psychology of dementia

The heterogeneity of dementia observed in people sharing the same pathology illustrates the complexity of the relationship between neuropathology and the clinical presentation. The biopsychosocial model needs to be adopted and practitioners must bring this understanding to the assessment of dementia [1–3]. Whereas Stokes and colleagues [4,5] argued that the origins of behaviour in dementia implicate a person's psychology, biology and life setting, and developed the concept of needs-led behaviours that carers may find challenging [2,6], Kitwood challenged the 'standard paradigm' by describing a dynamic interaction first between neurology and negative social relationships ('malignant social psychology'), before expanding the interplay of variables to encompass psychological, neurological, health, social, and environmental influences too [3]. The origins of aggressive resistance, continence difficulties, 'wandering', noisemaking, and a host of other acts of commission that carers find challenging, as well as the state of being 'pleasantly confused', are multi-factorial, implicating not only pathology, but also life setting and (critically) the psychology of the person. Unfortunately, the 'standard paradigm' failed to acknowledge the presence of a 'person with dementia' and consequently dementia for most of the Twentieth Century was denied a human face.

Kitwood [3] considered the greatest challenge in dementia care was for people with dementia to continue to be seen and treated as people, and thus if we are truly to support a person living with dementia then preserving their psychology becomes a fundamental principle of care. Acknowledging the presence of a person with dementia means we strive to support and improve their well-being and quality of life though evidence-based psychosocial interventions. Interventions that meet people's psychological needs, affirm personhood, promote emotional well-being and uphold social value constitute what is called person-centred care [7] (see Chapters 24 and 25 in this volume).

Contemporary psychological interventions

When evaluating intervention approaches any change has to be meaningful for and of value to the person with dementia and their supporting families and carers. The pursuit of a few points on a psychometric test is of no consequence if there is no demonstrable change in function, well-being, or life quality. As dementia progresses supportive interventions increasingly take place in the 'here and now'. There is no natural flow, no underpinning narrative to provide continuity. Just disconnected experiences that are barely, if ever remembered. Consequently, if joy is found, it does not matter that the experience which produced laughter is not remembered, for in no way can that diminish the happiness that was felt at the time. Conversely, if at any time the immediacy of life is unspeakably appalling then this is all life comprises. To all intents and purposes the person eventually drops out of the passage of time. All that remains is what approximates to the 'here and now'. This is the therapeutic ground we occupy.

However, the evidence-base for psychological interventions remains meagre, but 'lack of evidence of efficacy does not mean lack of efficacy' [8]. Despite some dissenting voices, randomized control trials (RCTs) are seen as the gold standard in evaluating any intervention approach, but the human material in dementia is too complex and impure to be accommodated within the scientific method. Caution is also required because RCTs provide information on what is effective for the average person with dementia [9]. In terms of clinical practice it is important not to reject interventions because they do not work for everyone. Again we return to the principles of person-centred care.

Behaviour that challenges

Behaviours that challenge carers have traditionally been understood in terms of symptoms of disease. Referred to as Behavioural and Psychological Symptoms of Dementia [10], these acts of commission, such as repetitive questioning, walking with risk and nuisance, aggression, agitation, confusion, and screaming are regarded as symptomatic of neurological disease [11]. The consequences of this neurological interpretation are care settings that strive to 'manage' people's behaviour, therapeutic nihilism, and symptom control through the use of antipsychotic medication [12,13].

In contrast, many investigators hold that behaviours that are seen as invasive and distressing have multiple aetiologies [14]. Stokes [2,6] argues that behaviours that challenge are often attempts to communicate unmet need, and in most instances viewing these behaviours as symptoms of pathology is evidence of diagnostic overshadowing. The pursuit of explanation is known as functional analysis. The methodology of behavioural (ABC) analysis [6] establishes the environmental context – 'the setting event' – of a behaviour (i.e. where, when, and what happened before, during, and immediately after the event), while functional analysis explores the possible reasons why the behaviour occurred. Functional analysis considers the contribution of neurobiological factors, life history, 'unobservable antecedent private events', which may include thoughts, beliefs, and the meaning of the behaviour [15] and the interrelationships with the recorded 'setting event'. The hypotheses about the function of a person's behaviour lead to case-specific interventions. This replaces the 'one syndrome – one treatment model', which (it is argued) has little clinical utility. Moniz-Cook and colleagues used functional analysis to understand the role of superstition in the development, maintenance, and management of aggression and agitation in five residents living in care homes [14]. By examining the meaning behaviour possesses and systematically influencing trigger situations, agitated and aggressive behaviour was reduced. Similarly, functional analysis has been used to explore the effects of person-centred individual-ized care plans formulated within the framework of emotional and interpersonal needs as determinants of challenging behaviour [16].

There is a growing evidence base in dementia care around the concept of needs-related behav-iours that challenge [1], and narrative-based evidence to illustrate that such behaviours are often driven by enduring psychological need [17]. A dementia care clinical guideline states that 'Health and social care staff should identify the specific needs of people with dementia . . . understanding behaviour that challenges as a communication of unmet need' [18].

Functional displacement

Functional displacement is an approach consistent with the understanding that challenging behaviours can be meaningful acts and, consequently, intervention may consist of providing the person with functionally equivalent but more socially appropriate ways of meeting their needs [16]. The provision of functional equivalents can be seen as a variant of the constructional approach to problem behaviour, which concentrates on building new patterns of behaviour [19]. However, for functional displacement to work the alternative action must be functionally equiva-lent to the challenging behaviour not just socially appropriate; the new behaviour cannot be more 'effortful' [20]; and in dementia care the functionally equivalent alternative must be either a feature of the interaction between caregivers and the person with dementia, or the functionally equivalent response must be the only behaviour available, or at the very least the most readily obvious and available [17]. The latter consideration explains why in dementia care the evidence-base for functional displacement is weak.

Simulated presence therapy

Simulated Presence Therapy (SPT) was first described by Woods and Ashley, who reported how twenty-seven people with dementia living in a care home were played a tape of their caregiver's voice using a personal stereo [21]. By simulating their presence it is proposed that the voice of a significant attachment figure serves to reduce the separation anxiety experienced by the person living with dementia [22], thereby alleviating distress-related aggression and agitation. A number of studies have shown that SPT can successfully alleviate 'problem behaviours' [21,23,24]. However, studies have shown that SPT does not work for everyone [25,26]. On balance, the evi-dence suggests that SPT may provide some people with a time-limited calming influence during episodes of distressing separation anxiety.

Engagement and activity therapy

Activity approaches in dementia care stem from findings that understimulation is the norm and knowledge that sensory deprivation experiments have shown that understimulation causes cogni-tive and perceptual disturbances [27]. To address the monotony of care, pioneering interventions focussed on the introduction of social and occupational activity to improve purposeful and appropriate behaviour [28]. Nowadays, a subjective indicator of good practice in care settings is the provision of recreational and social activities. These include physical exercise sessions that not only require gentle movement but task attention. Unsurprisingly, not only improvements in fitness have been reported, but improvements in cognitive function have also been recorded [29]. A Cochrane Review of reality orientation found, however, that in RCTs social groups appeared to be of no benefit for cognition [30]. Of late, the Talking Mats approach, a low-tech communication aid, has been introduced with promising results to support social engagement by helping people express themselves at all stages of dementia [31].

More recently passive and multi-sensory stimulation interventions have been used to improve the quality of life for people with severe dementia. Music, aromatherapy, massage and pet therapy have all been advocated, and the benefits of music have been shown [32,33]. Bearing in mind the value of working in the moment, in a comparison of three types of activity – music, puzzle exercises, and recreational activities, i.e. drawing and painting – it was found that music elicited the greatest degree of enjoyment, pleasure and engagement [34], although there is no evidence of lasting benefits for either music or multi-sensory stimulation [8].

Although the exact mechanism of action of aromatherapy remains unknown it is considered that the essential oils exert both psychological and physiological effects, with reviews reporting encouraging evidence [35]. However, responses seem to be individual. A recent review identified 11 prospective RCTs of aromatherapy in people with dementia [36]. The aromatherapy oils used, the methods of administration and outcome measures employed varied greatly, and the data supporting efficacy were meagre with both negative and positive effects being reported. The same review also draws attention to the potential toxicity of the oils and the need to be vigilant for side effects, concluding that the same standards should be applied to aromatherapy as to conventional medicines.

Multi-sensory rooms, known as Snoezelens, have subdued lighting and comprise relaxing music, visual stimulation from optic fibres, kaleidoscopes and lava lamps, tactile stimulation, and at times aromatherapy. Presenting as an overspill from the psychedelic youth culture of the 1960s there are reports that exposure is associated with mood improvement and a reduction in behavioural disturbance [37]. A study in nursing homes evaluated an 18-month programme of individualized exposure to Snoezelen integrated into a resident's 24-hour plan of care and showed an improvement in depression, a reduction in apathy, and less disturbed behaviour [38]. However, these interventions are affected by non-specific effects such as the presence of the carer who engages with the person in a way that is invariably intimate, patient, and encouraging. Is this interaction the essential therapeutic ingredient? What is commonly observed is that, when unaccompanied, a person with dementia finding they are alone in a Snoezelen invariably walks out! Consequently, activity needs to reflect personal preference and stimulation needs to be calming and not a source of over-arousal. A 'reduced stimulation unit' and its effects on people with Alzheimer's disease has also been described [39].

Cognitive stimulation therapy

Cognitive stimulation therapy (CST) is an intervention that has a strong evidence base [40]. The approach draws on the practice of the once-popular group reality orientation [41], an early attempt to engage people with dementia in psychological activity. CST has a similar social format but also includes non-cognitive and cognitive exercises, reminiscence and multi-sensory stimulation. In a controlled trial, cognitive stimulation therapy resulted in significant improvements on two measures of cognition, with associated improvements in quality of life for people with mild to moderate dementia [42]. It has been argued that the improvements in quality of life are mediated by the improvements in cognition and are not simply a result of improved social engagement [43]. There were, however, no changes in behaviour and function, although it has been suggested that behavioural outcome measures are often not sensitive enough to detect the functional impact of cognitive stimulation [44]. One conclusion is that if therapy gains are to be maintained then cognitive stimulation therapy needs to continue on a regular basis [42,45]. Studies have also suggested that CST is cost effective [47] and that it may enhance the effects of acetyl cholinesterase inhibitors [40]. Dementia care guidance recommends cognitive stimulation approaches for people with mild to moderate dementia [18]. However, expectations must be tailored to the findings that there is little evidence that CST positively affects day-to-day behaviour and performance [40].

Reality orientation

Reality orientation was in many ways the first psychological support to enter dementia care [47]. Growth in the use of reality orientation throughout the 1960s and 1970s led it to be considered the major therapeutic intervention employed in dementia care in the United States and in the United Kingdom between 1975 and the early 1980s until it began to fall into disrepute because it was not a 'miraculous cure', but was anti-therapeutic being preoccupied with 'hyper-cognitivism' [1], rather than attempting to understand the personal experience of dementia. Reports of its limitations and 'adverse effects' [48] led practitioners to question whether there was a place for reality orientation in contemporary dementia care [49].

The answer is that group reality orientation has evolved into cognitive stimulation therapy, which provides not only the opportunity for social exchange, but also exposure to a greater range of intellectual pursuits and emotionally-relevant activity than was observed in reality orientation sessions. The evidence-base for the benefits of reality orientation with people in the earlier stages of dementia laid the foundations for the recommendation that cognitive stimulation therapy be introduced into the care of people with mild to moderate dementia [50].

The social disability model of dementia argues that it is as much the social and built environments that disable people with impairments as the impairments themselves. Consequently, orienting people to their environment, both social and built, offers valued support and common sense dictates the need to use environmental cues, such as signage and directional information, as well as verbal orientation to help people find their way.

However, to maintain the motivation of carers and supporters, reasoned aspirations must prevail and, consequently, 24-hour reality orientation is acknowledged as a prosthetic therapy that cannot resolve the underlying inability to learn. However, in advanced dementia the prosthetic value of cues is questionable because the required associations are not acquired. For example, a blue arrow is a blue arrow, not an indication as to the way to the toilet. For this reason the results of reality orientation in counteracting the more disabling consequences of disorientation, have been generally disappointing [51]. Despite some evidence to the contrary, the weight of evidence is that behaviour does not improve. However, if addressing the challenge of disorientation in this way spares just one person the indignity of roaming around a care setting wet and soiled, then it remains a worthwhile intervention. One study found that orientation designs improved wayfinding and helped foster independence, but 'the most important aspect . . . [was] the enthusiastic and positive attitudes of all the staff' [52]. Contemporary 24-hour verbal orientation does not, however, have to be a dehumanizing prosthetic memory therapy solely concerned with behavioural functioning, it can be the means by which the fears of a person living with dementia can be acknowledged, the accuracy of their observations affirmed, and empathic emotional support offered [6].

If 24-hour reality orientation remains part of the supportive care offered to people struggling with disorientation, it has little or no role to play in the management of confusion. The focus of our attention, therefore, needs to be not on a person's factual errors, but on the feeling experience that flows from what constitutes their personal truth – a world of small children to be found, jobs to go to, a home to return to, and parents and partners to find – for empathy must take precedence over any approach or technique [49].

Validation

In contrast to reality orientation, validation therapy disputes the need to orientate and argues that we accept 'whatever reality they are in, in order to ease distress and restore self-worth' [53]. Happening in small groups or as an aspect of individual caring relationships, validation therapy does not concern itself with factual errors, but acknowledges that the emotion underlying a person's words and actions is true and real, and this is the material for therapeutic intervention. 'Validation works so much on the feeling level' [54]. It is at this point that we need to distinguish validation therapy from validation.

Validation therapy has been described as theoretically incoherent and unconvincing, offering little to our understanding of dementia [4] while the evidence in support of effectiveness is anecdotal [51]. A Cochrane review identified only three studies of group validation therapy that warranted inclusion in the review and the results from these studies were inconclusive [55].

Validation is the acceptance of the reality and 'personal truth' of another's experience [56]. Feil's methods of engagement enabled practitioners to appreciate the benefits of validation when caring for people living with confusion [57]. Feil combined a respect for the subjectivity of the confused person with a concern for their emotional welfare by maintaining that whatever the facts are, their emotions possess their own validity. Stokes [6] describes validation in practice.

Reminiscence therapy

The use of reminiscence with people with mild to moderate dementia is of potential benefit because it taps into a well of distant memory that may resonate with feeling. Moreover, faced with the destruction of recent memories the past may be all that remains. In groups, reminiscence also offers the opportunity for social engagement, while completing individual life story books enables professional carers to learn about those they care for. Reminiscence aids such as music, photographs, archive recordings, household paraphernalia, and foods are used to evoke memories, while memory boxes are to be found in care homes adjacent to residents' bedrooms as an aid to personalized orientation, and a stimulus to personally relevant conversation. Woods and Clare [40] describe the use of life story work in the development of meaningful and rewarding individualized care plans, which include activities that relate to the person's interests and experiences, and the creation of an environment individualized according to the person's own preferences [58].

A comparison of the sequential use of reality orientation and reminiscence therapy, demonstrated improved orientation and communication, with some evidence of long-term effects [59]. Conceivably the most significant finding was that staff reported they got to know the group participants better. Others have shown higher levels of well-being during reminiscence [60]. However, there has been little outcome research and the role of reminiscence work is doubtful [40]. It seems best regarded as a diversionary activity [61]. Without doubt, while the practice of reminiscence is to be found in most care settings, as is the use of 'nostalgia' interior designs, research is needed regarding the outcomes of the different types of reminiscence activity.

Psychological therapy

Recently we have seen the use of psychological therapies with people who are at the beginning of dementia with encouraging results. The National Dementia Strategy [62] for England emphasizes the need for early diagnostic investigations, and as more and more people receive a diagnosis within months of noticing first symptoms they will not only have insight into their cognitive failings, but they will also appreciate the implications of a diagnosis of dementia. As such there is a need for pre- and post-diagnostic counselling to help with feelings of insecurity, hopelessness and loss of efficacy and control. Groups for people at the early stages of dementia can focus on such questions as: 'what's it like when your memory is not as good as it used to be?' [63]. Group interventions, sometimes involving family supporters, sometimes addressing issues of advocacy and practical support, have reported reduced isolation and improved well-being, while attendance has been positively evaluated by participants [64,65]. Such psychological support may help to address the high levels of depression and anxiety observed in dementia. While there is no convincing evidence that cognitive-behavioural therapy for people with dementia is effective, it may be beneficial for people with mild dementia [66,67], although the presence of cognitive impairment requires therapists to modify the intervention [40]. There is evidence that relaxation therapy can improve sleep and reduce anxiety. Results suggest that progressive muscle relaxation is the favoured intervention method as this relies more on procedural memory which is less impaired in dementia, compared to relaxation techniques that use imagery which are more reliant on cognitive functioning [68].

Behaviour and cognitive rehabilitation

Viewing dementia as an intellectual disability yields the prospect that supportive care may incorporate rehabilitation. Traditionally there is a low expectation of any recovery of skills when working with people with dementia. However, personal recovery can be about restoring the person in the eyes of others, maximizing potential, and living a satisfying, contributing life within the limitations caused by disability.

A recovery-based approach for people with dementia focuses on the strengths that remain, defines dependency in terms of needs to be met (e.g. 'Mrs Walcott keeps wetting herself' is redefined as 'Mrs Walcott needs to toilet appropriately'; or 'Mr Wilshire loses everything' is expressed as 'Mr Wilshire needs to remember where he puts things'), understands why the need cannot be met, and implements assisted learning programmes to achieve needs-led goals [6]. Thus, we progress from lifeless statements of fact to working statements of intent.

In the area of skills training the timing of the intervention and the need for realistic expectations are most pertinent, for it is in mild to moderate dementia that skills are more likely to be re-learned, while the gains achieved by supporting independence will inevitably dissipate over time as a person's dementia becomes progressively severe. Consequently the aims of rehabilitation must change over time [69].

Behavioural training and memory aids can improve activities of daily living and self-care [70]. However, there is little evidence of improvement in toileting skills. Despite the availability of supportive interventions to help people regain or maintain continence [6,71], and occasional success using cued recall of behaviour [72] success has been limited [73]. Perhaps this can be attributed to the complexity of toileting behaviour [40,51], which relies upon cognitive and physical competence, environmental design, as well as staff attitudes: changing a soiled pad may be easier than devoting effort to preserving continence. Systemic interventions may be required [51].

Cognitive retraining involves people with dementia practising specific tasks to improve functions such as memory, attention, or problem-solving. However, there is a risk of exacerbating frustration and depression [74]. Hence, cognitive training is not supported by the evidence [40].

A positive development is cognitive rehabilitation, which helps people living with dementia to improve cognitive functioning in order to improve their well-being, occupational function, and social engagement, and is not designed merely to bring about marginal improvements on cognitive testing. Most rehabilitation work has been with people in the early stages of dementia. Cognitive strengths and weaknesses are assessed, preserved strengths supported, and limited demands placed on areas of deficit as efforts are made to help people with difficulties that are pertinent to their real lives [75]. Woods and Clare define interventions as restoration, compensation, or external environmental modification, all of which are individually-tailored to meet the specific needs of people with dementia and their carers [40].

Conclusion

Within the contemporary culture of person-centred care there is interest and enthusiasm for the use of psychological interventions to support and restore levels of functioning and well-being. However, caution is required. There must be realism as to what can be achieved, especially when dementia is characterized by severe cognitive impairment and frailty. The temptation to believe that, simply because interventions resonate with the term 'person-centred' and are 'non-pharmacological', they must automatically be ascribed value and that success is all but inevitable, must be resisted.

At present there is face-validity to support what is delivered under the guise of psychological interventions but little empirical evidence. We cannot afford to replace one set of interventions with a poor risk-benefit ratio for another that is equally unevaluated. However, effectiveness will not be determined by RCTs, but through an evaluation of individual-centred, supportive interventions that are predicated upon an assessment of each person's psychology, strengths, and needs, as well as an appreciation of whether the culture of care is able to deliver rehabilitative change. Then we will know what works for whom, in what settings, and for how long, until a regard for the person says now is the time to desist and revise what is being done in pursuit of recovery. To do otherwise would mean person-centred supportive care becomes simply another feature of institutional practice, albeit dressed in more contemporary clothing.

References

1. Downs M, Clare L, Anderson E (2008). Dementia as a biopsychosocial condition: implications for practice and research, in Woods R, Clare L (eds) *Handbook of the clinical psychology of ageing*, 2nd edn, pp. 145–159. Chichester: John Wiley.

2. Stokes G (1996). Challenging behaviour in dementia: a psychological approach, in Woods R (ed) *Handbook of the clinical psychology of ageing*, pp. 601–628. Chichester: John Wiley.

3. Baldwin C, Capstick A (eds.)(2007). *Tom Kitwood on dementia: a reader and critical commentary*. Maidenhead: Open University Press.

4. Goudie F, Stokes, G (1989). Dealing with confusion. *Nurs Times*, 20 September, 20.

5. Stokes G, Allen B (1990). Seeking an explanation, in Stokes G, Goudie F. (eds) *Working with dementia*, pp. 59–65. Bicester: Winslow Press.

6. Stokes G (2000). *Challenging behaviour in dementia: a person-centred approach*. Bicester: Winslow Press.

7. Brooker D (2007). Person-centred dementia care: making services better. London: Jessica Kingsley.

8. Livingston G, Johnston K, Paton J, Lyketsos C (2005). Systematic review of psychological approaches to the management of neuropsychiatric symptoms of dementia. *Am J Psychiatry*, **162**, 1996–2021.

9. Woods R (2003). Evidence-based practice in psychosocial intervention in early dementia: how can it be achieved? *Aging Ment Health*, **7**, 5–6.

10. Finkel S (2003). Behavioural and psychological symptoms of dementia. *Clinical Geriatr Med*, **19**, 799–824.

11. Cummings JL (2003). Toward a molecular neuropsychiatry of neurodegenerative diseases. *Ann Neurol*, **54**, 147–154.

12. Ballard C, O'Brien J (1999). Treating behavioural and psychological signs in Alzheimer's disease: the evidence for current pharmacological treatment is not strong. *BMJ*, **319**, 138–139.

13. Ballard C, Margallo-Lana, ML (2001). The relationship between anti-psychotic treatment and quality of life for patients with dementia living in residential and nursing home care facilities. *J Clin Psychiatry*, **65**(11), 23–28.

14. Moniz-Cook E, Wood R, Richards K (2001). Functional analysis of challenging behaviour in dementia: the role of superstition. *Int J Geriatr Psychiatry*, **16**, 45–56.

15. Samson DM, McDonnell AA (1990). Functional analysis and challenging behaviours. *Behav Psychother*, **18**, 259–272.

16. Moniz-Cook E, Stokes G, Agar S (2003). Difficult behaviour and dementia in nursing homes: five cases of psychosocial intervention. *Clin Psychol Psychother*, **10**, 197–208.

17. Stokes G. (2008). *And still the music plays: stories of people with dementia*. London: Hawker Publications.

18. National Institute for Health and Clinical Excellence and Social Care Institute for Excellence (2006). *Dementia: supporting people with dementia and their carers in health and social care, clinical guideline 42*, paragraph 1.1.9.2. London: National Institute for Health and Clinical Excellence.

19. Goldiamond I (1974). Toward a constructional approach to social problems: ethical and constitutional issues raised by applied behaviour analysis. *Behaviourism*, **2**, 1–84.

20. Carr EG (1988). Giving away the behavioural approach. *Behav Psychother*, **16**, 78–84.

21. Woods P, Ashley J (1995). Simulated presence therapy: using selected memories to manage problem behaviours in Alzheimer's disease patients. *Geriatr Nurs*, **16**(1), 9–14.

22. Miesen BML (1993). Alzheimer's disease the phenomenon of parent fixation and Bowlby's attachment theory. *Int J Geriatr Psychiatry*, **8**, 147–153.

23. Camberg L, Woods P, Ooi W *et al.* (1999). Evaluation of simulated presence: a personalised approach to enhance well-being in persons with Alzheimer's disease. *J Am Geriatr Soc*, **47**(4), 446–452.

24. Garland K, Beer E, Eppingstall B, O'Connor DW (2007). A comparison of two treatments of agitated behaviour in nursing home residents with behaviour: simulated family presence and preferred music. *Am J Geriatr Psychiatry*, **15**, 514–521.

25. Peak JS, Cheston RIL (2002). Using simulated presence therapy with people with dementia. *Aging Ment Health*, **6**(1), 77–81.

26. Cheston RIL, Thorne K, Whitby P, Peak JS (2007). Simulated presence therapy, attachment and separation amongst people with dementia. *Dementia*, **6**(3), 442–449.

27. Holden UP, Woods R (1995). *Positive approaches to dementia care,*. 3rd ed. Edinburgh: Churchill Livingstone.

28. Cosin LZ, Mort M, Post F, Westropp C, Williams, M (1958). Experimental treatment of persistent senile confusion. *Int J Soc Psychiatry*, **4**, 24–42.

29. Hopman-Rock M, Staats PGM, Tak ECPM, Droes RM (1999). The effects of a psychomotor activation programme for use in groups of cognitively impaired people in homes for the elderly. *Int J Geriatr Psychiatry*, **14**, 633–642.

30. Spector A, Orrell M, Davies S, Woods, R (1998). Reality orientation for dementia: a review of the evidence for its effectiveness. *Cochrane Library*, **4**, Oxford Update Software.

31. Cox S, Murphy J, Gray C M. (2008). Communication and dementia: how effective is the talking mats approach? *J Dementia Care*, May/June, 35–38.

32. Norberg A, Melin E, Asplund K (1986). Reactions to music, touch and object presentation in the final stage of dementia: an exploratory study. *Int J Nurs Stud*, **23**, 315–323.

33. Goddaer J, Abraham IL (1994). Effects of relaxing music on agitation during meals among nursing home residents with severe cognitive impairment. *Arch Psychiatr Nurs*, **8**(3), 150–158.

34. Lord TR, Garner JE (1993). Effects of music on Alzheimer's patients. *Percept Mot Skills*, **76**, 451–445.

35. Burns A, Byrne J, Ballard C, Holmes C (2002). Sensory stimulation in dementia. *BMJ*, **325**, 1312–1313.

36. Nguyen Q, Paton C (2008). The use of aromatherapy to treat behavioural problems in dementia. *Int J Geriatr Psychiatry*, **23**, 337–346.

37. Baker R, Dowling Z, Wareing LA, Dawson J, Assey J (1997). Snoezelen: its long-term and short-term effects on older people with dementia. *Br J Occup Ther*, **60**(5), 213–218.

38. Van Weert JCM, Van Dulmen AM, Spreeuwenberg PMM, Ribbe MW, Bensing JM (2005). Behavioural and mood effects of Snoezelen integrated into 24-hour dementia care. *J Am Geriatr Society*, **53**, 24–33.

39. Cleary TA, Clamon C, Price M, Shullaw G (1988). A reduced stimulation unit: effects on patients with Alzheimer's disease and related disorders. *Gerontologist*, **28**, 511.

40. Woods R, Clare L (2008). Psychological interventions with people with dementia, in Woods R, Clare L (eds) *Handbook of the clinical psychology of ageing*, 2nd edn, pp. 523–548. Chichester: John Wiley.

41. Taulbee LR, Folsom JC (1966). Reality orientation for geriatric patients. *Hosp Community Psychiatry*, **17**, 133–135.

42. Spector A, Thorgrimsen L, Woods R *et al.* (2003). Effectiveness of an evidence-based cognitive stimulation therapy programme for people with dementia: randomised controlled trial. *Br J Psychiatry*, **183**, 248–254.

43. Woods R, Thorgrimsen L, Spector A, Royan, L, Orrell, M (2006). Improved quality of life and cognitive stimulation therapy in dementia. *Aging Ment Health*, **10**, 219–226.

44. Zanetti O, Frisoni GB, deLeo D, Dello Buono M, Bianchetti A, Trabucchi M (1995). Reality orientation therapy in Alzheimer's disease: useful or not? A controlled study. *Alz Dis Assoc Dis*, **9**, 132–138.

45. Orrell M, Spector A, Thorgrimsen L, Woods RA (2005). A pilot study examining the effectiveness of maintenance cognitive stimulation therapy (CST) following CST for people with dementia. *Int J Geriatr Psychiatry*, **20**, 446–451.

46. Knapp M , Thorgrimsen L, Patel A, Spector A, Hallam A, Woods R *et al.* (2006). Cognitive stimulation therapy for people with dementia: cost-effectiveness analysis. *Br J Psychiatry*, **188**, 574–580.

47. Folsom JC (1968). Reality orientation therapy for the elderly mental patient. *J Geriatr Psychiatry*, **1**, 291–207.

48. Dietch JT, Hewett LJ, Jones S. (1989). Adverse effects of reality orientation. *J Am Geriatr Soc*, **37**, 74–76.

49. Woods R (1994). Reality orientation. *J Dementia Care*, **2**(2), 24–25.

50. Spector A, Orell M, Davies S, Woods R (2001). Can reality orientation be rehabilitated? Development and piloting of an evidence-based programme of cognition-based therapies for people with dementia. *Neuropsychol Rehabil*, **11**(3/4), 377–397.

51. Bleathman C, Morton I (1994). Psychological treatments, in . Burns A, Levy R (eds) *Dementia*, pp. 553–564. London: Chapman & Hall Medical.

52. Bignall A (1996). Look and learn: designs on the care environment. *J Dementia Care*, **4**, 12–13.

53. Morton I, Bleathman C (1991). The effectiveness of validation therapy in dementia – a pilot study. *Int J Geriatr Psychiatry*, **6**, 327–330.

54. de Klerk Rubin V. (1994). Misunderstandings about validation. *J Dementia Care*, **2**(2), 14–16.

55. Neal M, Barton-Wright P (2007). Validation therapy for dementia (Cochrane review). *The Cochrane Library*, 2. Chichester: John Wiley.

56. Kitwood T (1996). A dialectical framework for dementia, in Woods R (ed) *Handbook of the clinical psychology of ageing*, pp. 267–282. Chichester: John Wiley.

57. Feil N (1993). *The Validation Breakthrough: Simple Techniques for Communicating with People with 'Alzheimer's Type Dementia'*. Baltimore: Health Professions Press.

58. Gibson F (1994). What can reminiscence contribute to people with dementia? in Bornat J (ed) *Reminiscence review: evaluations, achievements, perspectives*, pp. 46–60. Buckingham: Open University Press.

59. Baines S, Saxby P, Ehlert K (1987). Reality orientation and reminiscence therapy: a controlled cross over study of elderly confused people. *Br J Psychiatry*, **151,** 222–231.

60. Brooker D, Duce L (2000). Wellbeing and activity in dementia: a comparison of group reminiscence therapy, structured goal-directed activity and unstructured time. *Aging Ment Health*, **4**(4), 287–296.

61. Thornton S, Brotchie J (1987). Reminiscence: a critical review of the empirical literature. *Br J Clin Psychol*, **26**, 93–111.

62. Department of Health (2009). *Living well with dementia: a national dementia strategy*. London: HMSO.

63. Cheston R, Jones K, Gilliard J (2003). Group psychotherapy and people with dementia. *Aging Ment Health*, **7**, 452–461.

64. Zarit SH, Femia EE, Watson J, Rice-Oeschger L, Kakos B (2004). Memory club: a group intervention for people with early-stage dementia and their care-partners. *Gerontologist*, **44**, 262–269.

65. Pratt R, Clare L, Aggarwal N (2005). The 'talking about memory coffee group': a new model of support for people with early-stage dementia and their families. *Dementia*, **4**, 143–148.

66. Kipling T, Bailey M, Charlesworth G (1999). The feasibility of a cognitive behavioural therapy group for men with mild/moderate cognitive impairment. *Behav Cogn Psychoth*, **27,** 189–193.

67. Scholey KA, Woods R (2003). A series of brief cognitive therapy interventions with people experiencing both dementia and depression: a description of techniques and common themes. *Clin Psychol Psychother*, **10**, 175–185.

68. Suhr J, Anderson S, Tranel D (1999). Progressive muscle relaxation in the management of behavioural disturbance in Alzheimer's disease. *Neuropsychol Rehabil*, **9**, 31–44.

69. Clare L (2003). Rehabilitation for people with dementia, in Wilson BA (ed) *Neuropsychological rehabilitation: theory and practice*, pp. 197–215. London: Swets & Zeitlinger.

70. Josephsson S, Bäckman L, Borell L, Bernspång, B, Nygård, L, Rönnberg L (1993). Supporting everyday activities in dementia: an intervention study. *Int J Geriatr Psychiatry*, **8**, 395–400.

71. Colling J, Ouslander J, Hadley BJ, Eish J, Campbell E (1992). The effects of patterned urge-response toileting (PURT) on urinary incontinence among nursing home residents. *J Am Geriatr Soc*, **40**(2), 135–141.

72. Bird M, Alexopoulos P, Adamowicz J (1995). Success and failute in five case studies; use of cued recall to ameliorate behaviour problems in senile dementia. *Int J Geriatr Psychiatry*, **10**, 305–311.

73. Stokes G (2002). Psychological approaches to bowel care in older people with dementia, in Potter R, Norton C, Cottenden A (eds) *Bowel care in older people: research and practice*, pp. 97–109. London: Royal College of Physicians.

74. Zarit SH, Zarit JM, Reever KE (1982). Memory training for severe memory loss: effects on senile dementia patients and their families. *Gerontologist*, **22**(4), 373–377.

75. Bourgeois MS. (1990). Enhancing conversation skills in patients with Alzheimer's disease using a prosthetic memory aid. *J Appl Behav Anal*, **23, ** 29–42.

Chapter 18

Supportive care: social care and social work approaches

Jill Manthorpe

Introduction

In England, the Department of Health White Paper, *Our Health, Our Care, Our Say* [1] declared that personalized services would be the way forward for social care. Indeed, policy in England speaks of the need to transform adult social care [2]. Everyone who receives health and social care support, whether from statutory services or through funding support for themselves, will in theory have choice and control over how that support is delivered. The goal is that they will be confident that services are of high quality, are safe, and promote individuals' independence, well-being, and dignity. Central to these aspirations are people with dementia. The *National Dementia Strategy* [3] reflects this same approach, being produced as part of the *Putting People First* policy [2], which is the cross-departmental commitment to this move to personalizing social care. If supportive care is to be at the heart of mainstream social care for people with dementia in England, then its proponents will need to understand this ethos of personalization and to decide whether its value base fits with an orientation to supportive care. Dementia care practitioners have an important role in shaping personalization and responding to its ambiguities [4].

This chapter explores these relationships, and, in doing so, takes a critical look at ideas of 'supportive care'. Social work and social care have long experience of terminology being used rather indiscriminately and as cloaks to cover substantial changes. Previous policy documents and discussions have used the term 'community' to mean a number of things for example. Likewise, 'care' too is a term that conveys political and gendered undercurrents and values [5]. Thus the current fashion for the replacement of 'care' by 'support' may signal shifts in values, responsibilities, and roles of great depth or superficiality.

A brief note on practice terminology may be helpful. This chapter uses the term social work when referring to the activities of social workers in England and Wales, where they have responsibilities under community care and mental health legislation to assess, arrange, and monitor support for adults in need, through local government structures in the main. Social workers may also work in multi-disciplinary teams, such as memory assessment services in the National Health Service (NHS) (specialist or secondary care), or in Community Mental Health Teams, jointly run by the NHS and local government (primary care level). There is always a contingency about what social work is and what it should be [6], illustrated in recent overviews of practice with people with dementia presented by Marshall and Tibbs in the United Kingdom (UK) [7] and Cox in the United States (US) [8]. The term social care is used to refer to a broader set of activities, largely undertaken in the non-statutory sector in the UK that includes residential care and home care provided by the commercial and voluntary sectors [9]. Dementia affects many older people using social care services as well as being a factor that brings older people into social care for the first time.

Personalization is an umbrella term employed across government to promote the development of public services to respond better to individual needs and requirements. In social care, it is being used to convey many laudable aims, among which are enabling people to have greater choice, control, and independence in their lives. There are many threads to personalization, but this chapter focuses on personal budgets to illustrate how care and support are changing in practice and to ask if these shifts fulfil the criteria of 'supportive care' for people with dementia.

Support and care

Person-centred planning, person-centred care, and the notion of support and support working, all underpin the construction of social care for people with dementia and for older people more generally. Standard 2 of the *National Service Framework for Older People* [10], for example, covers 'person-centred care', translating this term from dementia-related services to a near universal 'mission statement'[11]. The repeated emphasis on the need to make services more personal, or tailored, and practice more person-centred or personalized, is an explicit critique of social provision for people with dementia, as with other parts of social care. The Department of Health has asserted 'people who use social care services say the service is only as good as the person delivering it. They value people who have a combination of the right human qualities as well as the necessary knowledge and skills'[12]. As many accounts from people with dementia and carers together with a range of practitioners and commentators acknowledge, much is lacking in current social care arrangements and delivery [13].

The process of person-centred planning has been influential for over 20 years in social care services for people with learning disabilities in particular [14]. In this area of work, which has many similarities with dementia care, the development of an ethos of person-centred planning and care demanded that services become clearer about their purpose and effectiveness; and that they meet the needs of the people they serve, rather than other mere goals of containment and economy. The positive outcomes of working in such a way have influenced social care services delivered by the public sector for wider groups of people [15], for example, although a careful look suggests that the word 'support' is not so often used as terms such as 'independence' and 'rights'.

In social care support for people with dementia, the influence of person-centred planning can be detected in:

1 Greater attention to communication and biographical detail in assessment to ensure that support plans relate to individuals' needs, choices, and wishes

2 Specific focus on the resources and contributions of social networks; notably family and friends, but also community based facilities and peer support

3 Individualized social care support, with particular attention to activity, stimulation, enjoyment, and safety from harm

4 Efforts to ensure that if plans are made they are reviewed and adapted.

However, unlike other service sectors, publicly funded social care services in England are means-tested and work within very high eligibility criteria [16]. While trying to be supportive, social workers have to establish a person's eligibility for publicly funded social care and if the person does not meet local criteria of need or risk then the role of the social worker may be to put the person in touch with other support services in the health, voluntary, or community sectors. As social workers often comment, it is hard to work under the constraints of high eligibility criteria, and although many may be able to offer advice, their own skills and expertise can be under-utilized [17].

Levels of eligibility (commonly, in ascending order, moderate, severe and critical)[16] are connected to a policy entitled Fair Access to Care Services (FACS). This requires social service departments to standardize eligibility criteria for access to adult social care services by assessing people in terms of need and risk [18]. In essence, FACS provides local authorities with guidance about the ways they should review, revise, and use their eligibility criteria for access to adult care services in order to achieve greater equity in their provision of social care services to local people. While a person may have needs for support in many circumstances, if these do not reach the level decided upon by the local authority, then signposting to other agencies is what is likely to happen. For many people, a need for early support, perhaps at a time of diagnosis or when a person is finding it difficult to do housework or to shop, is therefore not likely to be met by local government social services directly, although the local authority may be funding a voluntary group or a housing-related service to provide such support.

The need for practitioners and people with dementia and those supporting them to know more about what support arrangements work best and for whom, and why, is important. The local context is also important because:

1 There is some discretion for local authorities about service levels, patterns, and types and how they keep within budgetary constraints [19]

2 Changes are occurring in the organization of services, including the merging or integration of social and health care services where eligibility systems and charging rules may need to be aligned [1]

3 The tradition of social work assessments of older people walks a fine line between advocacy and resource gate-keeping,[20] and between clinical and intensive care management models [21].

Support is thus localized in the UK, meaning that dementia care practitioners need to have a 'map' of services, support, and information points. Specialist team members often 'embody' this map and their functions in localities can be to acquire and provide sophisticated understandings of access, approaches, and capacity among local support organizations and personnel.

Providing social care support

Having noted the high eligibility levels in publicly funded social care, many people with dementia do have high levels of need and so meet these criteria. Evidence is that larger sums of social care resources are spent supporting people with very high levels of need, providing, in many cases, unprecedented levels of support, which enable people to stay living at home if this is what they want [16].

Individualized care and support are possible, but several factors conspire to undermine the supportive role of social work assessment. The first is that assessment becomes a matter of routine in social work; with pressures on social workers to meet targets of efficiency and throughput of cases. The second danger is that a number of professionals become involved and do not communicate, leading to duplication and confusion all round. The third is that matters of finance can become overwhelming; with social workers having to complete financial assessments early on and thus giving the impression that this area is their main interest. Lastly, is the question of the funding for social care services. As explained, eligibility or thresholds are high and this may lead to a siege mentality in some cases. The lack of social care funding means that social workers can be wary of raising expectations.

The care and support gap

As several of the chapters in this volume have commented, the phrase 'person-centred care' is used fairly often to summarize what is currently thought of as good and increasingly evidence-based practice [22]. The clinical outcomes of person-centred care, as established by interventions and outcome studies are emerging only now. What works and how much it costs (cost-effectiveness evidence) are largely unknown. Few tools measure person-centred care or its outcomes and clinically valid, reliable, or useful measures are not often relevant to social care settings, interventions, or proxy respondents. Far greater understanding of person-centred care is available from studies and practice development in settings such as care homes (e.g. the Alzheimer's Society's [23] set of person-centred standards for care homes) than elsewhere. For others working in social care settings, the influence of relationship-based care may currently be more prominent [24].

The word 'support' similarly reflects desires to be effective. However, social work and social care debates have sometimes adopted a more critical perspective, noting that the language of 'support' can be used as a way of substituting professional activity for work by non-professionals and by informal carers (usually families) and thus can be a form of cost containment or even reductions in services. Calls for 'support' for carers may be a way of transferring responsibility to them and enrolling them in the 'production' of care. Carers have drawn attention to the way in which they have felt put under pressure to care, and to the withdrawal of practical help for them[25]. Over a decade ago, researchers such as Twigg and Atkin pointed to the determined enlistment of family carers as 'care workers', being involved in the co-production of care with professionals [26]. Support for carers may be a matter of providing them with skills and confidence to take on care tasks, as substitutes for professionals, such as community nurses and home care assistants. Many carers have referred to the way in which support for them seems to be a matter of 'propping them up' to continue caring, and to the toll that this places on their own health and well-being [27]. Hospital discharge is one example of this – a time when carers often feel unsupported, when a great deal of work falls on them. For people with dementia there is the frequent complaint that more intensive community services, such as intermediate care, have largely been denied to people with dementia on their discharge from a hospital stay and the work of support falls on carers [3].

The reduction in publicly funded social care support for people with what are termed 'low level' needs occurred over the past two decades in order to provide greater support for people with more intense and immediate needs, as observed above [16]. This move has been hugely beneficial for many people, enabling care in the community to be realized, but, for those excluded from publicly funded social care, provision has been more threadbare. The 'care gap' has been a phrase coined to illustrate the predicament of not being eligible for support, but still having needs and feeling that things have to get worse before some assistance will be offered [28]. Social or community support may help fill these gaps, as do social security (financial) payments provided to meet additional costs of living for people with disabilities. Another feature of exclusion is the operation of the means test for social care which can mean that people with dementia and their support networks who have capital (savings) or higher than basic income are left on their own as 'consumers' of care, with very little advice and guidance about what to do for the best. The Commission for Social Care Inspection [16] made a very powerful critique of this; so elements of personalization policy are to ensure that advice, advocacy, and information are available to all [2].

These problems help explain the growing use of Direct Payments as a way of tailoring support to the individual. A Direct Payment is a payment in lieu of social care services given to people so they can arrange their own care and support in place of arrangements by local government social services departments. Over 50,000 people in England received Direct Payments in 2007. It is a mechanism to enable individuals to exercise greater choice and control over the social care services they receive and in the UK has been taken up by many younger people with disabilities. Direct Payments have been seen as a way to improve social care services [29], but they have not been an unqualified success in the support of people with dementia: first because they originally excluded older people; and secondly because people had to be able to consent to their receipt and be prepared to manage the 'business' of support.

Riddell and her colleagues [30] observed that the potential benefits of Direct Payments had been 'unequally distributed' among different groups of people with disabilities and suggested that these inequalities would deepen even further the more widely they are used.

Despite this frequent exclusion of people with dementia and their carers from Direct Payments, there is much to learn from them, since these have resulted in person-centred and personally controlled social care support. The experiences of many people who have accessed social care support in this way are that they often provide choice, flexibility, and support that meets people's own needs, choices and wishes. Carers, too, often find that they lead to positive outcomes [31].

The essence of a personalized approach to social care is not simply confined to Personal Budgets (Direct Payments are one form of this, and refer to direct passing of financial control to individuals, while other options are available, such as asking a brokerage service to deal with administration for a fee). But these do provide people using publicly funded social care services with a clear understanding of the finance and potential supports that are available to them. Each local authority is developing a Resource Allocation System or similar to establish the financial basis of linking needs and social care outcomes within the authority's social care budget. While means-testing still applies, individuals are being told the sum available to them.

Lessons from Direct Payments have influenced the development of social care support for people with dementia. The importance of getting support planning right, the need for accessible information and its clarity, and the value of informing frontline practitioners in other agencies (nursing, therapists, and medicine) about the potential to meet positive outcomes for people with dementia and their carers [32] are changing the culture of social care.

However, there are some matters that older people and their carers (who are a very heterogeneous group) may find concerning, which may affect their well-being and confidence in these new methods of social care delivery and support. Information and advice services need to be commissioned so that people can understand what is available and how they will be treated in this more consumer-type system. Older people's representatives have welcomed the development of personalized support [33] but have pointed to the limited (although growing) take up of Direct Payments by older people. The risks of social exclusion from good quality advice and information for some older people are high, often compounded by long-standing inequalities [34].

One factor that is often overlooked is that there are often limited or modest expectations among older people [35] and people with dementia. Likewise, some practitioners may assume that older people wish to have a restricted lifestyle [32], and this ethos will need to be challenged, perhaps by more finely tuned assessment conversations. These may provide greater information about older people's wishes and priorities, or the 'outcomes' they wish. A recent series of discussion groups with older people in Essex [36] found that when asked what they might want in their hypothetical personal support plan, older people expressed widely different priorities and preferences. They were insistent that information and good communication were essential. This consultation concluded that older people would only gain from personal budgets if they had suitable help and advice to enable them to benefit from flexibility and control. Otherwise flexibility and control could be burdensome, and some groups of older people would be disadvantaged:

> There is a real fear that the introduction of the personal budgets will be used to decrease overall expenditure and cut costs. In particular, the most vulnerable were seen to be at risk of asking for less, receiving less help and being reluctant to spend funds on reducing risks they may not be aware of. In particular, those with mental health needs or learning disabilities will need expert and specialist help. [36; p. 8]

The National Dementia Strategy is considering the role of dementia advisers in primary care for people with dementia and these advisers may alert them to the expanding options of support and care[3].

Older people with cognitive impairment, such as a dementia, may be less able to make decisions than other people and this may give rise to particular concerns about consent and possible harm or neglect. The *Health and Social Care Act* extends the availability of Direct Payments to people who lack capacity, under the *Mental Capacity Act 2005* (MCA). A person, normally a court appointed person or family member, will be able to manage the Direct Payment on their behalf. Local authorities will retain their duties of care in these and other circumstances. This is likely to impact upon older people with dementia, in particular, enhancing their ability to benefit from more tailored or personalized support but with the safeguards that have been set in place through the MCA. The MCA emphasizes that the *Code of Practice* under the Act applies to non-professionals as well as professionals, and everyone acting on behalf of people without capacity to make decisions about care and treatment (broadly defined) must abide by the *Code*. Personalized support is thus not simply a responsibility for practitioners but should be informing the activities of carers and other supporters. Whilst many carers may be adept at providing supportive care, others may be highly influenced by custodial models of care or have views about dementia that reflect myths and stereotypes.

Not everyone with a dementia is an older person and people of working age who have a dementia may need to be included in efforts to personalize their support. There have been many justified complaints over the years that people of working age who have dementia find services particularly inappropriate for their needs and that this causes excessive distress at difficult times (see Chapter 6) [37]. There are some indications that 'younger' people with dementia may be able to benefit from personal budgets and similar initiatives to counter the problems they face in accessing support that might help maintain activities of ordinary living, such as sport or exercise. An account by a carer of the way in which a person (in her 50s) has been supported at home by flexible social care funding (an Individual Budget (IB), a forerunner of personal budgets) that enabled her to employ a live-in care worker illustrates this well:

> She had always loved her independence and this way (using IB) she was able to maintain some of it. [38]

People with dementia may have needs that fluctuate, including those arising from varying or declining abilities to make decisions, and they may be accustomed to social care support that has emphasized meeting personal care needs rather than activities of ordinary living, such as social, cultural, educational, and other goals [39]. Managing the financial aspects of person-centred support often falls to individuals and their carers, but recent studies have revealed how little real support over financial management is available to people with dementia and their carers [40]. Supportive care may therefore cover a very wide definition of support and the question therefore remains whether this term is almost too elastic, and is in danger of meaning all things to all people.

Supporting social care supporters

This brief section turns to the vexed issue of how to promote supportive care. This is not a medication or something that can be pulled off a supermarket shelf, for it rests largely on encounters between people and touches on elements of relationship-based care. Much will depend on the personal interactions of the individuals concerned. It is easy to say that social care staff must be more supportive. There is increasing evidence that they themselves do not receive sufficient back-up from professionals, including those working in specialist services for people with dementia. Even in residential care services, an Alzheimer's Society survey found [41]:

1 One third of care home managers reported no support or very limited support from local older people's mental health services

2   One quarter of care home managers listed getting advice from external services as one of their top three challenges in providing good dementia care.

Care home staff are the most numerically sizeable group of social care practitioners, but they often find their own needs for support from specialist services, through advice, support, and training, are unmet:

> The findings of this report paint a picture of very inconsistent care, whereby a fortunate group of care home residents with dementia experience good care that supports them to live enjoyable, fulfilling lives. For others, the failures of the system result in treatment that is in no way acceptable. Enabling the standard of dementia care in all homes to be consistently raised to that of the best must be an imperative for providers, health and social care teams and policy makers. Quality care makes a difference to people's lives [41].

Here too we may find that the elasticity of the term 'support' may not sufficiently convey some of the major changes that are needed to the structure of social care. While interpersonal encounters are the cornerstone of support, they take place in a care and support system that is under-funded in the UK and sometimes distant from other services and professionals. National dementia guidelines have been valuable in making connections across the whole system [42], but even the *National Dementia Strategy* has much more to say about health care interventions and far less to say about social care [3], save that it is under-resourced and that the eligibility criteria (FACS) mentioned above should be revisited.

Social work – promoting supportive care

This chapter returns at its end to social work practice. There is no certainty that social workers will be able to offer support to people with early dementia or to extend their support more widely in a therapeutic sense. Their role instead may be to support other practitioners who are working with particularly complex cases and to promote the commissioning of person-centred approaches from a variety of organizations and supporters. Lessons from social work practice around the globe reveal that while there are islands of good practice, in many cases social work with people with dementia is only undertaken at a time of crisis or care breakdown [43]. There is a widely held opinion that the preventive potential of social work is often missed and that crises might be averted if social work support were available earlier [44]. For example, the difficulties of caregivers struggling on unsupported until they become ill themselves might be alleviated by earlier support and advice from social workers. However, social work expertise in communication, problem-solving, assessment and care planning, monitoring and reviewing, and social networking and community development is not often available to people with dementia. Direct support of people with dementia is likely to be undertaken by carers, unqualified practitioners, and volunteers in long-term contact with people with dementia and carers, perhaps in settings such as peer support groups, care homes, or carers' centres. The professional role may be far more likely to be the support of the supporters. Skills development and professional education need to embed this in their activities.

Changing social care cultures

The strengths perspective is not commonly or explicitly considered in supportive care for people who have dementia, but it may be a way in which, while challenging the bias of resource allocations, social care services are able to focus on an individual's capabilities and potentialities, and encourage them to express and implement their hopes for the future [6]. Work with people with dementia implicitly draws on such perspectives by recognizing that people have abilities and resources; that they are usually able to determine what they want and what is best for them; and that supportive partnerships between practitioners and people with dementia can reinforce and build up strengths.

Building up support in social care is therefore not just the business of social care services alone. In many instances, social workers will work with other members of primary care and secondary health care teams to help a person identify their goals and work towards them, rather than be left to bring in social care after assessment and treatment have concluded. The need for a more integrated approach, with financial investment of course, has been proposed by the *National Dementia Strategy* for England [3]. It may be that social workers will adopt a more advisory role, offering support in complex cases or where there is conflict, say between family members, or concerns about neglect and mistreatment. Social workers often have lead responsibilities for investigating and responding to situations of alleged abuse and neglect.

Some professionals argue that social work should continue to play an important part in helping older people to make decisions about their lives. Other professionals may see this as part of their role, with social work involvement in a minority of cases. In contrast, social care services, whether based in community or care home settings, are central to the long-term support of people with dementia. In England, the current focus on personalization as an overarching framework for social care is open to influence by advocates for people with dementia. There is room for notions of supportive care to influence the ethos and values of personalization, but, to do this, greater clarity may be needed about the way in which supportive care differs from other 'strap lines' that have been implicitly critical of social care but have failed to provide it with the resources to change its orientation and effectiveness.

References

1. Department of Health (2006). *Our health, our care, our say: a new direction for community services*. London: The Stationery Office.
2. Department of Health (2007). *Putting people first: a shared commitment to the transformation of adult social care*. London: The Stationery Office.
3. Department of Health (2009). *Living well with dementia: national dementia strategy*. London: The Stationery Office.
4. Ferguson I (2007). Increasing user choice or privatizing risk? The antinomies of personalization. *Br J Soc Work*, 37, 3, 387–403.
5. Fook J (2004). *Care*. Cambridge: Polity Press.
6. Cree V, Myers S (2008). *Social work: making a difference*. Bristol: Policy Press.
7. Marshall M, Tibbs MA (2006). *Social work and people with dementia*. Bristol: Policy Press.
8. Cox CB (ed) (2007). *Dementia and social work practice: research and interventions*. New York: Springer Publishing Company.
9. Platt D (2007). *The status of social care – a review 2007*. London: Department of Health.
10. Department of Health. (2001). *National service framework for older people*. London: The Stationery Office.
11. Manthorpe J, Adams T (2003). Policy and practice in dementia care, in Manthorpe J, Adams T (eds) *Dementia care*, p. 44. London: Arnold.
12. Department of Health (2005). *Independence, well-being and choice*. London: The Stationery Office, p. 14.
13. National Audit Office (2007). *Improving services and support for people with dementia* (HC 604). London: The Stationery Office.
14. Dowling S, Manthorpe J, Cowley S (2007). Working on person-centered planning: from amber to green light? *J Intellect Disabil*, 11(1), 65–82.

15. Carr S (2008). *Personalisation: a rough guide*. London: Social Care Institute for Excellence.

16. Commission for Social Care Inspection (2008). *The state of social care in England 2006–07*. London: Commission for Social Care Inspection.

17. Manthorpe J, Moriarty J, Rapaport J *et al.* (2008). Older people researching social issues (OPRSI). 'There are wonderful social workers but it's a lottery': older people's views about social workers. *Br J Soc Work*, **38**, 1132–1150.

18. Glasby J, Littlechild R (2004). *The health and social care divide – the experiences of older people*. Bristol: Policy Press.

19. Tanner D (2003). Older people and access to care. *Br J Soc Work*, **33**, 499–515.

20. Richards S (2000). Bridging the assessment divide. *Br J Soc Work*, **30**(1), 37–50.

21. Challis D, von Abendorff R, Brown P, Chesterman J, Hughes J (2002). Care management, dementia care and specialist mental health services: an evaluation. *Int J Geriatr Psychiatry*, **17**(4), 315–325.

22. McCormack B, McCance T (2006). Development of a framework for person-centred nursing. *J Adv Nurs*, **56**(5), 472–479.

23. Alzheimer's Society (2001). *Quality dementia care in care homes: person-centered standards*. London: Alzheimer's Society.

24. Nolan M, Keady J, Aveyard B (2001). Relationship-centered care is the next logical step. *Br J Nurs*, **10**(12), 757.

25. Carers UK. Help with caring. http://www.carersuk.org/Information/Helpwithcaring (accessed on 31 March 2009).

26. Twigg J, Atkin K (1994). *Carers perceived: policy and practice in informal care*. Buckingham: Open University Press.

27. Carers UK. Back me up. http://www.carersuk.org/Newsandcampaigns/BackMeUp (accessed on 31 March 2009).

28. Walker A (1985). *The care gap: how can local authorities meet the needs of the elderly?* London: Local Government Information Unit.

29. Campbell J (2008). 'Social care an equality and human rights issue'. Speech at the IPPR 'Power to carers and users: transforming care services' event, 16 February 2008. http://www.equalityhumanrights. com/en/newsandcomment/speeches/Pages/socialcareequalityandhumanrightsissue.aspx (accessed on 31 March 2009).

30. Riddell S, Pearson C, Jolly D, Barnes C, Priestley M, Mercer G (2005). The development of direct payments in the UK: implications for social justice. *Social Policy and Administration*, **4**(1), 76–85.

31. Glendinning C, Arksey H, Jones K, Moran N, Netten A, Rabiee P (2009). *The individual budgets pilot projects: impact and outcomes for carers*. York: University of York.

32. Clark H, Gough H, McFarlane A (2004). *It pays dividends: direct payments and older people*. Bristol: Policy Press.

33. Age Concern (2008). *The age agenda 2008: public policy and older people*. http://www.ageconcern.org. uk/AgeConcern/Documents/Age_Agenda_2008.pdf (accessed on 17 March 2008).

34. Age Concern (2007). *Out of sight, out of mind*. London: Age Concern.

35. Helen Sanderson Associates (2007). *Person centred thinking with other people: practicalities and possibilities*. Cheshire: HSA Press.

36. Herbert G (2008). *Personalised budgets: what do older people want? A research programme to inform the introduction of personal budgets in Essex*. Chelmsford: Essex County Council.

37. Beattie A, Daker-White G, Gillard J, Means R (2005). They don't quite fit the way we organize our services: results from a UK field study of marginalized groups and dementia care. *Disabil Soc*, **20**(1): 67–80.

38. Lyall J (2008). Declaration of independence. *The Guardian*. http://www.guardian.co.uk/society/2008/ feb/06/8 (accessed on 23 July 2008).

39. Davey V, Snell T, Fernandez JL *et al.* (2007). *Schemes providing support to people using direct payments: a UK survey*. London: Personal Social Services Research Unit, London School of Economics.

40. Arksey H, Corden A, Glendinning C, Hirst M (2006). *Carers and the management of financial assets in later life: report of a scoping study*. York: Social Policy Research Unit, University of York.

41. Alzheimer's Society (2007). *Home from home: quality of care for people with dementia living in care homes*. London: Alzheimer's Society.

42. National Institute for Health and Clinical Excellence/Social Care Institute for Excellence (2006). *Dementia: supporting people with dementia and their carers in health and social care*. London: NICE/SCIE. http://www.nice.org.uk/CG042#documents (accessed on 31 March 2009).

43. Manthorpe J, Moriarty J (2007). Models from other countries: social work with people with dementia and their caregivers, in Cox CB (ed) *Dementia and social work practice: research and interventions*, pp. 229–247. New York: Springer Publishing Company.

44. Marshall M, Tibbs MA (2006). Social work and dementia care: reasons to be cheerful? *Journal of Dementia Care*, **14**(6), 24–27.

Chapter 19

Care homes and long-term care for people with dementia

Katherine Froggatt and Deborah Parker

Introduction

A significant proportion of people living with dementia will live and stay in long-term care settings. Consequently care homes have an important role to play in the provision of supportive care for people with dementia. For people with dementia who reside in care homes their experiences of living will be increasingly shaped by their dying. Supportive care therefore needs to address ongoing physical, emotional, social, and spiritual concerns for people living in care homes, as well as for their family members and care staff.

In this chapter we initially describe the care home context, as this shapes the experiences of living and dying for people with dementia residing in care homes. We draw on two recent studies, both considering the provision of palliative care for people who are living and dying in care homes: one from the UK (Froggatt) and one from Australia (Parker). From this empirical research we identify two key challenges that face care homes as they support people with dementia living in such settings: how do we, on the one hand, create a culture of openness to people's experiences of living and dying alongside, on the other hand, maintaining people's identities? These both require attention in the care home setting if person-centred supportive care is to be provided throughout a person's life unto their death.

Context for long-term care for dementia

Many people with dementia live in long-term care settings. These institutions have a number of names such as care homes (UK), nursing homes (US, UK, Scandinavia), residential aged care facilities (Australia). In this chapter we use the term care home to encompass all care facilities that provide communal care and support for people with long-term health and social care needs. These facilities are often categorized by the degree of functional impairment of, and consequently the degree of support required for, the residents living in them. This determines the extent and type of care provided. In Australia this distinction is reflected in the terms 'high' and 'low' care. This categorization is similar to nursing homes (high care), which provide nursing care, and residential care (low care), which provide only personal care in the UK. Care homes are an integral part of the service provision of care for frail older people, including people with dementia, so that in 2004, 410,000 older people lived in a UK care home [1].

In the UK, over half of all people with dementia live in care homes [2]. Unsurprisingly, a high proportion of residents in care homes live with a degree of dementia. In 1996, 42–48% of residents in a range of care home settings demonstrated mild impairment, and a further 19% to 44% of residents demonstrated severe impairment [3]. More recent research suggests that dementia prevalence within care homes is estimated at 62% [4]. Similar figures from Australia, in 2003, indicate that 67,650 (48%) of the permanent resident population had dementia. Of these 4.5% had mild dementia, 63.7% had moderate dementia and 31.8% had severe dementia [5]. Higher levels of cognitive and functional impairment are to be found in care homes where nursing care is provided. A higher proportion of residents in high care facilities live with dementia in Australia and Sweden: 83% of residents have dementia in high care facilities in Australia [5] and 66% in Sweden [6].

The emphasis in current health and social care policy in the UK is to support people to remain in their own homes. However, many people with dementia may experience a move into a care home. Reasons for admission include: following hospitalization for an acute illness, a breakdown in informal care support at home or the death of the carer (often because the primary carer at home is old themselves), and concerns for the person with dementia's well-being and safety [7]. Whilst care homes provide a home for people with dementia who have a need for support and care, they can also be the place where their dying occurs. Approximately, 20% of people aged 65 years and older in the UK die in care homes [8]. In Australia, age specific death rates for dementia for people aged less than 65 years are more than doubled for each progressive 5 year category from 10.1 deaths per 100,000 population at 65–69 to 952.3 at 85 years and over [5].

A number of challenges exist in the delivery of supportive care for people with dementia in care homes, related to the resident population, the culture of care, staff skills and relationships with primary care [9]. Although, as outlined above, a high proportion of people living in care homes live with dementia, it is likely they will also be living with a range of other conditions [10,11]. People's experiences of dying in care homes can differ greatly, with or without dementia. It has been estimated that in the UK, 42% of residents in all care homes, and 51% in nursing homes, die following a long period of general deterioration [12]. This long, often undefined process is also used to describe the experience of many people dying with dementia [13]. There is therefore a great deal of uncertainty present in terms of knowing when a person with dementia is actively dying.

The culture of care within care homes reflects different historical roots to other elements of end-of-life care provision [9]. The care sector is located in an interesting position in terms of its location across a number of boundaries with respect to the type of care provided, the financial basis for the service providers, the funding sources for care, and the regulatory processes [14]. Staffing issues relate to wider resource issues in the sector, but reflect a workforce that is fluid in terms of recruitment and retention [15], and whilst staff may be caring and enthusiastic, many lack specific knowledge and expertise regarding either dementia care and/or palliative care.

The provision of palliative care to older people with dementia in primary care is provided by a range of nursing services working in collaboration with general practitioners (GPs) and consultants in palliative medicine. However, older people generally in care homes have variable and often inequitable access to National Health Service (NHS) provision [16], and it can be surmised that people with dementia will similarly experience variable levels of service.

Whilst this chapter focuses upon the supportive care needs of people with dementia living in care homes, we need to place this specific focus in a broader context of societal attitudes towards ageing, dying and the care home sector. Small et al. [17] describe how meeting the needs of people with living and dying with dementia is problematic for a number of societal reasons related to understandings of personhood, the functional emphasis currently placed upon quality of care and life, and the extent to which dying and death are accepted in Western society. Whilst we continue to focus here on the experiences of individuals, their location in a broader system needs to be borne in mind.

Understanding supportive care in care homes

In the care home context no work has been undertaken that specifically considers the provision of supportive care, although much work has addressed the needs of and provision of compassionate care to older people, their family and friends, and staff from within gerontological and dementia frames [17]. Already present in discussions of palliative care and end-of-life care in care homes there is a recognition that this care needs to be concerned with more than just the last few days, weeks and months of a person's life. This complements the concept of supportive care promoted in this book. A longer term perspective on definitions of end-of-life care for older people [18] and palliative care in care homes have been articulated [19], which we will describe here.

Ross *et al.* provide a broad definition of end-of-life care that moves beyond the last few days of someone's life and encompasses all conditions including dementia [18]:

> End-of-life care for seniors requires an active, compassionate approach that treats, comforts and supports older individuals who are living with, or dying from, progressive or chronic life-threatening conditions. Such care is sensitive to personal, cultural and spiritual values, beliefs and practices and encompasses support for families and friends up to and including the period of bereavement. (p. 9)

Froggatt [19] proposed that in the care home context older people experienced a range of transitions from admission to death to bereavement. Three stages are identified: living with losses, dying, and bereavement. The period called living with losses concerns the time from when an individual moves into a care home and also encompasses the ongoing losses of ageing which can be physical, social, and/or emotional. A range of losses may be experienced by older people during this transition into a care home [20], including the move out of a person's own home, the loss of nearby friends and neighbours, and even an animal companion. The second stage of dying and death is characterized for many older people in care homes as one of uncertainty and deterioration over many months. The presence of dementia can compound people's experiences because of the challenges of communication for the person with dementia and the people around them [17]. The bereavement stage for older people in care homes is actually not a final sequential stage, as residents' experiences of bereavement may begin before their physical death as they are subject to a social death arising from their age and dementia [21]. The deaths of residents may lead to experiences of bereavement for other residents, family members, and staff.

Although not specifically concerned with the experience of people with dementia in care homes, these models still have relevance. We therefore propose that supportive care is an integral part of the care any person with dementia receives throughout their residence in a care home, from their move into until their departure. We present empirical findings from two studies that have considered end-of-life care in its broadest sense for people with dementia living in care homes, to identify what from the residents' and family perspectives is important about living and dying in a care home. From this we shall identify some challenges for the ongoing provision of supportive care for people with dementia in this care setting.

Living now with future dying: developing end-of-life care in care homes through action research

The first study was an action research study undertaken in the UK in two care homes. The aim of the study was to develop end-of-life care in the care homes through the involvement of residents, relatives, and the full range of staff. Participatory research was undertaken in two care homes providing personal care for older people. Cycles of analysis, planning, action, and review were undertaken in each home, mainly working with care staff. Resident and relative perspectives were integrated into the work. Further details of the method are described elsewhere [22]. One care home was registered to care for people with dementia; and the second care home, whilst not having this registration status, did care for people with mild levels of cognitive impairment. The findings presented here concern the resident and relative perspectives on end-of-life care and the implications of this for staff who work in this setting. The people with dementia involved in the study were those whose cognitive impairment did not preclude them from participating in conversations with staff, other residents or the researcher.

A tension was identified in the resident and relative accounts regarding about how to hold 'living now' with 'future dying'. In talking about their life in a care home, the residents with dementia chose not to talk about the future and focused on their present life. As one lady said: '*I just take it as it comes*'. Residents were better able to express future wishes in the group context, than in one to one conversations. The use of an informal discussion focused around tea and cakes led to conversations that began with the remembering of past experiences of bereavements and how people experienced these.

Family members, too, were concerned with the present life for their relatives living in the care home. In these care homes, care was perceived to be good and the family members expressed confidence in care provided and thought that their relative was known and understood by the staff. Where concerns were raised they were focused on the 'little things', such as the cleanliness of nails. A further need was also raised regarding the need for adequate stimulation and activities for their relative. These family members were aware of the future death of their relative, as they watched the decline and care of the other residents in the care home. They expressed mixed feelings about their relative's future death, describing it as both a loss and a relief. Continuity of care and ensuring their relative stayed in the care home towards the end of life was important to them. The staff in this care home were focused on meeting the needs of a diverse group of residents in terms of their physical and cognitive abilities. The staff knew that residents would die, but they were not always equipped to engage with the issues dying and death bring for them as carers.

This tension of holding the 'living now' with the 'future dying' requires attention within the care home, as we discuss later. This study did not specifically address the dying experience of any of the residents living in the care home and how this was managed, but this is considered in the second study.

Self-identity for dying residents in care homes

The second study we present is an ethnographic research study undertaken in two care homes in Australia to explore the construction of self identity for dying residents [23]. The study focused on the experiences of residents who required nursing and personal care and who had been identified by a senior nursing clinician as having a prognosis of approximately 6 months. Of the eleven residents included in the study, four had a medical diagnosis of dementia but a further three had cognitive impairment indicative of dementia. Residents with dementia were not separated into designated special units but were integrated throughout the care homes. Participant observation occurred over a 6-month period in each care home, and in addition data was extracted from resident case notes and informal conversations were conducted with the residents, their family members, and staff.

In the study, the view was taken that care homes are social institutions with discursive environments that mediate the social interactions of individuals [24]. A person's self identity is socially constructed and as such the settings in which people live and work provide contexts for the production and reproduction of different selves. Care homes as institutions shape who and what residents are, were, or can be. Of particular consideration to this discussion is the institutional identity of the dying resident: who qualifies, what are the expectations of residents who enter this role, what are the responses of the staff and family, and how do the practices within the care homes support dying residents and their family.

The discursive practices within the two care homes could be considered predominantly supportive of a palliative approach. Each care home had a philosophy and mission statement that supported the principles of person-centred palliative care. While this integration of palliative care was very positive, care practices were ultimately constrained by other biomedical and economic discourses present within these settings, which limited the options available to dying residents in maintaining or reconstructing their self-identity particularly as their physical and mental capacities diminished.

Four possible templates for self-construction for dying residents were identified. These were the *economic self*, reflecting the economic discourse present, the *embodied* and *dying* self, which were created to serve the economical and biomedical discourses, and the *other constructed self* for those whose resources of identity construction are limited. Most pertinent to the discussion of the care of people with dementia is the *other constructed self* (see also the discussion in this volume by Sabat in Chapter 24). Maintenance of self identity for the person receiving care assists the family to persist with the current relationship, despite often no recognition by that person [23].

The following example of one resident with end-stage dementia illustrates the importance of both family and staff in maintenance of self-identity as the individual's own resources to do so become extinguished.

Wilma's story

Wilma is a 91-year-old resident who had been in the care home for approximately two years. She was widowed but had a supportive daughter and extended family, the daughter visited at least once a day, often twice. Wilma had originally been admitted to the care home for palliative care having been transferred from the acute hospital following a stroke. Within a few weeks of arriving in the care home her condition stabilized, although her daughter described several episodes over the last 2 years where her mother deteriorated and she prepared for her mother's death. Wilma had been diagnosed with dementia several years prior to her entry into the care home. When I met Wilma she did not speak, but sometimes made screaming noises. She had severe contractures of her legs and arms, was confined to bed or a water chair and was doubly incontinent. She needed full assistance with eating and drinking, but her co-operation with staff or family regarding this fluctuated.

Wilma's case illustrates some of the uncertainty surrounding the dying of people with dementia in care homes, in that she was identified as 'dying' on admission, but then was no longer deemed to be dying, as she stabilized, so left this category and joined the 'living' again [25].

For all residents there is concerted effort to construct a biography of the individual's life prior to entry to the care home. For those residents unable to construct their own story this task fell to others, usually the family. Wilma's daughter took on this role creating for staff a picture of who her mother was, what she liked to do, eat, dress, and a detailed personal history. Wilma's daughter had instigated a number of mechanisms to ensure her mother's identity was clear: through what she wore and through the writing of a visitor's diary. She had an extensive range of clothes for her mother, which she took home and washed herself, having learnt that the care home laundry service was sometimes unreliable in losing items and that the use of industrial style machines was harsh on the style of clothes she wanted her mother dressed in. Wilma, each day, at the request of her daughter, was dressed in a pair of ironed casual pants with a coloured match blouse, stockings, shoes, with her hair done, makeup and jewellery.

The second mechanism by which Wilma's daughter maintained a sense of her mother's identity was through the use of a visitor diary. Located at the bedside all visitors were requested to write the time and day of their visit and what had occurred. Immediate family, Wilma's daughter in particular, would document in great details any words Wilma had spoken, reactions to discussion topics, whether she was in bed or the chair, outside or in any activity, and what Wilma had eaten and drunk during he visit. The staff were asked to use this diary to remind Wilma who had visited and what had gone on in the days events.

The daughter also described the use of the dairy as a record of her commitment to her mother. It enabled her to flip back through the years and provided a reminder of the progressive deterioration of her mother. It reminded her of the times when her mother was able to communicate and of conversations or jokes they had shared. This helped her to maintain a sense of who her mother was as she became increasingly less recognizable. This acceptance over time had led the daughter to indicate she was prepared for her mother's death. These two strategies that Wilma's daughter had employed were to maintain her mother's identity in the face of her mother's inability to maintain or communicate who she was. These strategies also provided the staff with parameters of what was expected from both Wilma and her family.

Providing person-centred supportive care

Care homes are institutions that provide supportive care for people with dementia up until their death. How can these organizations hold both the 'living now' with the 'future dying' as described in the English care home, whilst also ensuring individuals can maintain their self-identity? This is a particular challenge in the face of decreased cognitive and physical function and the presence of different institutional discourses that shape the culture of the care home and the particular biographies of each resident.

Creating an open culture of living and dying

A supportive organizational culture is required to create an open culture of living and dying in care homes. From these studies three processes were identified that encouraged a death accepting culture within the setting. These concern: overt notification of a resident's death to other residents; the celebration of the life of residents through the use of memorial services; and practices of remembering. Overt notification of a resident's death occurred in one of the care homes by the use of a board outside the dining area. This board had a space for a resident's name, accompanied by the words rest in peace and the date of the resident's death. This name remained until replaced by the name of the next deceased resident. Word of mouth among the more fit and mobile residents ensured that the news was distributed quickly around the care home. This overt communication provided residents with the opportunity to contact the family and pass on their regards and gave staff license to clearly speak with the residents and other family members about the death.

A further avenue for integrating an open culture of living and dying was the holding of memorial services. One Australian care home held these memorial services approximately every 3 months. Any resident who had died within that time was remembered and their family invited to attend the service. Again feedback from other residents indicated it was an opportunity for them to pay their respects for people they had shared their lives with, some for many years. Since resident's funerals were usually reserved for family (although sometimes staff members did attend), the memorial services provided an opportunity for residents, staff, and family members of other residents to attend and were seen as a mark of respect of the person's life.

In the English care homes the issue of remembering residents was approached in similar ways. In both care homes there was a recognition by staff that many residents passed through their care and sometimes it was hard to remember who had lived in the home. In one home the staff created a resident's book of biographies, in which a photograph and short account of that resident was contained. This enabled the staff to remember who had been a part of this particular community and held their presence beyond their death. In the second care home in this study, a similar book was created, but this was used following a person's death to record people's memories (staff and residents) of the person who had died. People also used this to write farewell messages to the resident who had died.

Maintaining the individual as a person

Some residents who enter care homes when still able to speak and interact can establish identities with the staff, beyond those related to the provision of technical biomedical care. For these residents self-identity is assembled by the weaving of personal history to make sense of their current situation. This was illustrated with Wilma's story and how her daughter worked to maintain her mother's identity for herself and for others, such as the staff who cared for her mother.

In the English care home, the staff undertook an informal discussion with a small group of residents to understand better their life experiences of bereavements as a way to lead into any expressions of current wishes about their own care. Interestingly, as the women recounted their stories of how funerals were undertaken in the past, it became apparent that two of them had grown up with mothers who had the role of 'layers out' of bodies. They had therefore been used to being around death in a way that subsequent generations were not used to. Understanding people's pasts and hearing residents express their desire to know when fellow residents were ill had helped staff to have confidence to talk about issues around dying, death and bereavement on later occasions. For one staff member this led her to feel confident to tell other residents about the death of a resident.

Family and staff have an important role to play in ensuring the identity of a person with dementia is maintained. However, for family and staff to be able to do this, and address the changing nature of the person with dementia, requires an environment of support and attention to their needs as well. The identities of family members – as husbands, wives, daughters, and sons – need to be acknowledged, just as the role of being a paid carer, and the relationships that are formed through this, need to be recognized.

Conclusions

Care homes are an important setting where many people with dementia will reside for longer or shorter periods of time. Consequently, an understanding of supportive care is essential for staff working in this setting and for practitioners external to care homes. We have identified two elements of practice that we would propose are important in the delivery of supportive care in care homes. The first concerns the establishment of a culture that encompasses both living and dying. This requires an acknowledgement of the dying that does occur in this setting, in order that living can be maximized. The overt communication about this, and acknowledgement of it, through the marking of resident's dying and deaths, before and after the event, is a part of this process. On a more individual level, the need to maintain a person's identity even as their condition deteriorates is about their living and could be seen to be about denying their dying. We propose that ensuring a person's identity is maintained is about good person-centred care, which continues throughout a person's life and death. It has the potential to counter an unhelpful fatalism about dementia that is both life and death denying. The values of person-centred care can also helpfully underpin engagements between family and staff to create a dynamic culture where living and dying is acknowledged and people passing through this transition can be valued in all ways.

References

1. Office of Fair Trading (2005). *Care homes for older people: a market study*. London: Office of Fair Trading.
2. MacDonald A J D, Carpenter G I (2003). The recognition of dementia in 'non-EMI' nursing home residents in South East England. *Int J Geriatr Psychiatry*, **18**, 105–108.

3. Darton R, Netten A, Forder J (2003). The cost implications of the changing population and characteristics of care homes. *Int J Geriatr Psychiatry*, **18**, 236–243.

4. Matthews F, Dening T (2002). Prevalence of dementia in institutional care. *Lancet*, **360**(9328), 225–226.

5. Australian Institute of Health and Welfare (2006). *Residential aged care in Australia 2004-05: a statistical overview. Aged care statistics series no. 22.* Canberra: Australian Institute of Health and Welfare.

6. Sandberg O, Gustafson Y, Brannstrom B, Bucht G (1998). Prevalence of dementia, delirium and psychiatric symptoms in various care settings for the elderly. *Scand J Soc Med*, **26**(1), 56–62.

7. Aneshensel C, Pearlin L, Mullan J, Zarit S (1995). *Profiles in caregiving: the unexpected career.* London: Academic Press Inc.

8. Office of National Statistics (2000). *Mortality statistics general series, DH1 no 33.* London: Office for National Statistics.

9. Field D, Froggatt K (2003). Issues for palliative care in nursing and residential care homes, in Katz J, Peace S (eds) *End of life in care homes*, pp. 175–194. Oxford: Oxford University Press.

10. Bowman CE, Whistler J, Ellerby M (2004). A national census of care home residents. *Age Ageing*, **33**, 561–566.

11. Maddocks I, D Parker (2001). Palliative care in nursing homes, in Addington-Hall JM, Higginson IJ (eds) *Palliative care for non-cancer patients*, pp. 147–157. Oxford: Oxford University Press.

12. Sidell M, Katz J, Komaromy C (1997). Death and dying in residential and nursing homes for older people: examining the case for palliative care, in *Report for the department of health*. Milton Keynes: Open University.

13. Murray S, Kendall M, Boyd K, Sheikh A (2005). Illness trajectories and palliative care. *BMJ*, **330**, 1007–1011.

14. Froggatt K, Davies S, Meyer J (2009). Research and development in care homes: issues and context, in Froggatt K, Davies S, Meyer J (eds) *Understanding care homes: a research and development perspective*, pp. 9–22. London: Jessica Kingsley Publishers.

15. Davies S, Seymour J (2002). Historical and policy contexts, in Hockley J, Clark D (eds) *Palliative care for older people in care homes*, pp. 4–33. Buckingham: Open University Press.

16. Jacobs S (2003). Addressing the problems associated with general practitioners' workload in nursing and residential homes: findings from a qualitative study. *Br J Gen Pract*, **53**, 113–119.

17. Small N, Froggatt K, Downs M (2007). *Living and dying with dementia: dialogues about palliative care.* Oxford: Oxford University Press.

18. Ross M, Fisher R, MacLean M (2000). *A guide to end-of-life care for seniors.* Ottawa: Health Canada.

19. Froggatt K (2004). *Palliative care in care homes for older people.* London: The National Council for Palliative Care.

20. Holman C, Meyer J, Cotter A (2004). The complexity of loss in continuing care institutions for older people: a review of the literature. *Illness, Crisis Loss*, **12**(4), 38–51.

21. Sweeting H, Gilhooly M (1997). Dementia and the phenomenon of social death. *Soc Health Illn.* **19**(1), 93–117.

22. Hockley J, Froggatt K (2006). The development of palliative care knowledge in care homes for older people: the place of action research. *Palliative Med*, **20**(8), 835–843.

23. Parker D (2007). The construction of identities for people dying in residential aged care facilities, in *Department of palliative and supportive services*. Adelaide, Australia: Flinders University.

24. Gubrium J, Holstein J (2001). *Institutional selves troubled identities in a postmodern world.* Oxford: Oxford University Press.

25. Froggatt K (2001). Life and death in English nursing homes: sequestration or transition? *Ageing Society*, **21**(3), 319–332.

Chapter 20

Assisted living programmes providing supportive care for dementia

Philip D. Sloane and Sheryl Zimmerman

Introduction

Supportive care is the multidisciplinary, holistic care of patients and their families across the continuum, from the time of diagnosis, throughout the treatment aimed at cure or prolonging life, and into the phase currently acknowledged as palliative care. It involves addressing the psychological, social, and spiritual concerns of the individual and family, providing symptom relief, recognizing and caring for the side-effects of active therapies, and addressing co-morbidities. It also values the role of family care providers and helps them in supporting the patient. Ideally, supportive care should be individualized and flexible, and should address the individual's needs along the entire course of ageing, chronic illness, and, eventually, death.

The patient with dementia presents unique problems and challenges in terms of supportive care. For one thing, the illness is insidious, slowly progressive over a decade or more, and accompanied by tremendous variation in the presentation and course of the illness. In addition, it is accompanied by a variety of behavioural symptoms that can dominate the care provider's efforts, thereby leading to a situation that may place controlling undesired behaviour, and the well-being of the care provider, in tension with supporting the quality of life of the affected individual. Finally, the individual's diminishing capacity to direct his or her own care and to make decisions means that family and professional care providers have to be especially proactive in identifying wishes, and that decisions regarding every aspect of care are complicated by the need to involve multiple persons, as well as an anxiety that the decisions may not be correct.

Assisted living is a form of residential long-term care that is less intensive and less medically focused than nursing home care. In the United States (US), assisted living has mushroomed from around 1990, and now serves approximately 1.4 million persons – making it nearly as large as the nursing home industry. Because of fewer regulatory constraints, and because assisted living is regulated largely by the states rather than by federal agencies, much more variation exists across facilities, including many novel models of care.

The aim of assisted living programmes in the US is to provide a stable place of residence for older people who would otherwise be unable to live independently. The hope is that quality of life will be maximized through meaningful activity and support. The intention is that assisted living should prevent the need for admission to hospitals or nursing homes, although, as we shall see, both of these outcomes occur quite frequently. Research shows that a good proportion of people in assisted living have dementia, and it seems possible in many cases to maintain relative independence even until the end of life.

Emergence of assisted living as a dementia care setting

Assisted living is a form of housing for older persons that has grown rapidly in the US in recent years. Despite wide variations, these residences have in common that they all provide room, board, 24-hour supervision, and assistance with medications and activities of daily living (ADL). Facilities also tend to provide some degree of coordination of and access to medical and nursing services, although the extent of services varies widely.

Initially, the term 'assisted living' referred to a specific model of care based on principles of individuality, independence, privacy, dignity, and choice. It focused on homelikeness and insisted not only on individual sleeping spaces but also on full baths, kitchens, doors that locked, individual temperature controls, and personal furnishings [1]. By the mid-1990s, however, the term had become applied broadly to refer to a diversity of facilities regulated by the states under a variety of designations including board and care, residential care, personal care, foster care, domiciliary care, and congregate care – not all of which subscribed to the same principles.

Assisted living facilities range from private, converted houses with a few beds to multi-level campuses with more than 1400 beds. Some have private apartments, whereas others have as many as four residents per room. Rates (in US dollars) range from less than $400 to more than $6000 per month. The majority of facilities are for-profit, but a number of non-profit groups also provide assisted living care.

Given this diversity, typologies to create an organizing framework for residential care/assisted living have been suggested. Some typologies address differences in structure and access (public housing, units in continuing care retirement communities, and freestanding facilities), differences in services (institutional board and care, housing and services, and purely service-oriented), differences in the combination of services and privacy (low/minimal privacy and service, high privacy and low service, high service and low privacy, and high privacy and high service), and differences across a combination of size and medical needs/services.

Dementia is ubiquitous in assisted living communities. One survey of 193 facilities in four states found that between 24% and 42% of residents had moderate or severe dementia [2]. The study identified three different types of facilities: small (<16 beds); new-model (built after 1987 and with features indicating increased ability to manage residents with high levels of physical impairment); and traditional (built before 1987 and/or without features of new-model facilities). This study also found that dementia prevalence rates varied by facility type [3]. Across all facility types, however, the majority of residents with dementia were female (78%–79%), white (83%–98%), and not married (79%–91%) [4]). Table 20.1 demonstrates the functional and behavioural status of these residents. From this table, it is apparent that functional dependency is quite common, and problem behaviours are exhibited by almost one-quarter of these residents.

Dementia in assisted living may, however, be even more common than these figures suggest. A recent study demonstrated that when neurologists evaluated assisted living patients without a diagnosis of dementia, they found that 38% met criteria for probable dementia, and all but 10% of the remainder had some kind of cognitive impairment, usually mild cognitive impairment of the non-amnestic type [5]. This means that problems with judgement, planning, and other higher level cognitive tasks are ubiquitous in assisted living, and that the prevalence of overt dementia may be as high as 50% or more. Consequently, assisted living has emerged as a prime setting in which persons with dementia receive housing and services.

Needs of persons with dementia in assisted living

As has been noted earlier (Table 20.1), persons with dementia in assisted living can vary widely in capabilities and needs. Virtually all need help with instrumental daily activities such as managing

Table 20.1 Prevalence of selected functional dependencies and problem behaviours among assisted living residents with moderate or severe dementia, by facility type

	< 16 Beds (%)	> 16 Beds	
		Traditional (%)	New-model (%)
Functional Dependency			
Personal hygiene	74	48	64
Transfer, bed to chair	36	20	29
Locomotion on unit	32	18	25
Eating	24	17	18
Incontinent, daily (urine)	58	38	55
Problem Behaviour (weekly or more)			
Constant requests	18	17	17
Repetitive calls	19	19	20
Resists assistance	18	13	25
Physical aggression	11	7	13
Wandering or pacing	24	23	33
Physical restlessness, agitation	20	20	19

Source: Based on a sample of 687 persons from 193 facilities in four states [4].

their finances, cooking, doing laundry, and maintaining a household. The vast majority need help with activities of daily living that tend to be lost early in the disease (early-loss ADLs), such as bathing and dressing, although the amount of assistance needed also varies widely. Between a third and a half need assistance with the mid-stage or late-loss ADLs, such as toileting, ambulation, transfer, and feeding, again, with actual service needs varying widely from person to person. Thus, supportive care must address these needs by providing assistance when needed and avoiding unnecessary dependency.

Especially characteristic of persons with dementia are the multiple behavioural symptoms that can occur. These symptoms can be divided into several categories.

- *Memory loss and disorientation-related symptoms.* These take the form of frequent repetition of questions, confusion about the date, time, and schedules, and lack of ability to initiate and follow-through on activities.

- *Anxiety and depression.* Particularly early in the disease, awareness of one's deficits may be accompanied by clinical depression and a high level of anxiety. Symptoms range widely and include anxiety while receiving care and withdrawal from social situations. Often, anxiety and depression underlie issues such as resistance to care, agitation, or aggression.

- *Delusions.* Cognitive deficits combined with frontal lobe abnormalities can lead to the person with dementia misinterpreting environmental cues and, therefore, having misperceptions or illusions, as well as delusions (i.e. fixed false beliefs). An example of a common delusion is someone who feels that they are being threatened or persecuted by another. Delusions tend to be fixed and limited; however, occasionally they are severe enough to interfere with care and quality of life.

- *Agitated behaviours.* These are common in dementia. Physical agitation includes such activities as repetitive mannerisms (e.g. repeatedly tapping on a table), pacing, and trying to exit the facility. Verbal agitation usually refers to repeated loud noises such as requests for attention or screaming.

- *Aggression*. Agression is agitation directed at another person or object, usually in a hostile manner. Examples include hitting (or attempting to hit) another person, biting, kicking, or throwing something at a person or object.

- *Resistiveness to care*. This term refers to a variety of behaviours that are not aggressive but that are designed to resist or refuse care. Examples include refusing to be bathed or toileted or physically holding on to the care provider or an object (e.g. a handrail) to resist the care provider's help. These behaviours typically reflect an underlying anxiety or discomfort.

- *Markedly antisocial behaviours*. Occasionally behaviours are encountered that are considered especially out of place in social or living situations. Examples include disrobing in public, grabbing at the breasts or buttocks of care provider, or smearing faeces on the walls of a room. These behaviours often reflect a complex interaction of cognitive deficits, emotions, and environmental challenges (see further discussion of behaviours that challenge in Chapter 17).

Quality supportive care in assisted living includes addressing these behavioural symptoms. To do so successfully requires patience, an analytical problem-solving approach, a non-blaming attitude, and development, and implementation of a consistent, individualized treatment plan. In addition to caring for the physical and mood/behavioural needs of a person with dementia, supportive care must address higher issues that comprise quality of life. Definitions of quality of life in dementia vary but commonly include such elements as engagement in meaningful activities, demonstrating positive affect, having few agitated or depressed behaviours, and maintaining physical health and independence to the extent this is feasible [6].

Finally, supportive care of persons with dementia requires supportive care of the family. In assisted living, a high level of family involvement is more common than in nursing homes. As with individual patients, the needs of family members vary widely. Particularly important are: having a staff member they trust and can turn to if they have a concern or problem, participating in key decisions about care, and meeting with health care providers upon admission and whenever there is a change in status.

Supporting daily living and quality of life

One of the most important changes evolving in the field of residential long-term care is the appreciation that those who live there are not merely waiting to die. Instead, they are able to experience joy, meaningful relationships, a sense of comfort, and other pleasures that together constitute quality of life. Thus, there is an emerging appreciation that the quality of care should be judged by the quality of life achieved by the residents, and now all long-term care settings are being called upon to help provide meaning to residents' lives. Consequently, the quality of long-term care is improving, in part a result of federal nursing home regulations and state residential care/assisted living regulations, as well as from grass roots efforts that emphasize consumer involvement, better physical environments, and care that is person-directed and focuses on caring for people and relationships, rather than solely on the task of care provision.

Supporting function at the care provider level

Most of the day-to-day interactions experienced by persons with dementia in assisted living are with direct care providers (sometimes called aides or nursing assistants). These individuals typically are women, from racial/ethnic minorities, have little training in dementia or the elements of quality care provision in dementia, and are generally paid wages low enough to place them at or near poverty. For these care providers, job satisfaction tends to be derived from relationships with the residents themselves, from feeling empowered to do well in their work, and from support from peers.

Supportive care, therefore, begins with training and supporting the direct care providers. Table 20.2 outlines a curriculum for direct care providers that was developed specifically to improve dementia care provision in assisted living [7]. Key elements of that curriculum include education about dementia itself, communication techniques, methods to approach behavioural symptoms successfully, methods of fostering pleasant events in the care recipient's daily life, self-management (so as to be calm and supportive in providing care), and team building (so as to work effectively in the assisted living organization).

One key element of supportive dementia care at the direct care level is understanding how to tailor the level of assistance provided to the needs of the person to whom the care is being given (see Figure 20.1). Persons with dementia generally prefer to do what they can rather than have others do things for them; when this is not possible they can become frustrated and agitated even by attempts to promote independence. Tailoring the level of assistance refers to providing just as much help as is needed to allow the person with dementia to be successful while maximizing his or her independence. As dementia progresses, the level of assistance required tends to increase, first with IADLs, then with the early loss ADLs, and then (often in an unpredictable order, depending on the disease manifestations and/or other conditions such as osteoporosis) with the later loss ADLs. A sensitive, informed care provider will approach each activity by assessing what the individual can do and by both allowing and fostering successful performance. In dressing, for

Table 20.2 Dementia care curriculum for direct care providers in assisted living

Understanding dementia and realistic expectations
Communication with and without words
Listening with respect
Communication during personal care
Comforting and redirecting
Communicating with families
Understanding, assessing, and manageing behavioural symptoms
How to observe and report behavioural events
The ABC (activator-behaviour-consequence) approach to understanding behavioural symptoms
Understanding the mood state or emotion underlying a behavioural symptom
Role of the environment in shaping behaviour
Changing behaviours by changing activators and consequences
Improving quality of life by Identifying, implementing, and encourageing pleasant events
Self-management
Identifying and addressing negative thoughts and behaviours
Developing and implementing care plans
Team building
Working together to make work easier and less frustrating
Communicating together and with leadership

Source: Adapted from [7].

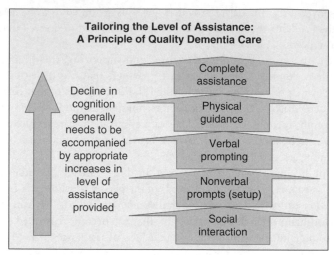

Fig. 20.1 Tailoring levels of assistance.

example, persons early in dementia may only need a reminder or two. Later on, being present to help them select their clothes may be enough. Later, the clothes will need to be selected and placed on the bed in the order in which they will be put on, often with the care provider standing by to provide reminders. Still later in the illness, the care provider may need to pick up certain articles of clothing and/or provide physical guidance, for example, touching the person's leg to indicate the need to lift it to begin the process of putting on pants. Late in the disease, the person may need to be completely dressed by the care provider, but still with explanation of what is happening and what is about to happen.

Supporting function at the institutional level

Assisted living facilities are complex organizations. Within them, individual care providers cannot be successful, and overall care cannot be maximally supportive, unless the organization's administration is supportive. The study of organizational competency and supportiveness in both nursing homes and assisted living is just beginning to mature. However, it is clear that administrative structures that do not maximally support the care providers are common.

The Pioneer movement, which began in nursing homes, has proposed a 'culture change' model that is appropriate for assisted living in encouraging supportive care through empowerment of direct care providers. Key characteristics of this culture change include: (a) fostering resident-directed care, for example, by allowing residents to determine their own daily schedules, providing resident-centered approaches to ADL care, and involving residents in decisions involving their care; (b) supporting a team approach to care; (c) cross-training staff; (d) making the organization less hierarchical; and (e) empowering direct care staff by placing them on management teams and providing them with decision-making abilities and opportunities [8].

Institutional policies can have a tremendous impact in supporting activities of daily living and preventing uncomfortable behavioural symptoms. Leadership is critical to providing optimal care and to improving care provision. Table 20.3 provides an example of how organizational changes at the facility level can improve the oral intake of persons with dementia; creative approaches can similarly foster supportive care in other areas as well.

Table 20.3 Examples of organizational changes at the facility level to improve food and fluid intake during meal times

Increase the number of persons available to offer assistance. Use the 'all hands on deck' approach.
Teach non-nursing staff (e.g. social workers, occupational therapists, business and office staff) to provide needed assistance at mealtimes.
Encourage, train, and support family members to visit during meals, to provide assistance and socialization.
Hold regular staff & resident meetings to discuss mealtime and food concerns.
Provide assistance in small groups for those who respond to verbal prompts.
Make food and fluid intake a quality improvement target. Create an interdisciplinary task force.

Supporting the person with end-stage dementia

Many assisted living facilities aim to provide services through the terminal phases of dementia, thereby allowing the resident to 'die in place'. Generally, this is accomplished by bringing in skilled care services, either through a home health agency or (more commonly) by engaging hospice services. Quality of life and quality of care during the dying process involves relieving physical symptoms, knowing and honouring the individual's wishes, assuring dignity, caring for spiritual needs, supporting involved family, and providing a dying experience that is satisfying for all involved (for an example of this approach, see Chapter 31).

In an examination of end-of-life care in both assisted living and nursing homes, our research team conducted 581 interviews with staff and 293 interviews with family care providers of persons who had recently died. The results indicated that residents dying with dementia in assisted living more often had a private room, received fewer non-palliative medical services (e.g. nutritional supplements, antibiotics, and calls for emergency services on the last day of life), used physical restraints less often, and communicated better with family members than was the case in nursing homes. Symptom care did not differ; however, skin ulcers occurred more commonly in the assisted living group. We concluded that quality of care was similar in the two settings and that assisted living facilities can provide quality end-of-life care [9].

Dementia-specific assisted living units and facilities

Alzheimer's specific facilities have been growing in number during the past two decades. Particularly rapid has been growth of larger (>15 bed) dementia-specific facilities. One typical example is the Claire Bridge facilities operated by Brookdale Senior Living, the largest provider of Assisted Living services in the US; as of 2009, there were 86 such facilities in operation in the US (http://www.brookdaleliving.com/alzheimers-dementia-care.aspx).

The typology developed by Davis et al. [10] is useful in understanding the variety of forms of dementia-specific care that have evolved in US assisted living. This typology is summarized in Table 20.4. Several examples and case studies are included in the US Alzheimer's Association's 1994 manual entitled *Residential Settings: An Examination of Alzheimer Issues* [11].

Debate rages on the relative value of dementia-specific care versus integration of dementia care into general assisted living facilities. Proponents of dementia-specific settings stress the need for specialized training and programming for persons with dementia, and the relative intolerance of cognitively intact persons of behavioural symptoms. Proponents of integrated settings assert that a good setting should be able to provide individualized care for all residents, regardless of needs, and note that persons with dementia are ubiquitous in assisted living settings. Little research has

Table 20.4 Types of dementia-specific assisted living settings

Type	Description of typical site	Comments
Dementia-specific small home	Less than 10–15 beds; owner-operator is small businessperson who lives on site	Least costly option; very homelike; quality is largely operator-dependent
Multiple dementia-specific small homes with a central administration	Several small, freestanding homes that are clustered nearby or on same property; standardized policies; professional staff (nurse, activities, social work) are shared and split time across multiple homes	Combines the personal, homelike nature of small settings with the professionalism of larger ones; similar to Green House model in nursing homes but evolved earlier
Dementia-specific large home	More than 10–15 beds; generally corporate owned/operated; built specifically for persons with dementia	Commonly are corporate owned; often in chains with standardized training and programmes; much attention to physical environment
Dementia-specific unit within a large assisted living facility	Dedication of one wing or area in a larger facility to persons with dementia	Particularly common in small towns or suburbs, or in large facilities. Dedicated staff, rather than staff recruiting across units, appears to be a key to success
Assisted living component within a nursing home	Beds integrated into a nursing home unit, but not certified by Medicaid or Medicare. Staffing, services, and quality of care tend to reflect the nursing home in which the beds are located	An aberration of the US certification process, whereby for years it was much easier to get beds certified as assisted living than as nursing home beds, thereby leading to nursing homes adding assisted living beds to increase the bed capacity of new construction. Tend to be operated as nursing home units

Adapted from [10].

been conducted comparing dementia-specific settings in assisted living. One small published study found no differences in health outcomes [12], a finding that mirrors results from nursing homes [13].

Conclusions and future directions

As assisted living has become an increasingly large provider of care for persons with dementia, providing quality care in this setting has become increasingly important. For assisted living providers desiring to provide optimal care for persons with dementia, the US Alzheimer's Association is developing a series of position statements and guidelines, which are available for free. Parts one and two of these recommendations cover food and fluid consumption, pain management, social engagement, resident wandering, falls, and physical restraint-free care [14]. Part three addresses end-of-life care [15]. The association plans to develop additional materials in the future.

Practically speaking, the main differences between assisted living and nursing homes are that assisted living employs fewer professionals, has fewer (though still many) regulations, and provides care at lower costs. All indications thus far are that the quality of care is equivalent, with the possible exception of persons who have severe medical problems requiring frequent physician and skilled nursing, monitoring, and care. Since nursing home care is by no means optimal, it follows that there is also room for improvement in assisted living. The challenges are imposing, as persons with dementia are complex and the resources in both nursing homes and assisted living are limited. Nonetheless, it is clear that quality of care is gradually improving, and that knowledge of effective management methods is growing. Clearly, assisted living has an important position in current and future dementia care, and so efforts should continue to identify best care models and to promulgate them throughout the industry.

References

1. Kane R, Wilson KB (1993). Assisted living in the United States: A New Paradigm for Residential Care for Frail Older Persons. Washington DC: AARP Public Policy Institute.

2. Morgan LA, Gruber-Baldini AL, Magaziner J (2001). Resident characteristics, in Zimmerman S, Sloane PD, Eckert JK (eds) *Assisted Living: Needs, Practices and Policies in Residential Care for the Elderly*, pp. 144–172. Baltimore: Johns Hopkins University Press.

3. Zimmerman S, Sloane PD, Eckert JK, *et al.* (2001). Overview of the collaborative studies of long-term care, in Zimmerman S, Sloane PD, Eckert JK (eds) *Assisted Living: Needs, Practices and Policies in Residential Care for the Elderly*. Baltimore: Johns Hopkins University Press.

4. Zimmerman SI, Sloane PD (1999). Optimum residential care for people with dementia. *Generations*, **23**(3), 62–68.

5. Zimmerman S, Sloane PD, Williams CS, *et al.* (2007). Residential care/assisted living staff may detect undiagnosed dementia using the Minimum Data Set Cognition Scale (MDS-COGS). *J Am Geriatr Soc*, **55**, 1349–1355.

6. Sloane PD, Zimmerman S, Williams CS, Reed PS, Gill K, Preisser JS (2005). Evaluating the quality of life of long-term care residents with dementia. *Gerontologist*, **45** (Special issue #1), 37–49.

7. Teri L, Huda P, Gibbons L, Young H, van Leynseele J (2005). STAR: a dementia-specific training program for staff in assisted living residences. *Gerontologist*, **45**, 686–93.

8. Doty MM, Koren MJ, Sturla EL (2008). Culture change in nursing homes: how far have we come? Findings from The Commonwealth Fund 2007 National Survey of Nursing Homes, New York: The Commonwealth Fund. Available at http://www.commonwealthfund.org/Content/Publications/Fund-Reports/2008/May/Culture-Change-in-Nursing-Homes--How-Far-Have-We-Come--Findings-From-The-Commonwealth-Fund-2007-Nati.aspx.

9. Sloane PD, Zimmerman S, Williams CS, Hanson LC (2008). Dying with dementia in long-term care. *Gerontologist*, **48**, 741–751.

10. Davis KJ, Sloane PD, Mitchell CM, *et al.* (2000). Specialized dementia programs in residential care settings. *Gerontologist*, **40**, 32–42.

11. Alzheimer's Association (1994). *Residential Settings: An Examination of Alzheimer Issues*. Chicago: Alzheimer's Disease and Related Disorders Association.

12. Samus QM, Mayer L, Baker A, *et al.* (2008). Characteristics and outcomes for assisted living residents with dementia: comparing dementia-specific care units with non-dementia-specific care units. *JAGS*, **56**, 1361–1363.

13. Phillips CD, Hawes C, Sloane P, *et al.* (1997). Effects of residence in Alzheimer's Special Care Units (SCUs) on functional outcomes. *JAMA*, **278**, 1340–1344.

14. http://www.alz.org/national/documents/brochure_DCPRphases1n2.pdf. [Accessed 1 April, 2009].

15. http://www.alz.org/national/documents/brochure_DCPRphase3.pdf. [Accessed 1 April, 2009].

Chapter 21

Spiritual care of people with dementia and their carers

Stephen Sapp

Preliminary considerations

For most of human history, physicians were unable to do anything truly meaningful to heal sick people; in the absence of the ability to *cure*, all that remained to them was to *care* for the ill. With the rise in modern scientific medicine, the ability to cure has progressed by leaps and bounds over the past half-century, but during the same period the medical establishment has received increasing criticism for its loss of caring, one of the major factors leading to the call for movements such as supportive care. Currently, dementias of the type addressed in this volume return medicine to its earlier situation of being unable to cure; in this situation, caring for the *whole* person, not just the person's body, once again becomes paramount, and this fact necessarily raises the spiritual question.

Attending to the spiritual needs of a person with dementia and his or her carers, in fact, is arguably the most important element in a truly supportive approach that aims to provide multi-disciplinary holistic care of patients and their families from diagnosis to death. Indeed, until very recently, religion and medicine have been inextricably linked for the reason just cited: in the absence of the ability to cure the body, people turned to those who offered the only help available when someone was ill – namely, the shaman, priest, or *medicine* man – who could prepare the person for death, the inevitable outcome of virtually all illnesses. In short, the *healer* has, for most part of human history, been seen to be the person who *cared* for people's souls, not the one who could realistically be expected to *cure* their bodies.

In the analogous situation created today by inevitably fatal dementias, it is, therefore, essential to recognize once again that a person's basic view of health and illness, life and death, and thus, of people who are ill and dying is not really a scientific matter at all, even though, obviously, the basic processes that bring about illness and death are. All that scientists *as* scientists can do is describe those processes. The question of attitudes towards illness and death – what it *means* to be sick and to die and how one should treat people who are sick and dying – is a philosophical/theological question, that is, a question of *value*. And finding the answer to that question demands a journey inwards (or perhaps outwards) to a place that science by its own admission cannot reach because that is not its goal or subject matter.

Modern medicine may be able to describe better and better the biological processes that bring about illness and death in the human organism, but the question of what being ill means, and how one should respond to it – both in oneself and in others – goes beyond any scientific description to a fundamental understanding of the nature and purpose of human life itself. And spirituality, broadly construed, serves as the source of values and of answers to such 'big questions'. Certainly, several of the biggest of these questions relate to illness, impending death, the meaning of growing old, and one's responsibilities to those who face these inevitabilities of human existence.

Serious illness and impending death focus one's attention on ultimate concerns, and these are precisely the issues that religion has always addressed. In short, scientific medicine may be able to provide us the *means* to live longer and healthier lives, but it is utterly powerless to offer us any *meaning* to live for. But that is precisely what spiritual care does offer and, therefore, why it is so crucial in supportive dementia care.

The problem of definition

Despite its critical importance, however, discussing the spiritual dimension of supportive care for persons with dementia and their carers is a more daunting task in some ways than examining the medical and even social aspects of the topic. Although it is true that the cause of the most prevalent form of dementia, Alzheimer's disease, is unknown and that many variations appear in the course of the illness as experienced by different people, medical professionals can, nonetheless, diagnose the illness with very high probability, anticipate the physical changes it will occasion and the consequent psychological and behavioural manifestations, and offer specific ways to manage the illness even if no cure is currently available. Similarly, although the particular situations in which persons with dementia and their carers find themselves vary widely, mental health professionals and social service providers have developed effective approaches and support systems that help those involved cope more or less effectively with the problems that they face in their daily lives.

When spirituality is the topic of conversation, however, speaking even this concretely becomes much more difficult. In the first place, to what is one referring? 'Spirituality' (and 'religion') defy precise, universally accepted definition because both words are very multi-faceted. A useful starting point is the suggestion that spirituality 'can be understood outside a specifically religious context as the human need to construct a sense of meaning in life'[1; p. 19]. An oft-suggested way to conceptualize this construction of meaning in life is to see spirituality as speaking of that which gives one a sense of *connectedness* – to oneself, to others, to the natural world, and to that which transcends all of these categories, a transpersonal source of power commonly called the sacred, the divine, or God, what Twelve-Step Programmes refer to as a 'Higher Power', however conceived by a given individual. Spirituality refers to the suprasensible 'something there' in human existence, which deals with an awareness of being part of something bigger than the individual self or even the entire material order:

> It is as if there were in the human consciousness a *sense of reality, a feeling of objective presence, a perception* of what we may call '*something there*,' more deep and more general than any of the special and particular 'senses' by which the current psychology supposes existent realities to be originally revealed [2; p. 61].

Human beings seem to need to know their place in the universe, how they 'fit in', how they are connected to everything else around them, and thus ultimately the meaning of their own existence – in short, why they are here and 'what it's all about'. Spirituality, therefore, is often especially associated with questions about finding 'meaning' and 'purpose' in human existence, particularly, in the last stage of a person's life when one's impending death renders unavoidable the question of what one's life has meant.

With this understanding of spirituality, 'religion' can be seen as offering specific concepts, symbols, norms, words, rituals, and the like with which to conceptualize, reflect upon, express, and understand this multi-dimensional connectedness and to formalize (some would say 'routinize') the 'Something There' that humans experience. In short, religion tends towards the 'institutionalization' or 'regularization' of the spiritual, that is, what is commonly associated with church, synagogue, or mosque. As it is sometimes put: 'Spirituality is God's reaching out to us and religion is our response'.

It should be noted that the two concepts are not opposed to each other, as common usage often implies – 'Oh, I'm not religious at all, but I'm very spiritual' – and for many people they overlap a great deal or are even identical. The eminent American religious historian Martin Marty, in fact, has coined the terms 'unmoored spirituality' (that which is not associated with formal religion) and 'moored spirituality' (that which is) to suggest that those who claim to be 'spiritual' in the current usage of the term do not have exclusive access to the commodity to the exclusion of the traditionally religious, who can also be very 'spiritual' within their own more formal traditions [3].

The matter of increased religious pluralism

Apart from the problem of simply defining the focus of a discussion of 'spiritual care', an examination of how to provide supportive spiritual care is complicated greatly by the many different spiritual paths people currently follow. Although in 'the West', it is tempting to start from a stance rooted in the traditionally dominant religions of Europe and North America (Christianity and Judaism), many factors have combined over the past half-century to render such an approach impossible. The three most obvious of these are the decline of the hegemony of Christianity, the large numbers of migrants from Africa and Asia who have created vibrant communities that practise their own non-Christian religions, and the rise of 'new religious movements', all of which have created a religious pluralism that makes very complex any attempt at a general discussion of spiritual care, essential as this component is in supportive care. Furthermore, several scholars of religion have argued that attempting to devise a generic approach to inherently 'religious' issues that is divorced from specific religious traditions renders it empty and meaningless, thus making any such discussion of 'spiritual' care of (at best) little use to clinicians and other care providers who want to take this dimension of experience seriously.

Basic principles of supportive spiritual care

Nonetheless, certain points can be made with regard to supportive spiritual care that apply to most of the situations care providers encounter, with a critical caveat: it is absolutely necessary to discover and respect each person's own distinctive and particular religious/spiritual preference to render truly supportive spiritual care. It goes without saying that those seeking to offer such care must respect the beliefs, values, concerns, and opinions of the person with dementia and not impose their own views. It is equally essential, however, to go beyond merely respecting individuals' beliefs and values to foster an atmosphere in which people can talk openly about concerns beyond the biophysical or even the psychosocial. They must be free to express and explore personal beliefs and disbeliefs, to ask for the input of others, to seek any source available to come to terms with their situations, and to be at peace with themselves. Helping this to occur is an important task for the physicians, nurses, chaplains, and other clergy, relatives, and friends. Because dementia and approaching death evoke inherently spiritual questions (about life and death, pain and suffering, why and why not), care providers must be prepared to offer resources and support people with dementia and their carers in their struggle to find meaning in their situation. When people who are struggling with dementia are unable to satisfy their *spiritual* needs, increased stress and suffering are as likely to occur as when physical or social needs are not met; pain is not limited to the physical realm.

James F. Drane makes the point clear in a reference that concerns the doctor–patient relationship specifically, but which is equally applicable to the role played by any member of the care team:

> But the fact is that both in doctors and in their patients, one will find non-scientific beliefs which stand at the center of who they are as persons. It is not required that every doctor–patient contact touch these deeper belief dimensions of personality, but there are times when ignoring these amounts to abandonment of the patient. Illness, especially serious illness, will call up every patient's belief system. Sometimes, his or her belief system may be adequate to handle what is happening, but not always. A particular patient may be struggling to make some sense out of illness, and the doctor may be the only person who can help. Sometimes, even secular doctors are forced to confront the deeper religious dimensions of life. [4; p. 123]

If this is the case with illness in general, how much more so when the illness is one like dementia; and if it is the case with physicians, how much more so with other carers who are likely to spend more time with the person.

The first task, then, for those who wish to provide supportive care to persons with dementia and their carers is to acknowledge that the spiritual dimension is essential to such care and to encourage exploration of it. Although this statement may seem unnecessary, given the accepted understanding of supportive care as the multi-disciplinary holistic care of patients and their families, it is all too easy for practitioners in some disciplines to dismiss, or at least to discount, the central role that spiritual concerns play in that holism, in dementia no less (and perhaps even more) than in most other illnesses. Indeed, it can be argued that far more than even cancer, say, dementia is inherently a 'spiritual disease' because it strikes at the heart of what most people today consider our very humanity, namely, our rational self-awareness and thus our sense of self. It has even been suggested that Alzheimer's is the 'Theological Disease' because it raises, 'theological and ecclesiological problems of enormous significance for all of us since they strike at the heart of who we are and what we may become' [5; p. 38]. As the disease progresses, a person's awareness of self, as that crucial concept is typically understood, with all that it connotes and means to us in terms of our personal identity and self-understanding, gradually declines and ultimately disappears (but see Chapter 23 for a challenge to this idea on the basis of good communication). It is also worthy of note that many people today find the prospect of dementia more terrifying than that of cancer, and for good reason: almost everyone knows someone who has survived cancer, often with no terrible long-term effects; no one, however, has ever been called a 'dementia survivor' and, given the progression that the malady follows and the inevitable outcome (as described elsewhere in this volume), it has a truly frightening prospect.

In light of the earlier discussion about spirituality as a sense of the self's connectedness with that which transcends it, however, the prospect of losing that self may appear to undermine the claim that dementia is an inherently 'spiritual' disease: if one no longer has a self to be connected to the 'Something There' (or the awareness of having one, at least), is spirituality even an issue? It is difficult to respond to this challenge without calling upon teachings of particular religious traditions that refute it, at least for those who adhere to those religions (but see the discussions of personhood by Dekkers in Chapter 27, and of selfhood by Sabat in Chapter 24). Still, even without citing explicit theological doctrines of a given religion, one can appeal to the broader cultural tradition that has been almost universally accepted in the West until quite recently and affirm: 'Human beings are much more than sharp minds, powerful rememberers, and economic successes' [6; p. 3]. If care providers remain constantly mindful of this, they are much more likely to treat everyone in their care in an appropriate way.

Although it is beyond the scope of this chapter to present an adequate discussion of a concept as complex as the Buddha's notion of 'no-self' (*anatman*), [7; pp. 122–124] it is instructive to mention it in this context to demonstrate that some spiritual traditions do not rely upon the highly refined sense of individuality, and thus, the all-important notion of 'self' that the religions more familiar in Europe and the United States put at their core. Indeed, the same can be said of the monism of classical Hinduism as well, in which the sense of separateness, and thus, the individual self-identity that the West holds so dear are, in fact, merely *maya,* part of the world of illusion that keeps us from realizing our true identity as the one, all-encompassing Brahman that is what really is and is in fact *all* that really is [7; p. 64]. If two major spiritual traditions can still affirm the value of human beings without basing it upon a doctrine of selfhood – indeed, in their traditional forms, each has been considerably more tolerant and open to various spiritual paths to liberation – perhaps the near-obsession of the Western tradition with individual identity as lodged in a rational, conscious entity called the 'self' is not so central in defining what it means to be human, and thus, its 'loss' is not so definitive of the worth and dignity of persons.

Supportive spiritual care of persons with dementia and their carers, therefore, means first and foremost, above all and beneath all, remembering that they are fellow human beings who should be respected and treated with all the dignity due to them. This is easier to do with regard to the carers; ignoring them and neglecting to provide the support of all kinds they desperately need demonstrates a failure to value them adequately. Not treating people with dementia in this way, however, is an all too common practice. An excellent illustration is an anecdote told by the eminent social worker/researcher Elaine Brody about a very old woman admitted to the Philadelphia Geriatric Center with advanced dementia. She had been unable to communicate for some time, but her only real behavioural problem was that she screamed without letup every time she was bathed. The staff, concerned about her obvious distress, talked to her family members, who could offer no explanation. So, they tried changing the temperature of water, playing soft music, and talking to her in a soothing way, but nothing helped. Then, during one of her baths, a staff member came into the room to tell the nurse's aide something she didn't want the other residents to overhear. As soon as she closed the door, the woman stopped screaming. From then on, as long as the door was closed, she accepted her daily bath with no protest; if the door were inadvertently left open, however, she screamed until the bath was over and she was dressed or the door was closed.

This story is important for two reasons: first, it challenges many assumptions about what persons with dementia can understand, even in later stages of their illness. Second and more important, it illustrates quite clearly that – even in conditions of severe mental and physical impairment – people hold onto their sense of dignity and suffer if that dignity is violated. The truth is that it is impossible to know what a person with dementia is comprehending or aware of, and reports abound about people who have been totally non-communicative for some time but suddenly join in the singing of a favourite hymn or the recitation of a familiar prayer. Indeed, providing spiritual care for those who have lived their lives in a particular religious tradition often involves moving beyond the verbal and into the symbolic because even when such people can no longer engage in higher level interactions or discussions of religious concepts, they often still respond to music (especially 'old favourite' hymns), familiar prayers and rituals, and physical symbols (a clergy collar, crucifix, communion chalice, or icon). As the disease progresses, those caring for people with dementia need to move more towards the familiar and the less cognitive. Instead of trying to explain or describe – for example – God's grace and love, they must embody it, demonstrating it in their own actions and through familiar rituals and symbols. And though from the limited human perspective of contemporary science people with late-stage dementia appear to have little capacity for conscious spiritual expression, if spirituality is seen as a sense of connectedness with something beyond oneself as suggested earlier, normal human interactions of tender touches, gentle words, and familiar faces and places (to the extent possible) certainly remain essential in truly supportive spiritual care.

A good illustration of the power of symbols to provide spiritual comfort for people with dementia is the story of the woman with Alzheimer's who asked an aide in her long-term care facility what her own name was. When the aide told her, she replied, 'You know, half the time I don't know my own name'. Then she pointed to a crucifix on the wall and said, 'But that's OK because he does, and that's all that matters'. And the continuing importance of familiar religious practices for people with dementia is shown by the woman with dementia who constantly hid her clothes, could not tell sugar from salt, and demanded potatoes for every meal. She also insisted, however, that she and her husband would kneel beside their bed every night and say 'Our Father'. She was able to go no farther, but her husband finished the prayer, whereupon she would get up and go to bed.

This story illustrates another important principle in spiritual care of persons with dementia if genuinely supportive care is the goal, especially care that recognizes and honours the spiritual dimension in human existence: carers must become 'memory keepers' for those they care for and remember for them when they are no longer capable of doing so. This is also an example of how a person's narrative unity can be maintained, even in dementia, as discussed by Baldwin in Chapter 26. In fact, one way to respect the humanity of persons with dementia and recognize the 'Something There' that goes beyond the physical that modern society values so highly is to treat them always as if they are fully conscious of how they are being treated, as did the man who prayed with his wife every night.

This basic principle of supportive spiritual care can be amplified by something that my pastoral psychology professor in seminary constantly told the class: 'The individual and not the problem is the focus'. Unfortunately – true to the 'modern' way of approaching practically any issue – we have come to focus so much on the *problem* of dementia that we have in many ways lost sight of the *individual* who has the problem. It is, therefore, especially important in supportive spiritual care of people with dementia and their carers to remember, in words attributed to Sir William Osler, 'It is much more important to know what sort of a patient has a disease than what sort of a disease a patient has'. If care providers strive to learn all they can about who the individual was before the onset of the illness, including the person's tastes and preferences in all of those small things that constitute the real fabric of human life, then they can truly remember for that person and respect his or her humanity by honouring preferences as much as possible. It is true that (as far as can be known) the person may reach the point of not being aware of whether he or she is served vanilla or chocolate ice cream, but if his or her life-long love of chocolate is known and respected, a powerful message is sent that the 'Something There' matters.

In many ways, of course, the predominant medical model of dementia as a progressive and incurable illness that robs people not only of their cognitive ability but of their humanity and dignity as well – indeed, of their very selves – has served contemporary society's values well, making it much easier to deal with people with dementia in a perfunctory, superficial way. After all, if the object of attention is not really a *person* – at least one who is a rational, subjective being with awareness of self and others – why take the time and energy to go through all those motions usually associated with appropriate caring interaction with *persons*? But clearly, this model fails to recognize the essential dignity and worth of every human being that all spiritual traditions affirm, and the approach to 'care' it fosters can hardly be called 'supportive'.

Contemporary society tends to *dismember* people with cognitive deficits, to remove such persons from the organic entity that is society, and thus, to hide them from the public eye, all the while rationalizing doing so by arguing that such beings are not really 'persons' – or at least they are not really *human* – at all. A constant awareness of the spiritual dimension of human existence – perhaps especially as embodied in traditional religions of the West with their central doctrine that every human being is created *imago dei*, in God's own image – serves as a buffer to prevent people with dementia from suffering this dismembering, this removal from the social body and consequent isolation. Indeed, by refusing to accept the currently dominant view, supportive carers can be said to *remember* people with dementia by bringing them back into the community of persons; which makes a link with the idea, in Christian theology, of the 'timeless intercommunion' of the Trinity, where 'the importance of the Trinitarian concept of the person is that we are not alone' [8; pp. 215–216]. This might include among other things, for example, ensuring that people with dementia continue to be included in worship and other types of community activities as long as they are physically able [9].

One final comment on supportive spiritual care of persons with dementia: obviously, the major obstacle to maintaining one's own spiritual life in the face of dementia is the loss of cognitive ability, which our society assumes means that the person can no longer experience God (or the 'Something There') because of the current assumption that everything meaningful in human life depends on a functioning neocortex. In terms of the earlier definition of religion as consisting of the formal structures in which humans try to capture and express their spiritual awareness and experience, thus regularizing it, and giving it substance, it may well be the case that people with dementia reach the point where they can no longer find such forms meaningful. It cannot be said with certainty, however, that they cannot still experience spirituality even after they may not be able to participate in religion. To put it in traditional religious terminology, 'God never forgets', even if people might when they suffer from dementia or when others (all too often) want to act on the maxim 'out of their mind, out of our sight'! [10] No one, however, can say (in a theistic context) that God cannot continue to speak to even the most severely demented person if God so chooses (or that some sense of the 'Something There' cannot endure, to put it less theistically), whatever the current scientific understanding of the brain asserts about a person's ability to comprehend human communication.

Conclusions

It has long been accepted among those working with dementia that this particular malady is a 'family illness' [11,12], meaning that care providers' attention must focus not only on the person with dementia but also on other members of the family, especially the person(s) providing on-site care. Beyond the truly significant challenges of everyday living that the progressive deterioration associated with dementia raises for carers, many more issues that can only be characterized as 'spiritual' also arise. Among the most widely noted of these are loss, grief, guilt, anger, and a sense of helplessness and hopelessness, all of which concern matters that touch the spirit and that religious traditions have long addressed. Again, the importance of discovering where each carer is in his or her personal spiritual journey is essential to bringing to bear all the resources available to respond to such issues (and if doing so is beyond the competence or comfort level of any given care provider, that person must be willing to enlist the assistance of those who are able to meet such needs).

A particularly promising approach to supportive care for people with dementia and their carers has been articulated thus: '. . . consider a new way of thinking: what if you were to approach car-*egiving* not as a two-step dance ("I give and you receive"), but as a dance of care*sharing* with multiple partners where each person is giving and receiving?' [13; p. 2]. (Once again, interestingly, we might recall that the early Greek word for the Trinity was *perichoresis*, or 'round dance'. [8]) Caresharing is a specific application of the view more broadly applicable to genuinely supportive care in general advocated by the late Tom Kitwood, a trailblazer in caring for people with dementia in a way that truly honours the spiritual dimension as set forth in this chapter:

> Care is much more than a matter of individuals attending to individuals. Ideally, it is the work of a team of people whose values are aligned, and whose talents are liberated in achieving a shared objective. It is unlikely that this will happen just by chance. [14]

In sum, carers have two fundamental needs from a supportive care perspective: they need to be encouraged that – despite the inevitable outcome – the care they are providing is not in vain; and they need to hear that the care recipients' lives are ultimately meaningful despite the unavoidable decline and death that accompany dementia. And as the 'things of this world', which the modern world has come to rely upon for meaning, necessarily diminish in importance and begin to disappear, if carers for persons with dementia are to maintain hope and a sense of the meaningfulness of life, as is the case with those for whom they care, the source of that hope and meaning must increasingly be that which transcends the earthly dimension, namely, the things of the spirit.

And so, this chapter concludes as it began, with the affirmation that far from being peripheral or even unnecessary in supportive care for people with dementia and their carers, spiritual care may well be the most important component of truly supportive care.

References

1. Payne BP, McFadden S (1994). From loneliness to solitude: religious and spiritual journeys in late life, in Thomas LE, Eisenhandler SA (eds) *Aging and the religious dimension*, Westport, CT: Auburn House.

2. James W (1958). Lecture III: the reality of the unseen, in *The varieties of religious experience: a study in human nature*. New York: Penguin Books.

3. Marty M (2006). in Kliewer SP, Saultz JW (eds) *Healthcare and spirituality*, pp. 14–15. Oxford and Ashland: Radcliffe Publishing.

4. Drane JF (1995). *Becoming a good doctor: the place of virtue and character in medical ethics*, 2nd edn. Kansas City, MO: Sheed & Ward.

5. Keck D (1996). *Forgetting whose we are: Alzheimer's disease and the love of god*. Nashville, TN: Abingdon Press.

6. Post S (1993). *The moral challenge of Alzheimer disease*. Baltimore, MD: Johns Hopkins Press.

7. Ellwood RS, McGraw BA (2009). *Many people, many faiths: women and men in the world religions*, 9th edn. Upper Saddle River, NJ: Pearson Education.

8. Allen FB, Coleman PG (2006). Spiritual perspectives on the person with dementia: identity and personhood, in Hughes JC, Louw SJ, Sabat SR (eds) *Dementia: mind, meaning, and the person*, pp. 205–221. Oxford: Oxford University Press.

9. Pohlman E, Bloom G (eds). *Worship services for people with Alzheimer's disease and their families: a handbook*. Troy, NY: Eddy Alzheimer's Services; Albany, New York: Northeastern New York Chapter of the Alzheimer's Association (85 Watervliet Avenue, Albany, NY 12206).

10. Sapp S (1997). Memory: the community looks backward, and hope: the community looks forward, in McKim D (ed) *God never forgets: faith, hope and Alzheimer's disease*, Louisville, KY: Westminster John Knox Press.

11. Cohen, D, Eisdorfer, C (2002). *The loss of self: a family resource for the care of Alzheimer's disease and related disorders*, rev. edn. New York: W.W. Norton.

12. Mace N, Rabins P (2001). *The 36-hour day: a family guide to caring for persons with Alzheimer's disease, related dementing illnesses, and memory loss in later life*, 3rd edn. New York: Warner Books.

13. Richards M (2009). *Caresharing: a reciprocal approach to caregiving and care receiving in the complexities of aging, illness or disability*. Woodstock, VT: Skylight Paths Publishing.

14. Kitwood T (1997). *Dementia reconsidered: the person comes first*. Philadelphia, PA: Open University Press.

Chapter 22

Anticipatory and disenfranchised grief among dementia family caregivers: helping spouse and adult-child caregivers to cope

Jacquelyn Frank

Introduction

The progressive nature of Alzheimer's disease (AD) has been called 'the long goodbye' for one good reason: many losses occur throughout the course of the disease. Some of these losses, such as *psychosocial death* (i.e. the loss of interpersonal relationships with the affected person), may be more difficult to manage than the eventual bodily death. It has been suggested that the pre-death grief of caregivers of people with dementia has the same intensity and characteristics as post-death grief [1]. As grief occurs in response to these losses, an important component of grief-related support is normalization (i.e. 'it is OK to grieve'). Because many caregivers do not receive support in relation to their emotional losses, they may feel 'disenfranchised' in their grief and unsure how to respond to their feelings or to work through their on-going grief [2].

Drawing on data from qualitative and quantitative studies, this chapter will examine the grief and loss experiences among dementia caregivers in order to offer new directions for supportive care. Of special note will be the differences between the grief experiences and coping mechanisms displayed by adult-child versus spouse caregivers. The variation in their coping mechanisms has implications for the types of support that will help to alleviate grief and loss among caregivers, thereby helping the person with dementia as well.

Prior to beginning a discussion on caregiver grief and loss, it is critical to note that people with dementia also experience anticipatory grief and loss as they battle with their illness. While the present chapter will focus on caregivers, it is essential to remember that the person with dementia can also face these same feelings and should not be overlooked.

Caregiver burden, anticipatory grief, and ambiguous loss

Feelings of loss and grief are frequent companions for current dementia family caregivers. Increased acknowledgement and understanding of caregiver grief amongst researchers have led to more comprehensive explorations of the multi-faceted nature of caregiver grief and loss. The investigation of caregiver grief and loss has grown out of the research on caregiver burden.

The concept of caregiver burden is now widely used to refer to physical, psychological or emotional, social, and financial problems experienced by family members caring for impaired older adults. Alternatively, physical health, mental health, social participation, and financial resources have also been viewed as dimensions of well-being [3]. Researchers studying caregiver burden have examined a number of different dimensions including depressive symptoms, effects of care recipient behaviour on the caregiver, role strain, self-esteem, emotional distress, life satisfaction, time spent on social activities, relationship strain, and physical health [4–6]. Because of the cognitive impairments and behavioural changes caused by the progression of the disease, individuals with AD often require 24-hour supervision, even during the early stages of the disease. As a result, Alzheimer's caregivers often experience shifts in family role dynamics, loss of intimacy, and feelings of isolation. The impact that such intensive caregiving can have on family and daily life is a primary reason why caregiver burden has received so much attention in the Alzheimer's literature and why caring for someone with AD has been referred to as a 'career'. It is important to note that caregiver burden and well-being research also show that some caregivers report positive outcomes from their caregiving experience (i.e. a sense of competence, satisfaction, a sense of meaning, etc.). This point will be re-examined later in the chapter when discussing adult-child caregiving experiences. Closely linked to burden is the experience of grief and loss while caregiving.

Anticipatory grief is the concept first presented by Erich Lindemann in 1944 and was further defined by Rando as [7]:

> The phenomenon encompassing the processes of mourning, coping, interaction, planning, and psychosocial reorganization that are stimulated and begun in part in response to the awareness of the impending loss of a loved one and the recognition of associated losses in the past, present, and future. (p. 24)

Such losses can become particularly profound with dementia as both the person with the disease and the family caregiver must constantly readjust their reality and expectations for functioning, communication, and interaction. The losses that accompany dementia are experienced as *ambiguous losses*. Boss defined ambiguous loss as 'an unclear loss – a loved one missing either physically or psychologically' [8; p. 237]. There are two major types of ambiguous loss. First is 'physical absence with psychological presence' and is exemplified through the loss felt by family members when a solider has gone missing in action [9]. The second type of ambiguous loss is 'psychological absence with physical presence' and is epitomized by the experience of caring for a family member with dementia. Boss *et al.* (1988) also refer to this form of ambiguous loss as *boundary ambiguity* [10; p. 125].

Ambiguous loss is an ongoing process that can be seen as having three phases [11]. The first phase is 'anticipatory loss' which centres on the losses that *can be expected* to be felt as the disease progresses. Phase II is 'progressive loss', and it is distinguished by the pain and anguish that family members feel as they watch the deterioration of the family member they are caring for (and truly experiencing the psychosocial loss). Phase III, 'acknowledged loss', usually occurs during the later stage of caregiving and takes one of two main paths: acceptance or avoidance. If acceptance accompanies acknowledged loss, then this means that the caregiver or family member is accepting the changes that have occurred in the person they are caring for, acknowledging they feel these losses, and then, dealing with the situation (and care recipient) as they now are – not as the person they used to be. However, acknowledged loss does not always come with acceptance. Instead, some take the path of avoidance. For Dupuis [11], this means that the caregiver knows the loss has occurred and does acknowledge it – but he or she avoids dealing with the full reality of the changed family dynamic and relationship. These two divergent paths can certainly have implications for the types of interventions and assistance that caregivers might seek out.

In the realm of dementia caregiving, anticipatory grief and ambiguous loss naturally weave closely together. Ambiguous loss can result in unresolved grief because caregivers (and other family members) experience the 'psychosocial death' of the person with dementia, meaning that 'the persona of the individual is so changed that others experience the loss of that person as he or she previously existed' [12]. This sense of loss can be severe and result in ongoing grief for the caregiver during the course of the disease. In fact, a study conducted by Frank [13] of over 400 dementia family caregivers revealed that aspects of grief and loss are the major difficulties they face in caring for their loved ones.

Disenfranchised grief

Dementia family caregivers not only experience burden, anticipatory mourning, and ambiguous loss, but they are also in the unusual position of experiencing *disenfranchised grief* often.

> Disenfranchised grief refers to losses that are not appreciated by others. In effect, the individual has no perceived 'right' to mourn. The loss is not openly acknowledged or socially sanctioned and publically shared. Others simply do not understand why this loss is mourned, and they may fail to validate and support the grief. [2; p. 143]

Disenfranchised grief can happen because of three reasons: (1) the relationship is not recognized by others because it is not based on kin-ties; (2) the loss itself is not recognized because it is not socially defined as significant; and (3) the griever is not recognized. Dementia caregivers most often experience the second type of disenfranchised grief where they deal with the psychological death of the person they knew and mourn the relationship they have lost as the dementia progresses. Disenfranchised grief is a paradox because it creates additional grief for the sufferer while limiting or eliminating sources of support because such grief is often not acknowledged or understood by others [14]. Caregivers' grief can be disenfranchised by their own family members and close friends as well. Some family members may be in denial that anything is wrong or simply not understand the full impact dementia has on the person and his or her family. Thus, even though the person with dementia is still alive, the caregiver might be experiencing intense grief, but those around the caregiver do not necessarily understand that a 'loss' is taking place.

In recent years, organizations such as the Alzheimer's Association have become more aware of the symptoms of grief and are attempting to educate caregivers on this vast issue. At first, grief can be difficult to detect because of the numerous ways it can manifest itself. Denial, periods of helplessness and despair, withdrawal from activities, anger, frustration, and guilt are all signs of grief. It is only recently that these symptoms have been acknowledged as signs of *grief* among caregivers rather than categorized as stress or depression. One of the major reasons why this grief has come to our attention is because of the scholarly attempts to measure it. A particularly significant tool in grief research is the Marwit-Meuser Caregiver Grief Inventory (MM-CGI).

The three dimensions of the MM-CGI: a tool to help measure caregiver grief

The MM-CGI is an empirically derived instrument used to measure grief among dementia family caregivers [15]. The model developed is important because it is sensitive not only to the differences in grief experiences between adult-child and spouse caregivers but also to the stage of AD experienced by the care recipient. The MM-CGI is a psychometric inventory consisting of 50 items and is designed to measure levels of grief in current Alzheimer's family caregivers. It consists of three factors (or subscales) that capture the different grief-related issues that caregivers might be experiencing. The first factor (or subscale), 'personal sacrifice burden', takes into account what the caregiver gives up because of the caregiver role such as 'loss of personal freedom, loss of sleep, compromised health, and loss of energy'. 'Heartfelt sadness and longing' is the second factor, and it revolves around the emotional and intrapersonal aspects of caregiving, such as longing for how life used to be, feelings of loss, and difficulty with accepting the present situation. The third factor, 'worry and felt isolation', focuses on the inherent uncertainty regarding how things will turn out, coupled with isolation caregivers often feel from others, including other family members as well as the wider society.

A study conducted by Frank [13] showed clear links between the three dimensions of the MM-CGI and caregiver's subjective experiences. For example, one spouse caregiver from the study shows the personal sacrifice burden she is experiencing through the following statement:

> Sometimes it's very difficult when you can't get away from your spouse – and they get mad at you when you're gone – and then you spend two hours after that coping with it.

A caregiving daughter also expressed burden in trying to juggle family life with caregiving. She said:

> Balancing time dealing with my husband and my daughter and taking care of my father [is very difficult].

Heartfelt sadness and longing are also experienced both by spouses and by adult children. When asked what the biggest difficulty in caregiving is that she faces, one wife said:

> Loneliness, I see good years of my life slipping by: no traveling, little shopping, little golf games – and guilt for my feelings.

One daughter reflects not only heartfelt sadness but also ambiguous loss when she talks about:

> The sadness of losing mom, but still having her to be cared for.

Expressions of worry and felt isolation are also shown by spouses and adult-child caregivers. One wife said that she is,

> . . . not able to talk to my husband because he can't talk any more. So there is no one to talk over your problems with.

A son caring for his mother said that he,

> . . . feels trapped by the disease. Knowing that I am the only person my mom has there for her. [13]

Because each caregiver experiences loss and grief differently, the inventory is intended to be used either one-to-one with a clinician, or as part of a group to help caregivers gain a better understanding about the nature of their grief, and to analyze how this grief relates to their present life situation. The MM-CGI subscales highlight which domain(s) may be causing the highest emotional stress for individual caregivers (e.g. one caregiver may experience very high scores under the heartfelt sadness and longing factor, whereas another caregiver may be experiencing increased grief in the domain of worry and felt isolation). Such variation in scores illustrates that grief and loss can be experienced quite differently among Alzheimer's family caregivers.

Grief differences among adult-children and spouse caregivers

When trying to help adult-child and spouse dementia caregivers handle their anticipatory grief, it is important to be aware of the differences in grief experienced between these two groups of caregivers.

On the basis of studies of grief using the MM-CGI and the MM-CGI Short Form (SF) [13,16–18], it is evident that spouses and adult children often experience different levels of grief intensity than their counterparts. The studies that have used the MM-CGI illustrate interesting grief differences between adult-child and spousal caregivers. For example, spouses experience an escalation of grief as the disease progresses [19,20]. Spouses are also more likely to experience stronger grief reactions related to changes in their relationships with friends and family than their adult-child counterparts [21]. Frank and Johnson [22] also found that personal sacrifice burden and heartfelt sadness and longing were significantly interrelated among spouse caregivers, but not among adult-child caregivers.

The place of residence of the person with AD is also correlated with grief among spousal caregivers. Research reveals that grief increases among spouses after placement in a nursing home, while the same is not the case for adult children [16,19]. Specifically, significantly higher levels of guilt and sadness were expressed among spouses after their partners were placed in a long-term care facility.

By contrast, adult children were more likely to experience anger and frustration as part of their grief experience. Differences can also be found among spouse and adult-child caregivers in relation to stage of the disease, meaning that as the disease progresses, the shape and form of the grief reaction and expression may change – but change on different trajectories for adult children versus spouses.

Coping mechanisms: how caregivers deal with grief

Two recent studies illustrate some interesting differences in coping mechanisms between adult-child and spouse caregivers [13,16]. These differences can help shed light on the types of interventions and programmes that may be best suited for these two different categories of caregivers. As part of a statewide study of 414 adult-child and spouse caregivers, Frank designed a quantitative instrument that included a section on the coping mechanisms caregivers might use to deal with stress and emotional aspects of caregiving, including grief [13]. Table 22.1 contains the 18 questions from this segment of the survey instrument.

The questions were examined statistically to discern differences between adult-child and spouse caregivers. They were also analysed in relation to MM-CGI scores. Three major themes emerged from the data. First, adult children were twice as likely to talk to or spend time with friends in order to cope with the emotional aspects of caregiving than spouses. Adult children were also more likely to talk to family members to help them cope. This finding was supported by a study that found adult children appeared to have more social outlets for support through friends in contrast to spouses, who were more likely to attend support groups to help them cope with feelings of grief and loss [21]. A second theme to emerge from the Frank study was that spousal caregivers perceived that they had much less social support than adult-child caregivers. Caregivers in the study repeatedly lamented the feeling that friends had disappeared since their spouse's diagnosis, and this led them to greater feelings of isolation. Sanders and colleagues also noted:

> The spouses in this study expressed that they had relied on their husband or wife for the majority of their socialization, emotional support, and well being during the course of the marriage. Thus, the onset and decline of dementia had triggered in these spouses a great deal of loss related to the changes in their relationship with their husband or wife, but also other friends and family. [21; p. 515–516]

In addition, Ott et al. [16] found that adult children were more likely to use substances, vent, reframe, and use humour to cope with the grief and losses of caregiving than their spousal counterparts. Coping mechanisms employed by both groups of caregivers who experienced high levels of grief included spiritual faith and pets.

A third theme emerging from the Frank study was not related to coping per se but rather the rewards of caregiving. Various studies show similar results that need to be highlighted [16,23,24].

Table 22.1 Example of instrument to measure coping with stress and emotional aspects of caregiving [13]

Answer key:
1 = never // 2 = rarely // 3 = sometimes // 4 = frequently (about once a week) // 5 = more than once a week

60.	I attend church/synagogue or other religious services to help me cope with the stress of caregiving.	1 2 3 4 5
61.	I pray or read the Bible to help me cope with the stress of caregiving.	1 2 3 4 5
62.	I exercise to help me cope with the stress of caregiving.	1 2 3 4 5
63.	I read books to help me cope with the stress of caregiving.	1 2 3 4 5
64.	I watch movies to help me cope with the stress of caregiving.	1 2 3 4 5
65.	I use respite care services to help me cope with the stress of caregiving.	1 2 3 4 5
66.	I eat to help me cope with the stress of caregiving.	1 2 3 4 5
67.	I drink alcohol to help me cope with the stress of caregiving.	1 2 3 4 5
68.	I attend support group meetings to help me cope with the stress of caregiving.	1 2 3 4 5
69.	I write in a journal or diary to help me cope with the stress of caregiving.	1 2 3 4 5
70.	I use adult day care services to help me cope with the stress of caregiving.	1 2 3 4 5
71.	I listen to music to help me cope with the stress of caregiving.	1 2 3 4 5
72.	I see a psychologist or counselor to help me cope with the stress of caregiving.	1 2 3 4 5
73.	I talk with other family members to help me cope with the stress of caregiving.	1 2 3 4 5
74.	I talk with a friend to help me cope with the stress of caregiving.	1 2 3 4 5
75.	I spend time with my friends to help me cope with the stress of caregiving.	1 2 3 4 5
76.	I attend cultural programmes to help me cope with the stress of caregiving.	1 2 3 4 5
77.	I have hobbies that help me cope with the stress of caregiving.	1 2 3 4 5

Among the study of over 400 caregivers, Frank and Johnson [22] found that adult children experience a much stronger sense of reward from their caregiving experience. Ott *et al.* [16] measured perceived personal growth among spouse and adult-child caregivers and found that adult children scored significantly higher on personal growth than did spouses through a two-way analysis of variance. The difference in experienced reward and personal growth can have implications for potential grief interventions and remind practitioners that not all family caregivers feel negative emotions about caregiving.

Steps towards supportive care for anticipatory grief and ambiguous loss

Currently, there exists a rich body of literature on dementia caregiver interventions, covering important issues such as stress, burden, depression, and coping [25–29]. However, with a few notable exceptions [17,21,30,31] at present, there is little published research focussing on the efficacy of pre-death loss and grief interventions for dementia caregivers, and there is an absence of research exploring the relationship between post-intervention caregiver grief and caregiver well-being over time. In addition, while research has shown that anticipatory grief exists among dementia caregivers [2,30,32], and even serves as a barrier to caring for the person with dementia [13], Zarit and Femia [33] caution researchers against jumping into interventions as if this might provide a panacea.

Specifically, Zarit and Femia point out that researchers cannot assume that all caregivers will benefit from interventions that target a particular risk factor because not all caregivers will have a particular risk factor. Applying this advice to the case of anticipatory grief, unless the caregiver is actually experiencing high levels of grief, it should not be assumed that caregivers want or need a grief intervention. The intervention must be generated on the basis of the caregivers' expressed needs, not on someone else's perception of those needs.

Next, if caregivers are aware that they are experiencing feelings of loss and grief, then avenues need to be provided to help normalize the feelings of grief [2]. The avenues or supports that help normalize feelings of grief and loss should be directed towards the types of coping mechanisms used by these two separate groups of caregivers.

For example, existing caregiver interventions fall into two general categories: (1) interpersonal peer–peer support and (2) instruction-based support. Peer–peer support involves learning from others in an informal, discussion-oriented setting. Most Alzheimer's Association support groups are built around this experience. Instruction-based support, in contrast, involves focussed and organized discussion around an instrumental or psychoeducational topic or theme. Effective grief-related support for caregivers is likely to require both types of intervention, as the loss-grief experience in this population is quite complex [1,10,34,35]. However, perhaps the proportion of the intervention or programme dedicated to instruction-based support versus peer support could be shaped on the basis of the information gleaned about coping mechanisms. Because spouses have been shown to have less support from friends and family members than adult-child caregivers, spouses might benefit from an intervention that relies more heavily on a peer-support model than instruction-based support.

Several other recommendations regarding caregiver grief support should be noted. The first question is – how much sharing and talking is good for the caregiver? One study [17] revealed that dementia caregivers reported 'a significantly higher desire to talk about their loss' than the corresponding cardiac family caregivers. But it needs to be noted that processing and venting are two different things. Ott *et al.* [16] noted the conflict:

> Although suppression of grief-related distress may be maladaptive . . . , increasing evidence suggests that rumination over grief-related distress is also maladaptive. . . . On the basis of results from this study and the accumulating body of knowledge on emotional disclosure, health care providers need to consider providing a balance between emotional disclosures about their circumstances that cannot be changed and a positive reframing of one's life experiences that ultimately may result in personal growth. (p. 806)

The findings from the study by Ott and colleagues also reveal that venting of emotions did not reduce grief among the caregivers [16]. If anything, it increased it.

Based on findings from various recent studies [13,16–19,36], the MM-CGI has emerged as a very valuable tool to begin to assess and address grief and loss among dementia caregivers. Therefore, a starting point to aid caregivers in coping with grief and loss would be to administer the MM-CGI in clinical or therapeutic settings to discern if the caregiver is experiencing high levels of grief. If so, then this tool can also gauge the depth of the grief experience, as well as the quality of that grief through the domains of personal sacrifice burden, heartfelt sadness and longing, and worry and felt isolation. Regardless of the strength and value that the MM-CGI instrument has for identifying and measuring grief, the data it gathers must then be applied to outreach services and programmes for caregivers so that grief can be normalized for both spouses and adult-child caregivers [17,21].

> What is currently missing is the recognition of and support through a true and unique grief process that is present in varying forms for an extended period of time. What is needed is an awareness of the true value of processing, understanding, and supporting the long journey of anticipatory grief [17; p. 19].

References

1. Meuser TM, Marwit SJ, Sanders S (2004). Assessing grief in family caregivers, in Doka KJ (ed) *Living with grief: Alzheimer's disease*, pp.169–195. Washington, DC: Hospice Foundation of America.

2. Doka, KJ (2004). Grief and dementia, in Doka KJ (ed) *Living with grief: Alzheimer's disease*, pp. 139–151. Washington, DC: Hospice Foundation of America.

3. Chappell NL, Reid RC (2002). Burden and well-being among caregivers: examining the distinction. *Gerontologist*, **42**(6), 772–780.

4. Gallagher-Thompson D, Coon DW, Rivera P, Powers D, Zeiss AM (1998). Family caregiving: stress, coping and intervention, in Hersen M, Van Hasselt B (eds) *Handbook of clinical geropsychology*, pp. 469–493. New York: Plenum Press.

5. George L, Gwyther L (1986). Caregiver well-being: a multidimentional examination of family caregivers of demented adults. *Gerontologist*, **26**, 253–259.

6. Zarit SH, Reever K, Bach-Peterson J (1980). Relatives of the impaired elderly: correlates of feelings of burden. *Gerontologist*, **20**, 649–655.

7. Rando TA (1986). A Comprehensive analysis of anticipatory grief: perspectives, processes, promises, and problems, in Rando TA (ed.), *Loss and anticipatory grief*, pp. 3–37. Washington, DC: Lexington Books.

8. Boss P (2004). Ambiguous loss, in Walsh F, McGoldrick M (eds) *Living beyond loss*, 2nd edn, pp. 237–246. New York: W.W. Norton & Company.

9. Boss P (1999). *Ambiguous loss: learning to live with unresolved grief*. Cambridge, MA: Harvard University Press.

10. Boss P, Wayne C, Horbal J (1988). Alzheimer's disease and ambiguous loss, in Chilman C, Cox FM (eds) *Chronic illness and disability, families in trouble series, vol. 2*, pp. 123–140. Newbury Park, CA: Sage.

11. Dupuis SL (2002). Understanding ambiguous loss in the context of dementia care: adult children's perspectives. *J Gerontol Soc Work*, **37**(2), 93–115.

12. Doka KJ (2000). Mourning psychosocial loss: anticipatory mourning in Alzheimer's, ALS, and irreversible coma, in Rando TA (ed) *Clinical dimensions of anticipatory mourning*, pp. 47–92. Champaign: Research Press.

13. Frank J (2008). Evidence for grief as the major barrier faced by Alzheimer caregivers: a qualitative analysis. *Am J Alzheimers Dis Other Demen*, **22**(6), 516–527.

14. Doka KJ, Aber R (1989). Psychosocial loss and grief, in K J Doka (ed) *Disenfranchised grief: recognizing hidden sorrow*, pp. 187–198. Lexington, KY: Lexington Book.

15. Marwit SJ, Meuser TM (2002). Development and initial validation of an inventory to measure grief in caregivers of persons with Alzheimer's disease. *Gerontologist*, **42**(6), 751–765.

16. Ott C, Sanders S, Kelber S (2007). Differences in the grief and personal growth experience of spouses and adult children of person's with Alzheimer's disease. *Gerontologist*, **47**, 798–809.

17. Ross A, Dagley J (2009). An assessment of anticipatory grief as experienced by family caregivers of individuals with dementia. *Alzheimer's Care Today*, **10**(1), 8–21.

18. Sanders S, Adams KB (2005). Grief reactions and depression in caregivers in caregivers of individuals with Alzheimer's disease. *Soc Work Health Care*, **30**, 287–295.

19. Meuser TM, Marwit SJ (2001). A comprehensive, stage-sensitive model of grief in dementia caregiving. *Gerontologist*, **41**(5), 658–670.

20. Ponder RJ, Pomeroy EC (1996). The grief of caregivers: how pervasive is it? *J Geron Soc Work*, **27**, 3–21.

21. Sanders S, Ott C, Kelber S, Noonan P (2008). The experience of high levels of grief in caregivers of persons with Alzheimer's disease and related dementia. *Death Stud*, **32**(6), 495–523.

22. Frank J, Johnson DK (2008). *Spouse and adult child differences in grief while Alzheimer's caregiving.* Paper presentation, 11th International Conference on Alzheimer's Disease, July 26–31, Chicago, Illinois.

23. Arden S, Elmstahl S (2005). Family caregivers' subjective experiences of satisfaction in dementia care: aspects of burden, subjective health, and sense of coherence. *Scand J Caring Sci*, **19**, 157–168.

24. Cohen C, Pushkar Gold E, Shulman KI, Zucchero CA (1994). Positive aspects in caregiving: an overlooked variable in research. *Can J Aging*, **13**, 378–391.

25. Gallagher-Thompson D, Lovett S, Rose J *et al.* (2000). Impact of psychoeducational interventions on distressed family caregivers. *J Clin Psychol*, **6**(2) 91–110.

26. Gitlin LN, Belle SH, Burgio LD *et al.* (2003). Effect of multicomponent interventions on caregiver burden and depression: the REACH multisite initiative at 6-month follow-up. *Psychol Aging*, **18**, 361–374.

27. Gwyther L (1994). Service delivery and utilization: research directions and clinical implications, in Light E, Niederehe G, Lebowitz B (eds) *Stress effects on family caregivers of Alzheimer's patients: research and interventions.* New York: Springer Publishing Company.

28. Schulz R, O'Brien A, Czaja S *et al.* (2002). Dementia caregiver intervention research: in search of clinical significance. *Gerontologis*, **42**, 589–602.

29. Thompson LW, Gallagher-Thompson D, Haley WE (2003). Future directions in dementia caregiving intervention research and practice, in Coon DW, Gallagher-Thompson D, Thompson LW (eds) *Innovative interventions to reduce dementia caregiver distress: a clinical guide,* pp. 3–22. New York: Springer.

30. Kasl-Godley J (2003). Anticipatory grief and loss: implications for intervention, in Coon DW, Gallagher-Thompson D, Thompson LW (eds) *Innovative interventions to reduce dementia caregiver distress: a clinical guide,* pp. 210–222. New York: Springer Publishing.

31. Sanders S, Sharp A (2004). The utilization of a psychoeducational group approach for addressing issues of grief and loss in caregivers of individuals with Alzheimer's disease: a pilot project. *J Soc Work Long-Term Care*, **3**, 71–89.

32. Loos C, Bowd A (1997). Caregivers of persons with Alzheimer's disease: some neglected implications of the experience of personal loss and grief. *Death Stud*, **21**, 501–514.

33. Zarit SH, Femia EE (2008). A future for family care and dementia intervention research? Challenges and strategies. *Aging Ment Health*, **12**(1), 5–13.

34. Austrom M, Hendrie G (1990). Death of the personality: the grief responses of Alzheimer's family caregivers. *Am J Care Relat Disord Res*, **5**, 16–27.

35. Theut SK, Jordan L, Ross L, Deutsch S (1991). Caregiver's anticipatory grief in dementia: a pilot study. *Int J Aging Hum Dev*, **33**, 113–118.

36. Sanders S, Marwit S, Meuser T, Harrington P (2007). Caregiver grief in end-stage dementia: using the Marwit-Meuser caregiver grief inventory for assessment and intervention in social work practice. *Sol Work Health Care*, **46**, 47–65.

Chapter 23

Communicating with people with dementia

Kate Allan and John Killick

Introduction

> I'm losing my mind – but the essence of a person is their heart. I hope as I grow older I'll still be able to laugh – and to hug – and to know love.
>
> (Fran Noonan Powers, quoted in [1; p. 21])

Why look at communication? We will state our position simply, and then, explain our reasons: we believe that communication should be central to how we think about dementia and how we work with those who live with it. As for the emerging concept of 'supportive care' for people with dementia, we offer some thoughts about this idea generally, and about where communication should fit in.

In considering the subject of communication, we are adopting a broad understanding of this term, encompassing the use of language, non-verbal channels, and the range of ways in which people can express themselves and connect with others through creative activities. One of the challenges in working with people with dementia, especially those whose disabilities are profound, is that our commonplace notions of what counts as communication may be brought into question. It is vital that we maintain an open mind on this, adopting an inclusive approach which views sometimes tiny and ambiguous acts – a sound, gesture, or movement – which might easily be overlooked or dismissed, as being potentially highly significant.

Although the nature of dementia itself has been discussed in detail elsewhere, it seems important for us to say that we understand dementia as arising out of a complex and, for each person, unique combination of factors. As Kitwood (1997) described, in addition to neurological change, these include psychological and interpersonal factors, the individual's life history, and their physical health status [2]. To this we add the effects of the environments in which the person spends time. Looking beyond the immediate situation and thinking about the Western world, we need to locate this interplay within a wider social and political context where older people, and those identified as ill or disabled, occupy a devalued status and have drastically reduced access to resources. A final and crucial caveat here is to emphasize that none of us fully understands the nature of the condition and how it affects the individual, their relationships with other persons, and their way of being in their world. We need to recognize this incompleteness, to identify and question our assumptions, and to consider the possibility that things might, in fact, be quite other than they seem.

Finally, on the use of words, we tend to favour the words 'support' and 'supporters' over 'care' and 'carers' as the latter seem to cast the person at the centre in a more passive role, connoting a system which positions people primarily as recipients of care or users of services and obscures their many and complex roles in life outside of the system. To us, terms related to the word 'support' carry a greater sense of encouraging the other person to utilize their own resources, a subject we will revisit at some length. But our use of the word 'support' does not arise directly from the term 'supportive care'.

Why is communication important?

We stated at the beginning of the chapter that we believe that communication needs to be at the centre of how we think about dementia. There are various reasons for this. The first is that as social animals, relationships based on communication with others have always been vital for our survival as a species and as individuals. Our brains have developed with this need as a basic organizing principle and this affects the way they function at a fundamental level.

The second reason relates to the concept of personhood, which is of central relevance to dementia. Against a prevailing theme in Western philosophy which allies the quality of personhood to sophisticated cognitive functioning, Kitwood argued that what makes each of us a person, as distinct from an object, is not a function of an intact brain and is not even something any of us can 'possess' as individuals [2]. Instead he argued that it is constructed and maintained through our relationships with others, which in turn are built on communication. This means that whenever we attempt to communicate with another person, we are making real their status as a person. Disregarding communication, for example by ignoring someone or treating them like an object, is damaging for us all, but for an individual with dementia, who is already facing a whole range of profound changes, it is especially deleterious. Persons in this situation have a heightened need of genuine communication that has the potential to strengthen their sense of self and foster resilience to the challenges they face.

This latter point leads directly into another reason why communication is so fundamental. If things go badly in this respect, for example if a person experiences brain changes which make it difficult for them to use familiar channels of communication, and if they then lose confidence and become anxious about trying, then they are at an enormous disadvantage in terms of how things are likely to develop from there. If others are not disposed to try hard to find ways of connecting with the individual, to understand their experiences and needs and to foster opportunities for them to enjoy things and use their strengths, then it is very likely that there will be more a more rapid and steep deterioration in the person's overall functioning. This, combined perhaps with the appearance of behaviours that others find offensive or irritating, may well be attributed to the severity of the individual's brain damage, further reducing the chances for positive change. We know that people who are seen by others as being unable to communicate are regarded as being much more disabled generally, are likely to experience poorer quality of care, and have fewer opportunities for positive experiences. They are also at risk of having unrecognized and untreated physical problems, and experience poorer health overall.

If, on the other hand, a person who encounters problems with expressing themselves and understanding others, finds alternative ways of connecting with those around them, perhaps through nonverbal means like physical contact and facial expression, and in turn finds those others responsive, then the whole scenario can be completely different. Such individuals are more likely to have opportunities for communication which strengthen their otherwise threatened sense of self, to find ways of expressing their needs and experiences, to continue to be involved in decisions about their lives, and to remain within the network of relationships which may have sustained them over a lifetime and can continue to do so.

What happens to communication in dementia and why

With the broader changes in our understanding of dementia in the last 20 years or so, we have come a long way in our appreciation of the place of communication. We are now able to see that far less of what happens is a 'given', determined purely by neurological deterioration. Although studies from the fields of neuropsychology and neurolinguistics have described a set of changes, which typically occur in the way persons with dementia use language, a properly broad understanding of communication must recognize that communication is about far more than how we use words, and acknowledge a greater diversity and degree of unpredictability in what happens to the individual.

Several works have drawn attention to the variety of ways people with dementia communicate, including the creative use of language [3], and the role of nonverbal channels such as touch, movement, and eye contact [4,5]. We have come to understand how people find new ways to express themselves when old ways become obstructed. There is an inherent creativity and resourcefulness that demands a commensurate response from those around the individual. Appreciation of a universe of hitherto unsuspected possibilities has ushered in a recognition that creative activities of all sorts – dance, collage, puppetry, for example – can be powerful ways for people with dementia to share their experiences, express their views and communicate their needs.

Happily it is now possible to cite many examples of innovative and inspiring practice in the area of communication, including work on ways of involving persons with dementia in decisions about their lives [6], exploring the use of specially designed board games [7] and photography [8] to stimulate interaction and promote well-being.

A particular interest of ours is the role of creative activities in nurturing communication. It is difficult to select single examples from the many available, but one of our favourites comes from musician Maria Mullan [9], who uses music in a range of ways to encourage the person to share their thoughts and feelings. With one man she sits at a table where there are a number of different percussion instruments within reach. She encourages the man to choose one, and he goes on to tap out a rhythm showing real concentration and absorption in the activity. Maria then echoes the sequence. He proceeds to create another longer and more complex sequence. Again Maria echoes it. This continues until the dialogue seems complete.

But despite the encouragement we can derive from such excellence, we cannot afford to be complacent. Recent research, carried out by Richard Ward and colleagues in a variety of services in the southeast of England [10], has demonstrated that, in the normal course of service provision the quality of communication between care staff and persons with dementia is very poor indeed. By analysing many hours of video recordings they found that an individual had direct contact with a member of care staff for an average of only 2% of a day, and that most of this was limited to carrying out routine care tasks characterized by impoverished communication. For a variety of complex reasons it seemed that many staff actually seemed to avoid direct contact with those in their settings. The details of the study are beyond the scope of this chapter, but the message is clear: we are very far from realizing our communication ideals in current practice.

Communication within supportive care

In what follows we explore three main ideas about what this thing we are calling supportive care might look like, and where communication fits. We will provide illustration with examples, quotations and stories in order to try to bring our thoughts into sharper and more lively focus.

Focussing on strengths

When we made reference to the terms we have used in this chapter, we suggested that the word 'support' has different connotations to that of 'care', carrying a sense of acknowledging and building upon what is already there. This is about focussing on and working with *strengths* as opposed to identifying and compensating for deficits and losses.

The idea of working with strengths is not very familiar in mainstream health and social care, which tends to focus on problems and attempt to fix them and, where there is no prospect of a fix, to institute routines of 'care' to meet needs. Perhaps the discipline of occupational therapy with its concentration on the person's remaining resources and how they can use these to achieve goals and meet needs comes closer than most. An emphasis on identifying and working with the strengths of a person, family or organization is a major theme within the relatively new branch of psychology called 'positive psychology' [11].

In our view a fundamental principle of supportive care should be to assume that no matter how disabled the person with dementia is, they continue to have strengths, and that those in a supporting role should seek to discover and work with these strengths to the greatest possible extent. This applies both broadly in working with the person, and specifically in relation to communication.

A focus on the person's strengths means noticing and valuing different things, actively looking for hidden abilities and interests, and searching for meaning in actions which may more usually be seen as problems or challenges. We will have to look more closely at what the person does and maintain a more open mind on its significance. And we will very likely have to question our own values, at least at times, about what constitutes a strength. Once we have identified strengths we will have to alter our way of working with the person to support them or even go out of our way to create new situations in which the person can use them.

The following example comes from 'A walk with Gordon' by drama therapist Paul Batson [12]. Gordon is a tall, gaunt man in his late sixties, who lives in a long-stay ward for people with advanced dementia. He says nothing and wears a mask-like expression on his face. Paul learns that Gordon likes to walk, and begins spending time with him regularly, taking him out into the hospital grounds. They walk hand in hand, with Paul pointing out features of interest on the way. Sometimes Gordon seems to look in the direction indicated by Paul, but there is never any other response from him. He never speaks and his facial expression never changes.

At one point on the path, there is a post. As they approach Paul lifts both their hands over it and they pass on either side. Soon after doing so Paul asks himself why he automatically took this decision on behalf of both of them. It seems to have arisen out of an assumption that Gordon would have been incapable of doing the same. They retrace their steps, and this time it is Gordon who lifts their hands over the post. Paul thanks him. They continue to take this walk weekly over the next few months, and every time the same thing happens. Paul comments:

> Gordon taught me never to make assumptions about people living with dementia. He reinforced my belief that if we are on the look-out and offer sensitive opportunities for interaction, then we can connect with people living with dementia, even when their illness is severe. On our walks together, Gordon gave me a helping hand, far more than he ever knew. [12; p. 115]

This was an apparently unpromising situation but a sensitive and reflective approach, which invested in Gordon's only obvious strength (walking), revealed more awareness and ability than was expected. We do not have any information about whether this learning was fed back into the wider situation, perhaps leading to others approaching Gordon in different ways and discovering hidden strengths, but the use of learning from one context in the wider picture should be an important facet of working in this way. Looking for strengths and supporting the person in using them may well lead to further discoveries and opportunities becoming apparent.

The following is another example from John's work that bears on the subject of strengths. It involves recognizing and celebrating how much the person with dementia still has to give:

> When I enter she is over the other side of the room. She sees me and walks slowly towards me pointing. I do the same. When we meet we intertwine our little fingers and say 'Oh you!' over and over. This is a game she has invented.

These are the only words of Mary's that I understand. She talks a good deal, to herself, and to me. I nod and smile encouragingly. I can tell the tenor of her communications by the tone of her voice and her body language.

We are always exploring our environment, and the residents, staff and visitors who inhabit it. However many times we encounter the same person or object it is always fresh for Mary, and therefore new-minted for me.

Supporting the supporters

Our second point relates to the aspiration of supportive care not only to respond to the needs of the person with the condition, but also those around him or her. We have already argued that our very sense of being a person depends on our relationships with others. It therefore makes sense that the focus of supportive care is extended to the others involved, whether in a professional or family capacity. It also potentially includes those who come into contact with persons with dementia in the course of their lives beyond the world of services. This touches on the issue of public education and stigma, which is beyond the scope of this chapter, but nevertheless deserves mention.

This more inclusive focus has particular relevance for the area of communication. In arguing for an approach which places communication at the centre of the way we think about the individual and their condition, we are asking a great deal of those in a supporting role. We are asking them to engage their very personhood – their emotions, their life experiences and their vulnerability – in this activity. As well as enjoying encounters characterized, perhaps, by humour, gratitude or companionship, they may be called upon to tolerate ambiguity, be close to someone who is in deep distress or take the risk of uncovering such distress, and they may find themselves confronting their own anxieties and griefs. There is also the potential that in the course of engaging with an individual experiencing dementia the supporter will need to deal with an issue which runs contrary to their own deeply-held values, potentially raising ethical concerns.

In an article responding to the question 'Can we risk person-centred communication?', Faith Gibson is forthright in asserting that far more resources are required for genuine communication to take place than is generally recognized: 'Person-centred communication is not costless in terms of physical and emotional wear and tear' [13; p. 21]. We have numerous examples of what can happen when adequate support is not available, including John's own experience when after years of unsupported and intensive work he reached the point of exhaustion and saturation, and was forced to realize that his own mental health was on the line [14].

So what needs to happen in order to allow those around the person to engage in real communication without putting themselves at risk? Whilst we often think first of what we need to do differently, there is real benefit in helping the supporters to identify their existing strengths and knowledge, often in the course of exploring what already works well. Beginning from a starting point of success can give people who face a complex challenge a greater sense of pride and confidence in what they already do and in their capacity to enhance their resources further. The following quotations come from practitioners who participated in a project carried out by Kate, which explored ways of developing communication between care practitioners and persons with dementia:

> [The project] has shown us how much we already do unconsciously.
> It has given me confidence and I feel well able to pass on my experiences to other colleagues. [15; p. 89]

This study also demonstrated that a crucial part of the development process in terms of learning was the opportunity to reflect on work already undertaken. Whilst being actively engaged in face-to-face communication work (such as inviting conversation during intimate care or going for an outing) was necessary, having the time and encouragement to think and talk about what had happened was also essential. It was at these times that new connections were made, insights achieved and ideas for further development arose.

And this process links directly into another element which seems integral to what we think supportive care should attempt to do: the need for those around the person to develop a robust sense of meaning in what is happening to the person with dementia, which can ultimately connect with their own experience of being a person. The specific form such a sense of meaning might take would depend on the people involved; but having a wider framework within which to locate particular experiences seems essential.

We end this section with the following quotation from Deborah Shouse, whose mother had dementia [16]. To us this is an example of the depth and quality of communication that is possible even in the midst of profound change, and of the development in the sphere of spirituality which dementia can make possible:

> I sink into my mother's face like she is a meditation. We smile at each other for a half-hour, something we have never done before, something that would be too intense, too personal in our earlier, rational life together.
>
> Then her eyes gently flutter shut. I feel like I've been on a mystical retreat. I feel a rich sense of renewal and hope.
>
> . . .
>
> Mom's eyes are closed; her hands resting by her sides. I kneel on the floor and rest my head against her legs. I feel her warmth and the sureness of her breathing. Then I feel her hand on my head, tugging playfully at my curls, just as she used to do when I was a little girl. I smile, close my eyes and rest. [16; pp. 125–126]

Working with change

The third area we wish to explore is pertinent both to the subject of supportive care generally, and to communication more particularly, that of change. In attempting to conceive of a way of working with persons with dementia over what is commonly 10–15 years, we must grapple seriously with the reality of profound change in many domains of the individual's life, including in the way we can communicate with them.

Whilst changes in the way a person uses language have been studied most extensively, there is much more to communication than this. One of the focuses of change which has commonly been observed and has wide implications is that of a shift away from intellectually-based functioning to a fuller experience of emotion. On this Richard Taylor, a psychologist who has developed dementia, has said [17]:

> The locus of my attention is definitely shifting from my head to my heart. I feel and think about feelings more than I think about thinking. . . . Sometimes I am very happy, and sometimes I am very sad, and at all times I am aware of all my feelings. (p. 138)

This shift will have a variety of effects on the way people communicate, and it will be necessary for supporters to recognize and respond to these. Whilst the person is still using language, their speech may acquire a greater immediacy and vividness, often characterized by the use of imagery or taking the form of stories. In her novel, Elizabeth Cohen [18] describes the language of her father who has dementia in this way (Ava is his very young granddaughter):

> His own speech is pared down, skeletal, like he has become. And eloquent. He himself has begun to speak in poetry. When Ava walks into a room he says 'Here's the one that fills the room with hurricanes'. (pp. 54–55)

Another commonly-encountered change is an increasing reliance on non-verbal forms of communication, that matrix of subtle indicators including eye-contact, facial expression, touch, gesture, body movements, and use of voice. Again this shift demands a commensurate response from supporters, both in terms of recognizing these forms of communication and apprehending their significance, and also in engaging in non-verbally based communication themselves. To step out of one's 'comfort zone' in this way, putting aside a facility for words and turning instead, perhaps, to silence, touch, face-to-face contact, and rhythm as a way of connecting, takes courage and faith. The following vignette from John's experience illustrates the possibilities:

> Bronwen comes into the lounge of the nursing home. She seems to be looking for me and leads me to a chair. I ask her permission to sit. 'Yes' she says.
>
> Once we are seated, comfortable and face-to-face, I encourage her to continue: 'say anything you want'. A look of what could be interpreted as exasperation crosses her features, and her shoulders sink. But then she puts a finger to her lips, in a gesture commonly understood as an enjoinder to silence. I take the point and mirror it.
>
> The encounter then gets properly into its stride. Bronwen takes the lead. She grasps my right hand in what begins as a greeting and turns into a game of slow rhythmic shaking. She points to a vase of flowers and also to a scene outside the window. She moves her hand over the chair arm exploring its texture. She does the same with the back of my hand, a flower, and also touches my face. We have episodes of close eye contact throughout. The only word she uses during the interaction is 'yes', usually accompanied by an emphatic nod. I continue to mirror both actions and words.
>
> Eventually, after 8 minutes of intense interaction, she lets my hand drop. She appears exhausted. 'Wonderful' she murmurs.

Over the years a person lives with dementia it is highly likely that there will be both a slowing down in the way they communicate, together with a reduction in the magnitude and clarity of what they offer. The slower pace and the tendency towards more subtlety and ambiguity increases the risk that the person's actions and words will be overlooked altogether or dismissed as mere evidence of confusion. In a video [19], showing arts practitioners working with persons with dementia using humour, we see Tiny and Sweetie Pie, complete with their eccentric clothing and red noses, kneeling in front of Ann who is seated. Her gaze is focused on them but her face is inexpressive. It is impossible to tell what she is making of it all. Slowly she reaches out and touches Tiny's red nose. He laughs and says 'It's my nose. It's a bit red today!' Again slowly, Ann's face breaks into a smile and then a laugh. The practitioners are entirely comfortable with this pace and allow the encounter to unfold at its own pace.

And again from John's experience we share the following description of an interaction with Pat, a woman with very advanced dementia:

> This was our third meeting in her room. As on the previous occasions, though I held her hand, spoke her name, synchronized our breathing and attempted eye contact, she was unresponsive. For ten minutes her body was turned away in the chair, and she was silent.
>
> Then gradually she raised her head, spoke, though I could not follow her words, and smiled. For a further ten minutes we were clearly in communication. I played her some music and she expressed interest and pleasure with her face, her gaze and through nonverbal sounds. She then went on to engage in a sustained sequence of speech-like sounds, only a few of which were recognizable to me but which were very definitely spoken in an Australian accent! Again her tone, expression, and eye movements were obviously communicative.
>
> Then quite quickly it was over. Her body moved back into its former position, she ceased speaking, and was wholly unresponsive.

This brings us to what we believe is a capacity which acquires ever greater importance in interactions with persons with dementia, that of being *in the moment* with our attention fully and open-mindedly focused on the person and our encounter with them. So often our thoughts dart back and forth between the future and the past with the consequence that we miss the present, and its possibilities. Intimately related to this is the observation that dementia is a process which appears to alter the person's own sense of time, and intensifies the prominence of the here and now. Social worker Lisa Snyder describes her own experience in the following way [20]:

> ... for Bill the past is elusive and the future uncertain. A relationship with him can be demanding – but also deeply inspiring. Like a Zen master he exacts my conscious attention to each present moment and renews my appreciation for the unpredictable and spontaneous dimensions of life. (p. 56)

Part of responding to individual types of changes is having a perspective on how to think about change generally. It is surely true that we make sense of changes in people very differently depending on the context in which they occur. For an 18-month-old child, change is continuous and intense but is seen as part of a natural and desirable process of development. Change at the other end of the lifespan is usually regarded much more negatively, and changes associated with dementia have been almost universally framed as deterioration and loss. The kinds of changes seen within supporters are similarly seen as undesirable – stress-induced health problems, economic hardship, and grief.

So conditioned are we to see change in dementia within this frame, it takes a particular effort to conceive of it in different terms, perhaps as the development or emergence of new capacities, qualities and interests. But if an emphasis on the person's strengths, and those of their supporters, is part of the idea of supportive care, then this will involve looking for new possibilities amid a shifting picture. Again, a challenging thing to do but an approach which opens up much that is new and charged with potential. Finally on the subject of change, it seems important also to consider that part of having a sense of meaning regarding the process of dementia may be having a sense of what does not change. This links us to the subject of spirituality, which is beyond the scope of this chapter, but is dealt with in Chapter 21 of this book.

Towards a conclusion of our contribution here, we again suggest that communication, in all its diversity, ambiguity and still largely unexplored potential, must play a central role in this ambitious concept we are calling supportive care. If we can find a way for this approach to realize its potential, it will surely be by listening, reflecting, offering ideas, and taking creative risks.

References

1. Peterson B (2004). *Voices of Alzheimer's: courage, humor, hope and love in the face of dementia.* Cambridge, MA: De Capo Books.
2. Kitwood T (1997). *Dementia reconsidered: the person comes first.* Buckingham: Open University Press.
3. Killick J (2008). *Dementia diary.* London: Hawker.
4. Goldsmith M (1996). *Hearing the voice of people with dementia: opportunities and obstacles.* London: Jessica Kingsley.
5. Killick J, Allan K (2001). *Communication and the care of people with dementia.* Buckingham: Open University Press.
6. Allan K (2001). *Communication and consultation: exploring ways for staff to involve people with dementia in developing services.* Bristol: The Policy Press.
7. Benham L (2007). What shall we do today? *J Dementia Care*, **15**(4) 24–25.
8. Mitchell R (2005). *Captured memories.* Stirling: Dementia Services Development Centre.
9. Mullan M, Killick J (2001). *Responding to music.* Stirling: Dementia Services Development Centre.
10. Ward R, Vass A, Aggarwal N, Garfield C, Cybyk B (2005). What is dementia care? 1. Dementia is communication. *J Dementia Care*, **13**(6), 16–17.

11. Peterson C, Seligman M (2004). *Character strengths and virtues: a handbook and classification.* Oxford: Oxford University Press.

12. Batson P (2006). A helping hand: walking with Gordon, in Marshall M, Allan K (eds) *Dementia: walking not wandering*, pp.114–115. London: Hawker.

13. Gibson F (1999). Can we risk person-centred communication? *J Dementia Care*, 7(5), 33–37.

14. Killick J (1999). Pathways through pain – a cautionary tale. *J Dementia Care*, 7(1), 22–24.

15. Allan K (2001). *Communication and consultation: exploring ways for staff to involve people with dementia in developing services.* Bristol: The Policy Press.

16. Shouse D (2007). *Love in the land of dementia.* Kansas City, MO: The Creativity Connection.

17. Taylor R (2007). *Alzheimer's from the inside out.* Baltimore, MD: Health Professions Press.

18. Cohen E (2003). *The house on Beartown road: a memoir of learning and forgetting.* New York: Random House.

19. Red Nose Coming! (2003). Video produced by Stirling Dementia Services Development Centre, Scotland.

20. Snyder L (2000). *Speaking our minds: personal reflections from individuals with Alzheimer's.* New York: WH Freeman.

Chapter 24

Maintaining the self in dementia

Steven R. Sabat

Introduction

The selfhood of a person with dementia can be undermined not simply as a result of biological factors, but to a far greater degree, by psychosocial factors. In order to support and maintain the selfhood of the person with dementia to the greatest possible degree after the diagnosis is given and for the balance of the person's life, it is crucial to understand three fundamentally important and interrelated issues that affect the person with dementia as well as his or her formal and informal carers. Understanding these issues and their effects can shed light on the subjective experience of the person with dementia as well as the ways in which carers interact with him or her, and thereby affect the degree to which his or her selfhood can be maintained. These are:

1 Negative stereotypes, negative self-stereotypes, and stereotype threat

2 Malignant positioning

3 Aspects of selfhood that are affected by both of the above.

In this chapter, I shall address each issue in turn and attempt to convey the meanings of dementia to the person diagnosed, to the healthy others who are carers, and how those meanings can come to create a filter of sorts through which the world is seen by all involved. Once these 'filters' are in place, carers can easily engage in Malignant Positioning of the person diagnosed. This means that it becomes more and more likely that healthy others will interpret the actions of the person with dementia in ways that emphasize pathology such that what might actually be healthy, adaptive behaviour will, instead, be pathologized so as to validate the diagnosis. Once Malignant Positioning is in place, healthy others focus more and more attention on real and imagined effects of dementia, so that the person becomes defined increasingly by his or her diagnosis, while healthy, intact, admirable attributes are increasingly obscured from view. This process then leads to the person's social personae being confined more and more to that of the 'dysfunctional, burdensome patient', thereby creating what Goffman [1] called a 'spoiled identity'. Once we understand how the selfhood of the person with dementia can be undermined by psychosocial factors, we can then understand how to remedy the situation and thereby work to support and maintain his or her selfhood. Maintaining the person's selfhood thus becomes a crucial aspect of the work of supportive care.

Stereotypes, self-stereotypes, and stereotype threat

In a recent article, Scholl and Sabat [2] examined some of the above issues as they pertain to people with Alzheimer's disease (AD). It is clear from research conducted over the past 3 decades that, consciously and unconsciously, people in the developed Western world hold negative stereotypes about ageing *per se* and these may be disconnected from what they explicitly say they believe [3–5]. In other words, people can hold negative stereotypes about ageing even though they do not outwardly indicate anything of the sort. Indeed, when they finally identify with being a 'senior citizen' they see those negative stereotypes as applying to themselves. This process is known as negative self-stereotyping and it can have powerful effects. For example, the mere perception of one's memory as being poor as a consequence of ageing can lead to dependency, unnecessary medical attention, depression, and anxiety [6]; indeed, negative self-stereotyping has been found to have a detrimental effect on performance on tasks requiring recall [7]. Interestingly enough, Levy [8] used the following words as negative stereotype priming cues (ways to make a person think about ageing in negative ways) in her experiments: 'Alzheimer's', 'senile', 'forgetful', and 'dying', while other researchers [9] employed 'Alzheimer's', 'decline', 'dependent', 'senile', 'misplaces', 'dementia', 'confused', 'decrepit', and 'incompetent'. These researchers, then, provide clear support to the notion that negative stereotypes about ageing are associated with these very attributes. Therefore, if such words are laden with negativity, it is reasonable to consider the possibility that people (1) who have been exposed to decades of negative connotations associated with ageing and with dementia and (2) who are now themselves older and diagnosed with dementia are now susceptible to the effects of negative self-stereotyping and the associated deleterious effects on performing many different tasks in everyday life. The major implication of all this is that, in the absence of negative self-stereotyping, the same people would be able to perform better on the very same outcome measures.

Support for the above logic can be found in the recent work of Corner and Bond [10]. The authors discuss the case of Rose and Ron, who had been married for decades when Rose began to have some memory problems. Although their family physician assured them that she was experiencing 'normal ageing', Rose subsequently saw another physician who recommended further tests at a hospital, where they were told that it was likely that Rose had mild early stage dementia. The meaning of this diagnosis can be found in Ron's reaction:

> When we were told that Rose had this dementia we were just devastated. . .our world came crashing down on us and . . . we cried for days. We couldn't bring ourselves to talk to . . . the kids . . . or anyone about it. It was too shameful for Rose. She didn't want anyone to know. . . . You picture these people who are vegetables. (pp. 7–8)

For her part, Rose said in response to being given standard tests of cognitive function,

> I was always good at maths and that at school. I came in the top per cent . . . But it threw me those tests, I felt such a . . . failure and it really knocked me. (p. 8)

Indeed, Rose went further and said, 'I can't think of anything worse to be told. . .I wouldn't wish it on anyone. And it's changed everything' (p. 9). Thus, the meaning of dementia was consummately negative to both partners, even shameful, leading Rose to stereotype herself negatively.

That Rose's performance on subsequent testing was affected negatively by her reaction to the diagnosis, is an example of 'stereotype threat' [11,12]: the notion that the negative stereotypes about a group of people can have adverse effects on the ability of individual group members to perform particular tasks if they are put into a situation in which they might confirm the negative stereotype. Thus, Rose experienced stereotype threat because of her fear that she would, in her performance on tests, confirm the negative stereotype about the group to which she now belonged (people with dementia). Indeed, research has predicted precisely what Rose reported regarding her performance on mathematical tests: stereotype threat is greatest for those who placed the greatest value on the trait being stereotyped [13,14]. Thus Rose, who had always been good at maths and had placed a clear positive value on that attribute, was especially threatened when she had to take math tests in the clinic once she had been diagnosed with dementia. To bring this matter full circle by demonstrating that the psychosocial factors being discussed herein are critical, Hess *et al.* report that the impact of stereotype threat-related factors was minimized when research subjects were informed that memory decline was not inevitable and when they were given effective coping strategies [14]. Thus, the authors showed that performance was facilitated when participants felt less threatened. It follows that poor performance on standard tests is not necessarily a result of neuropathology alone.

Malignant positioning

Positioning is a way by which people make their actions intelligible as social and help to define, strengthen, or weaken an individual's moral and personal attributes while helping to create narratives or story lines about the person. Through the use of positioning, people are able to explain their own behaviour and that of others [15]. If one were to explain another person's actions in a way that emphasized that person's negative attributes, one would be positioning that person in what might be a potentially malignant way because it can have a negative effect on that person's social selfhood. For example, in everyday life, Person A might position Person B in a negative way: person A sees Person B trip and fall, and asserts that Person B is clumsy. Person B might object to having been positioned in a way that is uncomplimentary, and might reject such positioning by saying, 'No, I'm not clumsy, I simply didn't see the crack in the pavement because I was carrying a large box in my arms'. In this way, Person B repositions him or herself in a way that is not uncomplimentary.

On another level, when Person A attributed Person B's tripping and falling to Person B's clumsiness, we can say that Person A explained Person B's actions in terms of something about Person B's disposition or nature – the way Person B 'is' by definition (clumsy). When Person B rejects Person A's 'dispositional' positioning, Person B attributes his or her tripping to something about the environment, the situation, that existed. Thus, Person B is saying, 'No, I didn't trip and fall because I'm clumsy, but because of the pavement's characteristics – the situation I was in'. There are two main points here: (1) persons can be negatively positioned in ways that emphasize uncomplimentary qualities inherent in them, but (2) they can reject such positioning and reposition themselves in ways that negate the existence of dysfunctional qualities in themselves, but rather explain their actions in terms of the environment's effects over which they had no control. Let us, now, apply this calculus to a situation confronted by a person with dementia.

Once people are diagnosed with dementia, they become vulnerable to malignant positioning immediately, such that many of their actions will be attributed to their disposition (having a diagnosis of dementia or, even worse, to the alleged fact that he or she is 'demented'), rather than to the situation in which they find themselves. In my experience of administering standard neuropsychological tests to people with dementia, it was not uncommon for a person being tested to become extremely upset upon failing to answer what might be thought of as rather simple questions. Indeed, some people would begin to cry, others became angry and adamantly refused to continue with the testing, or went so far as to leave the room and refused to return. It was common to hear such reactions labeled as 'catastrophic' and exemplary of 'emotional lability' caused by the dementia. In this interpretation, the person's behaviour is attributed to 'the disease' (the way the person 'is') and is considered symptomatic of the pathology of dementia. In other words, the 'filter' through which the observer is interpreting this behavior is one that places pathology in a privileged position such that any behaviour that seems 'out of the ordinary' will be viewed as a species of pathology and the person will be positioned accordingly so as to validate the original story line that places dementia in the forefront of the person's behaviour. There is at least one other way in which to view this behaviour and one other way to position the person in question.

One could position the same person as a semiotic subject: a person whose behaviour is driven by the meaning of the situation at hand [16]. More specifically, persons who become very upset when confronted with their failure on such test items (a) are aware that there is a difference between what they can do now as opposed to what they could do in healthier times; (b) have evaluated correctly the meaning of the difference as being terribly negative; and (c) are reacting more or less appropriately to the loss that is thus evidenced. Clearly, positioning the person as a semiotic subject would be appropriate under the circumstances and hardly pathological in nature. That people diagnosed with dementia in the moderate to severe stages can be semiotic subjects has been established in a number of cases [17]. Ironically, if the person did not react negatively at all, but seemed nonplussed in the face of such an obvious failure, it is quite likely that the same professional who interpreted the above behaviour as being 'a catastrophic reaction' or 'emotion-ally labile' would interpret the opposite reaction as a species of the diagnosed person being 'bliss-fully unaware' of his or her defects, yet another example of negative, potentially malignant, positioning. Indeed, it might just as well be the case that the person who did not become dis-traught was just as aware of the meaning of his or her failure on test items, but that the individual was not in the habit of revealing his or her significant emotions to what is, for all intents and purposes, a stranger. The only way to elucidate the full meaning of the person's reaction or lack thereof would be to investigate how that person dealt with adversity in the past and how he or she expressed emotions socially. This is to say, that one cannot make simplistic attributions of another person's behaviour (such as it's due to dementia) without knowing the larger context of that person's historic way of being in the social world and how that person has lived his or her life during healthier times [17,18]. To do otherwise, would be to believe tacitly that one can under-stand the nature and meaning of a person's actions without knowing anything significant about that person other than the fact that he or she has been diagnosed with dementia. It would mean that the health professional would feel (a) quite secure in being 'blissfully unaware' of the character of the person in question and (b) perfectly willing to engage in depersonalization of that individual.

The negative positioning described above becomes malignant when it leads to treatment that is depersonalizing and assaults the self-worth of the person with dementia. Such treatment has been outlined by Kitwood [19] and Kitwood and Bredin [20] and is called 'Malignant Social Psychology', examples of which are 'ignoring' in which the person with dementia is being spoken about in the presence of others as if he or she were not there at all, and 'invalidation' in which the subjectivity of the person with dementia is denied or overlooked. For example, if the person is anxious about something, the anxiety is viewed as a symptom of dementia and no attempt (other than, perhaps, dispensing medication) is made to interact with the person in a sensitive, supportive way, for the anxiety is not considered to be 'real'. If the person with dementia objects to being treated in these ways, the objection itself is viewed as yet another symptom of disease and the untoward behaviour of healthy others will persist indefinitely and will continue to have a negative impact on the person in question. Under such conditions, as the person with dementia becomes depressed, the depression is viewed as a worsening of the disease rather than a result of increasingly dysfunc-tional treatment from which the person with dementia has no escape. Thus, negative positioning becomes malignant very easily and, compounding the problem, its effects are not understood in social terms, but in biomedical terms, thereby condemning the person with dementia to social treatment that would never be accorded to him or her in healthier times. It is then innocently, tacitly, assumed that the person with dementia is oblivious to being treated in ways that are demeaning and depersonalizing which, itself, is an assumption guided by negative positioning in the first instance. When does such negative positioning begin?

Gleaned from the subjective experience of people with mild to moderate AD who attend sup-port groups that she leads, Snyder [21] offers some important insights into where negative and malignant positioning have their origins. Speaking about the experience of going through the testing that led to her being diagnosed, one of Snyder's group members called Bea commented,

> The last person who interviewed me was the neurologist. He was very indifferent and said it was just going to get worse. It wasn't professional as far as I was concerned. If he had just shown a little compassion. He was there to diagnose my problem, but he wasn't there to understand my feelings. He had no feelings for me whatsoever. I've hated him ever since. Health care professionals need to be compassionate (pp.17–18).

Thus, we have Bea being treated immediately as something of a non-person, someone who doesn't rate any compassion, understanding, interest, perhaps because she's already been positioned as being incapable of understanding, of needing understanding and compassion. Another of Snyder's support group members, Betty, a retired social worker, said of the health care professionals she met during the process of being diagnosed and treated:

> . . . they don't really accept the significance of illness for people. They know the diagnosis, but they don't take time to find out what it truly means for the person. This casualness with which professionals deal with people with Alzheimer's is so painful to see. . .You have to really be willing to be present with the person who has Alzheimer's. But there are some people who don't want to learn, and it's the looking down on and being demeaning of people with Alzheimer's that is hard to watch. (pp. 123–124)

Thus, we see, at least in these cases, that there is, *even at the time of initial diagnosis*, already an unwillingness or inability on the part of professionals to engage people diagnosed with dementia (herein of the Alzheimer's type) as people who have feelings, reactions, hopes, fears, and the need for affiliation and to be understood. That is, from the time of the diagnosis onward, people with dementia are frequently treated as non-persons not only by professionals, but by lay people as well, all of whom have been members of a culture in which negative stereotypes about ageing and dementia have been the rule rather than the exception, in which stereotype threat is clearly felt, in which malignant positioning is frequently imposed, such that the self worth of the person with dementia is assaulted far more frequently than it is supported. Indeed, the very selfhood of the person is assaulted as a result and it is to that aspect of the experience of dementia that I now turn.

Supporting the selfhood of the person with dementia

In order to understand how selfhood is assaulted and, thereby, how it can be supported in people with dementia, it is helpful to use a Social Constructionist approach [22] as a heuristic device. Although there have been allegations that dementia, especially of the Alzheimer's type, results in a loss of self due to the disease alone [23], there is ample evidence to the contrary that implicates dysfunctional social treatment as the root cause of the ways in which selfhood may be compromised [17,24–28]. From a Social Constructionist standpoint, there are three different aspects of selfhood, Self 1, Self 2, and Self 3. In what follows, I shall explore each in turn and indicate, where appropriate, the ways in which one or another aspect can be undermined or supported.

Self 1 is the self of personal identity and we experience it in terms of our singular, continuous point of view in the world (as opposed to having multiple personality disorder). We express our Self 1 via first person pronouns such as 'I', 'me', 'myself', 'our' (yours and mine), and the like, whereby we take responsibility for our statements and actions and indicate the source of autobiographical statements. Self 1 has been found to be intact even in the severe stages of AD [17]. Self 2 consists of physical and psychological attributes of the person, past and present. Thus, one's eye colour, skin pigmentation, height, are Self 2 attributes, as are being a college graduate, having a good sense of humour, a facility with crossword puzzles. Likewise, one's beliefs such as those in the political and religious spheres, are Self 2 attributes and one's beliefs about one's attributes are part of the Self 2. For example, one might take pride in some of one's attributes and one might be ashamed about or embarrassed by others. Being diagnosed with dementia is a Self 2 attribute and feeling aghast and deeply fearful about it is another. Having difficulty recalling recent events and feeling frustrated and angry about it are Self 2 attributes as well. By their very nature, Self 2 attributes cannot be completely erased by dementia, but it is in this aspect of selfhood that we can come to appreciate more fully how we can support or undermine a person who has been diagnosed.

It is unfortunately the case that from the moment of the diagnosis onward, there is an increased focus, on the part of the person diagnosed and healthy others, on the negative Self 2 attributes associated with dementia. Thus, failure to recall, inability to organize movements properly, word finding difficulties, and the like, are held more clearly in attention than are the person's positive attributes that remain intact. Thus, more and more of the person's positive qualities are obscured and, increasingly, attention is paid to the very attributes that are anathema to the person with dementia. I would ask the reader to imagine: how would you feel if all the significant people in your life saw you principally in terms of the characteristics you like least about yourself and if, furthermore, you were unable to change those characteristics for the better? Dr. M, with whom I had an association that spanned more than 2 years during the time she was in the moderate to severe stage of AD, provides a telling comment about the negative aspects of AD in the following extract [17]:

> SRS: When you walk around, saying to yourself, 'I can't stand the way things are going, I can't do this, I can't do that, I have trouble with this and that. . .'
> Dr. M: Ya, that's the issue. The issue is, what kind of life is that? (p. 119)

And later in the same conversation,

> SRS: Let me back up for a second because I think I'm missing your point. You don't want your life to be. . .
> Dr. M: Going always to see people to see what's wrong with me. (p. 120)

For the person with dementia, it's not merely a case of not wanting to go to see people who will, via tests and measurements, see what's wrong. It's being in situations in which healthy others, including one's family, increasingly define the person in terms of the diagnosis and symptoms both real and imagined.

The remedy is clear. It is vitally important that healthy others pay vigilant attention to the intact positive attributes that the person with dementia still possesses and that those characteristics are brought to the attention of the diagnosed person in order to show that she or he is valued and appreciated now just as in healthier times. One cannot have a strong sense of self-worth if others do not appreciate one's honourable and worthy qualities of character. If the person in question valued helping others, it's important to find ways in which that person can continue to do so.

Self 3 is comprised of the multiple social personae that one constructs with the cooperation of others in the social world. For example, being a loving spouse, a devoted parent, a loyal friend, a demanding supervisor, are all social personae and each has a unique pattern of behaviour. One behaves differently with one's child than with one's colleagues at work. It is the case, however, that any particular Self 3 persona is *jointly constructed* in that it is impossible for one to construct the persona of 'a loving spouse' if one's husband or wife does not recognize one as being his or her spouse. You cannot construct the persona of 'a devoted son or daughter' if your parents do not recognize you as their child. Likewise, if one's parents are deceased, one cannot construct the persona of 'a devoted child', for one lacks the necessary cooperation from the people who are critical in the joint construction of that persona. There are some limitations to this latter notion, for one can still observe the anniversaries of one's parents' deaths by going to the cemetery, praying in a house of worship, and such outward forms can be recognized by others as exemplary of one's devotion as a child.

For the person with dementia the situation can be dire. As more and more healthy others focus increasingly on one's dysfunctional attributes (Self 2), it is less and less likely that those same healthy others will cooperate with the person with dementia in constructing a healthy, worthy social persona. Indeed, from the point at which the diagnosis is rendered, the person with dementia is viewed more and more as 'the patient', than as the 'burdensome patient' and 'patienthood' becomes the central focus of one's social identity. A well-educated professional introduced me to her husband by saying, 'This is my husband. He's the patient'. Indeed, in relation to his physician, dentist, other health professionals, he was a patient, but he was most assuredly no more a patient in relation to everyone else in the social world than are you or me. The fact that he had a diagnosis does not confine his social identity (Self 3) to being 'the patient'. To impose this constricted social identity on a person is to imprison that person in ways that lead to increasingly dysfunctional treatment (malignant social psychology) and deepen the person's feelings of depression and lack of self-worth. It is pouring salt on an open wound.

Conclusion

It is possible, however, as research has shown, to cooperate with the person in the moderate to severe stage of dementia to construct worthy social personae such as 'research collaborator', 'day centre liaison', 'life of the party', 'sage advisor', and others [17], all in accordance with the person's wishes and long-standing dispositions and inclinations. In so doing, we continue to treat the person with dementia as a person first, and most assuredly not as 'the burdensome patient', all the while extending to that person the very same common courtesies that were so easily granted during the balance of the person's life in healthier times. The notion of supportive care suggests, at root and at best, an attitude towards the person as a unique, individual, and valued self. Whatever else it might be in practical terms, supportive care must ensure that the selfhood of the person is maintained. And, perhaps just as important, in supporting the selfhood of the person with dementia and thereby focusing on his or her humanity, we find more clearly our own positive attributes and social personae and, indeed, our own humanity as well.

References

1. Goffman E (1968). *Stigma: notes on the management of spoiled identity*. Harmondsworth: Penguin Books.
2. Scholl JM, Sabat SR (2008). Stereotypes, stereotype threat and ageing: implications for the understanding and treatment of people with Alzheimer's disease. *Ageing Soc*, **28**(1), 103–130.
3. Dijksterhuis A, van Knippenberg A (1998). The relation between perception and behavior, or how to win a game of trivial pursuit. *J Pers Soc Psychol*, **74**(4), 865–877.
4. Devine P (1989). Stereotypes and prejudice: their automatic and controlled components. *J Pers Soc Psychol*, **56**(1), 5–18.
5. Nosek BA, Banaji MR, Greenwald AG (2002). Harvesting intergroup attitudes and beliefs from a demonstration website. *Group Dyn*, **6**(1), 101–115.
6. Bandura A (1989). Regulation of cognitive processes through perceived self-efficacy. *Dev Psychol*, **25**(5), 729–735.
7. Levy B, Langer E (1994). Aging free from negative stereotypes: successful memory in China and among American deaf. *J Pers Soc Psychol*, **66**(5), 989–998.

8. Levy B (1996). Improving memory in old age through implicit self-stereotyping. *J Pers Soc Psychol*, **71**(6), 1092–1107.

9. Stein R, Blanchard-Fields F, Hertzog C (2002). The effects of age-stereotype priming on the memory performance of older adults. *Exp Aging Res*, **28**(1), 169–181.

10. Corner L, Bond J (2006). The impact of the label of mild cognitive impairment on the individual's sense of self. *Philos Psychiatr Psychol*, **13**(1), 3–12.

11. Steele CM (1997). A threat in the air: how stereotypes shape intellectual identity and performance. *Am Psychol*, **52**(6), 613–629.

12. Steele CM, Aronson J (1995). Contending with a stereotype: African-American intellectual test performance and stereotype threat. *J Pers Soc Psychol*, **69**(5), 797–811.

13. Leyens J, Désert M, Croizet J, Darcis C (2000). Stereotype threat: are lower status and history of stigmatization preconditions of stereotype threat? *Pers Soc Psychol Bull*, **26**(10), 1189–1199.

14. Hess TM, Auman C, Colcombe, SJ, Rahhal TA (2003). The impact of stereotype threat on age differences in memory performance. *J Geron: Psychol Sci*, **55B**, P3–P11.

15. van Langenhove L, Harré R (1999). Introducing positioning theory, in Harré R, van Langenhove L (eds) *Positioning theory*, pp. 14–31. Oxford: Blackwell.

16. Shweder RA, Sullivan M (1989). The semiotic subject of cultural psychology, in Previn L (ed) *Handbook of personality theory and research*. New York: Guilford.

17. Sabat SR (2001). *The experience of Alzheimer's disease: life through a tangled veil*. Oxford: Blackwell.

18. Hughes JC (2001). Views of the person with dementia. *J Med Ethics*, 27, 86–91.

19. Kitwood T (1998). Toward a theory of dementia care: ethics and interaction. *J Clin Ethics*, 9(1), 23–34.

20. Kitwood T, Bredin K (1992). Towards a theory of dementia care: personhood and well-being. *Ageing Soc*, 12(1), 269–287.

21. Snyder L (1999). *Speaking our minds: personal reflections from individuals with Alzheimer's disease*. New York: W.H. Freeman and Co.

22. Harré R (1991). The discursive production of selves. *Theory Psychol*, **1**(1), 51–63.

23. Cohen C, Eisdorfer C (2002). *The loss of self: a family resource for the care of Alzheimer's disease and related disorders*. New York: Norton and Co.

24. Sabat SR, Napolitano L, Fath H (2004). Barriers to the construction of a valued social identity: a case study of Alzheimer's disease. *Am J Alzheimer's Dis Other Demen*, **19** (3), 177–185.

25. Hughes JC, Louw S, Sabat SR (eds) (2006). *Dementia: mind, meaning, and the person*. Oxford: Oxford University Press.

26. Kontos P (2005). Embodied selfhood in Alzheimer's disease: rethinking person-centred care. *Dementia: The Int J Social Res Practice*, **49**(4), 553–570.

27. Kontos P (2006). Embodied selfhood: an ethnographic exploration of Alzheimer's disease, in Cohen L, Leibing A (eds) *Thinking about dementia: culture, loss, and the anthropology of senility*, 195–217. Cambridge: Cambridge University Press.

28. Sabat SR (2003). Some potential benefits of creating research partnerships with people with Alzheimer's disease. *Res Policy Plan*, **21**(2), 5–12.

Chapter 25

Person-centred care as supportive care

Murna Downs

Introduction

One of the most influential ideas in the field of dementia has been Tom Kitwood's notion of person-centred care. This approach has been credited with opening therapeutic potential in dementia care in contrast to the therapeutic nihilism characteristic of the traditional biomedical paradigm of dementia at the time of his writing. Kitwood described person-centred care as the 'new culture' of dementia care. A similar renaissance was championed by Saunders in the care of people who were dying. While the person who is dying may no longer be responsive to medical intervention, Saunders argued, there was much that could be done to improve quality of life by ensuring physical comfort and attending to the psychosocial and spiritual aspects of living with terminal illness. These two approaches, person-centred care and palliative care, can be readily compared; and there are also benefits to be derived from bringing the approaches together. This chapter explores how the notion of supportive care might encompass the ideals of person-centred and palliative care.

The person-centred approach to dementia care: key concepts

A philosophy of care

The person-centred approach to care for people with dementia is first and foremost a philosophy of care. It does not prescribe particular behaviours in particular contexts. Rather it seeks to ground its efforts in a respect for the dignity and well-being of the person with dementia. Its pioneer was Professor Tom Kitwood (1937–1998). Writing in the 1980s and 1990s, Tom Kitwood sought to improve the care of people with dementia by an emphasis on the essential humanity of the person, rather than on the disease and its associated deficits and dysfunctions. He was critical of the view that because there was no cure for neurological disease there was nothing that could be done to enhance the person's quality of life.

Dementia as dialectic interplay between biological, psychological, and social factors

The traditional biomedical paradigm of dementia attributed much of what a person did, or failed to do, to their neurological disease. Prior to the advent of anti-dementia drugs, a sense of therapeutic nihilism followed. It was felt that, as there was little that could be done to arrest neurological disease, there was little that could be done for a person with dementia. In short, people with dementia were viewed as being beyond the therapeutic potential of medicine. As we will see in our discussion of the hospice movement, in the eyes of a medical professional concerned with cure, people with dementia had much in common with those who were dying – both were seen as failures of a system designed for cure.

Much of Kitwood's interest in dementia was prompted by his disillusionment with this standard medical understanding of, and response to, people with dementia. In his view it neglected the psychological, social, and spiritual aspects of living with progressive cognitive impairment. He was highly critical of a health and social care system that attributed everything a person experienced to their neurology alone. For him, this had at least two interrelated and unfavourable consequences for people with dementia:

1 A sense of therapeutic nihilism, i.e. nothing can be done to help people with dementia.

2 A neglect of the important influences of life history, personality, physical and mental health, and social psychology on quality of life. This was of particular concern as he saw potential in interventions which addressed physical and mental health and the person's social and interpersonal environment [1].

The person-centred approach to dementia care provided the field with an alternative view of dementia. For Kitwood an exclusively neurological or biological view of dementia was not sufficient to explain the process of dementia [2]. He proposed a view of dementia as a dynamic interplay – or dialectic – between biological, psychological, and social factors [3–5]. Kitwood was by no means a lone voice. Around the same time, in the U.S. Karen Lyman wrote a seminal paper entitled *Bringing the social back in: a critique of the bio-medicalisation of dementia* [6], while Gubrium challenged us to consider the social construction of Alzheimer's disease [7].

The importance of the person with dementia's subjective experience

The person-centred approach assumes that the subjective experience of dementia is the starting point in dementia care. Kitwood considered that people with dementia were aware of their circumstance, if not in factual detail at least in emotional, lived experience [8]. Empirical support for awareness in dementia has since been demonstrated for those recently diagnosed [9,10] as well as for those with more severe dementia [11–20].

A key tenet of Kitwood's person-centred care for people with dementia is the importance of taking the person's perspective, being concerned with understanding their subjectivity [8]. He provided suggestions as to how this experience might be ascertained including traditional methods of interview and observation as well as less commonly used methods of role-play and the arts. Kitwood with his colleague Bredin developed an observational framework for measuring the quality of care, from the perspective of the person with dementia, Dementia Care Mapping (DCM) [21]. They proposed that such information be gathered on a regular basis and fed back to staff to prompt the development of person-centred action plans. This process has much in common with methods of continuous quality of improvement.

The importance paid to the person's perspective has grown enormously since Kitwood first mooted this idea. It is now recognized as being essential to both day-to-day care and to the development of appropriate service development and evaluation [22–25]. Indeed while remarkable when first established, collectives of people with dementia, whether meeting virtually (e.g. the Dementia Advocacy and Support Network International (DASNI) www.dasninternational.org) or in person (see e.g., Scottish Dementia Working Group (www.sdwg.org.uk)), are now relatively commonplace.

People with dementia are semiotic beings actively negotiating their world

Kitwood stressed that people with dementia actively sought meaning in their world and acted on the meaning they made of the world [26]. Sabat and Harré referred to people with dementia as semiotic or meaning-making beings [27]. Most notably from Sabat [28], we now have a wealth of evidence demonstrating that people with dementia actively strive to make sense of the world and their place in it. Kontos has since provided empirical support for the persistence of self and agency in dementia noting that for people with severe dementia this selfhood and agency is embodied [13]. Hughes and colleagues draw on Merleau-Ponty [29] and describe people with dementia as 'situated embodied agents'.

Personhood

For Kitwood the aim of dementia care was to enhance personhood [30–33]. Personhood was seen as being constructed in relationship with others [34], something 'bestowed' by the other. In Kitwood and Bredin's view the greatest threat to a person living with dementia is the loss of personhood [34] – no longer being seen as fully human in the eyes of others. Kitwood describes behaviours which bestowed personhood (e.g. validating, celebrating, holding) as 'positive person work' and those that diminished it as 'personal detractors' (e.g. ignoring, outpacing, banishment) constituting a 'malignant social psychology' [32,33,35]. Such malignancy was never considered to be intentional on the part of families or care staff but a benign adoption of the dominant culture [35]. In this relational approach to personhood, a person is a person among others [29]. What other people do or fail to do will enhance or diminish that person's personhood or standing as an individual. Kitwood questioned the extent to which some of the impairment observed could be attributable to the 'malignant' or 'iatrogenic' psychosocial context in which people with dementia lived. A malignant social psychology was thought to lead to a diminished sense of personhood, self and worth.

Kitwood imported concepts associated with symbolic interactionism [36] and social psychology [37] to argue that who we are and how we behave is a function of our relationships with others [30]. Thus therapeutic potential in dementia care lay within the interpersonal and social dimension of people's lives [26,38,39]. It was through human interaction and engagement that personhood and feelings of well-being were to be attained and maintained. Thus, by changing the nature of the interaction one could directly affect the individual's personhood and well-being. Kitwood was one of the first writers to emphasize the importance of the social environment in supporting personhood and meeting a person's psychological needs [32,33].

Psychological needs and well-being

In Kitwood's view [26], well-being was achievable for people with dementia, but it required that their needs be met, including, and perhaps most importantly, their need for love. Kitwood proposed that people with dementia had needs for:

1 Attachment – the need for secure bonds with carers
2 Comfort – the need for relief of pain, closeness and tenderness
3 Identity – the need to be known by others
4 Occupation – the need to be involved in the process of life
5 Inclusion – the need to have one's social standing as a person recognized,

with an overarching need for love and interconnectedness [26]. Thus, addressing these psychological, emotional, social and spiritual needs is at the heart of person-centred care.

Cohen-Mansfield, Stokes and others [40,41] argue that many of the 'behavioural symptoms' viewed as inevitable aspects of living with dementia are attempts to meet needs (see also Chapter 17). Indeed, an alternative paradigm for understanding behaviour is the needs-compromised paradigm from Algase *et al.* and Beattie and colleagues [42,43]. Over 20 years ago Rader and colleagues coined the term 'agenda behaviour' [44] to describe the phenomenon whereby people with dementia's behaviour was goal-directed and not just random. For Kitwood [26], distressed behaviour was seen, as an expression of ill-being (e.g. wandering, crying, shouting, and hitting), as legitimate responses to assaults on personhood, rather than as part of the disease process.

Moral worth and social action

The person-centred approach has been credited with reinstating the person as a valued human and social being with moral worth and human rights [45]. A key need was for the intrinsic value of people with dementia to become enshrined in public policy and to eradicate stigma and discrimination [46]. Kitwood's focus on personhood set a value base that people have moral worth and entitlement to social standing, regardless of degree of cognitive impairment [32,33]. Thus Kitwood emphasized the importance of the moral development of practitioners and professionals in order to ensure quality dementia care [47]. Post also highlights the 'moral challenge' of dementia care [48].

For Kitwood it would not have been enough to provide more and more services for people with dementia. His concern was not one of increasing the *quantity* of existing services. His concern was with a *qualitative* change in the way we conceptualize, and care for, people with dementia. As recently argued by Kellehear [49], this did not see the solution for people with dementia as lying within the domain of clinical medicine, although clearly this specialty had a key role to play. For Kitwood, as for Kellehear, a broader social change was required. As Kellehear argues, people with dementia spend many years living with dementia in community as well as in institutional settings. Thus community action and development is as important as the development of clinical services.

The palliative approach to people with terminal illness: key concepts

A philosophy of care

In common with the person-centred approach, palliative care is both a philosophy and an approach to care. The pioneer of palliative care was Dame Cicely Saunders (1918–2005). Cicely Saunders was driven to improve the care of people who she witnessed dying during the 1950s and early 1960s. People who were dying were poorly served by new advances in treatments for cancer that focused on cure. Death was seen as a failure rather than as a natural part of life [50]. Saunders was critical of the view that because there was no cure for cancer, nothing could be done to improve the quality of life of people dying from the disease [51].

Quality of life and dignity

Saunders focused on using new drug treatments to manage pain and other symptoms; improving dignity and quality of life, and identifying the importance of attending to the whole person, rather than the disease [52]. In her view much could be done to improve quality of life – to give quality to life – for someone whose condition is not amenable to medical cure or treatment. The palliative approach stresses the need to address the 'total pain' experienced by someone who is dying in order to ensure quality of life for that person. This includes attention to physical, psychological, social, and spiritual aspects of living with a progressive condition [50]. The palliative philosophy is person-centred, focusing on both the person's quality of life before death and the quality of his or her death when it happens. Originally stated by Dame Cicely Saunders:

> You matter because you are you. You matter to the last moment of your life and we will do all we can not only to help you die peacefully but to live until you die [53].

Saunders was not alone in influencing how we think about and care for those dying. Glaser and Strauss had drawn attention to the plight of those dying in hospitals where they experienced 'social death', or a neglect of them as persons, prior to their biological death [54]. Aries had pointed out how in society's view death was unacceptable and was something to be removed from social view [55]. Kubler-Ross testified in a similar vein to the U.S. Senate Special Committee on Ageing:

> We live in a very particular death-denying society. We isolate both the dying and the old, and it serves a purpose. They are reminders of our own mortality [56].

Inter-disciplinary team approach

The palliative approach requires one to adopt a holistic and inter-disciplinary approach for assessing and managing ongoing physical, psychological, social, and spiritual aspects of a person's life. Support may be provided by specialist palliative care teams if the person and their family are experiencing complex problems or require complex symptom management.

Supporting the family during the patient's illness and in their own bereavement

A palliative approach places emphasis on supporting families throughout the period between diagnosis and death and into bereavement. Support may be provided by different health and social care practitioners over time.

Applicability early in the course of illness

Palliative care commences from diagnosis and is guided by the main principles of holistic care and quality of life. Part of the help provided is to assist people in addressing their own mortality [57]. Care is provided by a range of health and social care professionals incorporating a range of different treatments or therapies used to support the person and to manage their condition as it changes over time.

Person-directed

A palliative approach sees the person with the illness as being in control of what care, support, treatment, and interventions are provided. The key component is open communication. There are a variety of tools used by hospice, hospital, and community practitioners to record the person's choices and to facilitate these [58,59].

Person-centred and palliative approaches within supportive care

Supporting the person as a living, human being

Both person-centred and palliative approaches stress the importance of engaging with the person who is living with, while dying from, a terminal condition [60–63]. This engagement includes affirming the value of life and enhancing the quality of life, as well as addressing the anticipated and actual losses faced by the person [64,65]. Such support should develop and strengthen one's family and community supports [49], keeping things 'normal' and non-stigmatizing for people with dementia, thus preventing the well documented, if unintentional, consequences of receiving psychiatric services [66].

From diagnosis to death and bereavement

Both person-centred and palliative approaches stress the importance of engaging with the person from diagnosis to death [62,63]. People early in the course of living with dementia may need support to prepare for, and adjust to, the diagnosis. While this support can be provided by health and social care specialists, it can also be provided by informal supports in the community. Group psychotherapy may be useful for some [67]. Adjustment to the implications of the diagnosis is also required of families. As most people with dementia live in the community, as the person's cognitive and functional impairment increases, family members carry most of the responsibility for their care. A significant percentage of people with dementia live in care homes originally designed for those with physical frailty. The potential of palliative [68,69] approaches in these settings are being realized. We now have an evidence base from the US [70], UK [71], and Australia [72] demonstrating the benefits of person-centred approaches in these settings. Support at the end of life is as important for people with dementia as it is for others dying with neurodegenerative conditions. While specialist palliative services may not always be required, there is much that can be done to promote personhood, comfort, and well-being at the end of life [3].

Support for physical needs

Physical care is an integral part of supportive care; person-centred and palliative approaches see physical care as integral to holistic care. Physical care – personal, nursing, and medical care – is inevitably care for the person as an embodied individual. Personal care includes assisting with eating, dressing bathing, toileting, and ensuring physical comfort. Personal care provides opportunities for engagement with and communicating respect for the person. Unfortunately these opportunities are often missed in care homes [73]. Twigg [74] describes the role of clothing in upholding the personhood and dignity for a person with dementia. The provision of timely medical (including dental) attention is as important for people with dementia as it is for those without dementia. Early diagnosis of infections ensures comfort and optimal well-being.

Support for emotional needs

It is self evident that the person with dementia is an emotional being having a physical dimension. Living with dementia requires a period of continual adjustment to, and integration of, loss [9]. Care for people with dementia requires that we attune to and address this experience of loss. This requires both emotional intelligence and empathy. As such, emotions are at the heart of living with dementia and are, therefore, at the heart of person-centred dementia care [72].

Support for social and spiritual needs

As Kitwood [32] argued, personhood is realized in relationship with others. As such, the loss of friends and community commonly associated with living with dementia puts people at risk. It is not just the social world of the person with dementia that shrinks, but families too become isolated at a time when they most need social support themselves. Person-centred care emphasizes the importance of social contact and relationships. It recognizes that those close to the person with dementia will need support. Regardless of particular (if any) religious persuasions a person is facing death and thus faces questions about the meaning of their own life. There is no reason to assume that cognitive impairment negates the need for such active resolution and meaning-making in one's life. Indeed, one could argue that the progressive neuro-degeneration associated with dementia makes such resolution even more compelling.

Conclusion

We need to transform the quality of the care we provide people with dementia and their families [75]. We have two guiding philosophies and many examples of these philosophies in practice to guide us. First and foremost, supportive care needs to have as its focus a living, human being, however impaired or ill. Secondly, care should be concerned with supporting all aspects of the person's experience of living with dementia – cognitive, emotional psychological, physical, and spiritual. Thirdly, those who provide care to people with dementia, whether as family or paid carers, in turn need support for doing so. We can no longer say there is nothing that can be done to support people to live well with dementia. Perhaps the most pressing concern is to put what we know into practice. There is now a compelling argument for bringing both person-centred and palliative approaches together to form the basis of supportive care for people with dementia and their families.

References

1. Livingston G, Cooper C, Woods J, Milne A, Katona C (2008). Successful ageing in adversity: the LASER–AD longitudinal study. *J Neurol Neurosurg Psychiatry,* **79**, 641–645.

2. Kitwood T (1990). The dialectics of dementia: with particular reference to Alzheimer's disease. *Ageing Soc,* **10**(2), 177–196.

3. Downs M, Small N, Froggatt K (2006). Person-centred care for people with severe dementia, in Burns A, Winblad B (eds) *Severe dementia.* London: Wiley and Sons.

4. Downs M, Clare L, Anderson E (2008). Dementia as a bio-psychosocial condition: implications for practice and research, in Woods R, Clare, L (eds) *Handbook of the clinical psychology of ageing,* 2nd edn. Chichester: Wiley.

5. Sabat S (2008). A bio-psycho-social approach to dementia, in Downs M, Bowers B (eds) *Excellence in dementia care: research into practice,* pp. 70–84. Maidenhead: Open University Press.

6. Lyman K (1989). Bringing the social back in: a critique of the biomedicalisation of dementia. *Gerontologist,* **29**(5), 597–605.

7. Gubrium J (1986). *Oldtimers and Alzheimer's: the descriptive organization of senility.* Greenwich: JAI Press.

8. Kitwood T (1997). The experience of dementia. *Aging Ment Health,* **1**(1), 13–22.

9. Clare L (2002). We'll fight it as long as we can: coping with the onset of Alzheimer's disease. *Aging Ment Health,* **6**, 139–148.

10. Moniz-Cook E, Manthorpe J, Carr I, Gibson G, Vernooij-Dassen M (2006). Facing the future: a qualitative study of older people referred to a memory clinic prior to assessment and diagnosis. *Dementia: Int J Soc Res Pract,* **5**(3), 375–395.

11. Clare L, Rowlands J, Bruce E, Surr C, Downs M (2008). 'I don't do like I used to do': a grounded theory approach to conceptualising awareness in people with moderate to severe dementia living in long-term care. *Soc Sci Med,* **66**(11), 2366–2377.

12. Clare L, Rowlands J, Bruce E, Surr C, Downs M (2008). The experience of living with dementia in residential care: an interpretative phenomenological analysis. *Gerontologist,* **48**, 711–720.

13. Kontos PC (2004). Ethnographic reflections on selfhood, embodiment and Alzheimer's disease. *Ageing Soc,* **24**(6), 829–849.

14. Norberg A (1998). Interaction with people suffering from severe dementia, in Wimo A, Jonsson B, Karlsson G, Winblad B (eds) *Health economics of dementia,* pp. 113–121. Chichester: John Wiley and Sons.

15. Norberg A (2001). Communication in the care of people with severe dementia, in Hummert ML, Nussbaum JF (eds) *Aging, communication, and health: linking research and practice for successful aging,* pp. 157–173. New Jersey: Lawrence Erlbaum Associates.

16. Norberg A, Melin E, Asplund K (2003). Reactions to music, touch and object presentation in the final stage of dementia: an exploratory study. *Int J Nurs Stud,* **40**, 473–479.

17. Normann HK, Asplund K, Norberg A (1998). Episodes of lucidity in people with severe dementia as narrated by formal carers. *J Adv Nurs,* **28**(6), 1295–1300.

18. Normann HK, Norberg A, Asplund K (2002). Confirmation and lucidity during conversations with a woman with severe dementia. *J Adv Nurs*, **39**(4), 370–376.

19. Phinney A (1998). Living with dementia from the patient's perspective. *J Gerontol Nurs*, **24**(6), 3–15.

20. Phinney A, Chesla CA (2003). The lived body in dementia. *J Aging Stud*, **17**, 283–299.

21. Kitwood T, Bredin K (1992). A new approach to the evaluation of dementia care. *J Adv Health Nurs Care*, **1**(5), 41–60.

22. Cantley C, Woodhouse J, Smith M (2005). *Listen to us: involving people with dementia in planning and developing services*. Dementia North: University of Northumbria.

23. Cotrell V, Schulz R (1993). The perspective of the patient with Alzheimer's disease: a neglected dimension of dementia research. *Gerontologist*, **33**(2), 205–211.

24. Harris PB (ed) (2002). *The person with Alzheimer's disease: pathways to understanding the experience*. London: Johns Hopkins University Press.

25. Litherland R (2008). Involving people with dementia in service development and evaluation, in Downs M, Bowers B (eds) *Excellence in dementia care: research into practice*, pp. 397–413. Maidenhead: Open University Press.

26. Kitwood T (1997). *Dementia reconsidered: the person comes first*. Buckingham: Open University Press.

27. Sabat SR, Harré R (1994). The Alzheimer's disease sufferer as a semiotic subject. *Philos Psychiatr Psychol*, **1**(1), 145–160.

28. Sabat S (2001). *The experience of Alzheimer's disease: life through a tangled veil*. Oxford: Blackwell.

29. Hughes JC, Louw SJ, Sabat SR (eds) (2006). *Dementia: mind, meaning and person*. Oxford: Oxford University Press.

30. Baldwin C, Capstick A (2007). *Tom Kitwood on dementia: a reader and critical commentary*. Maidenhead: Open University Press.

31. Brooker D (2004). What is person-centred care for people with dementia? *Rev Clin Psychol*, **13**, 215–222.

32. Kitwood T (1993). Towards a theory of dementia care: the interpersonal process. *Ageing Soc*, **13**(1), 51–67.

33. Kitwood T (1994). The concept of personhood and its relevance to a new culture of dementia care, in Miesen BML, Jones GMM (eds) *Caregiving in dementia*, vol. 2, pp 3–13. London: Routledge.

34. Kitwood T, Bredin K (1992). Towards a theory of dementia care: personhood and well-being. *Ageing Soc*, **12**(3), 269–287.

35. Kitwood T (1998). Toward a theory of dementia care: Ethics and interaction. *J Clin Ethics*, **9**(1), 23–34.

36. Mead GH (1932). *Mind, self and society from the standpoint of a social behaviourist (edited by Morris CW)*, Chicago: University of Chicago.

37. Harré R (1991). The discursive production of selves. *Theory psychol*, **1**(1), 51–63.

38. McCormack B (2004). Person-centredness in gerontological nursing. *J Clin Nurs*, **13**(3a), 31–38.

39. Zgola JM (1999). *Care that works: a relationship approach to persons with dementia*. Johns London: Hopkins University Press.

40. Cohen-Mansfield J (2008). Understanding the language of behaviour, in Downs M, Bowers B (eds) *Excellence in dementia care: research into practice*, pp 187–211. Maidenhead: Open University Press.

41. Stokes G (2000). *Challenging behaviour in dementia: a person-centred approach*. Bicester: Speechmark.

42. Algase DL, Beck C, Kolanowski A *et al.* (1996). Need-driven dementia-compromised behavior: an alternative view of disruptive behavior. *Am J Alzheimers Dis Other Dem*, **11**, 10–19.

43. Beattie ERA, Algase DL, Song J (2004). Behavioural symptoms of dementia: their measurement and intervention. *Aging Ment Health*, **8**(2), 109–116.

44. Rader J, Doan J, Schwab M (1985). How to decrease wandering, a form of agenda behaviour. *Geriatr Nurs*, **6**(4), 196–199.

45. Morton I (1999). *Person-centred approaches to dementia care*. Oxon: Speechmark Publishing Ltd.

46. Graham N, Lindesay J, Katona C *et al.* (2003). Reducing stigma and discrimination against older people with mental disorders: a technical consensus statement. *Int J Geriatr Psychiatry*, **18**(8), 670–678.

47. Kitwood T (1998). Professional and moral development for care work: some observations on the process. *J Moral Educ*, **27**(3), 401–411.

48. Post S (2000). *The moral challenge of Alzheimer's disease: ethical issues from diagnosis to dying*, (2nd edn). Baltimore and London: Johns Hopkins University Press.

49. Kellehear A (2009). Dementia and dying: the need for a systematic policy approach. *Crit Soc Policy*, **29**(1), 146–157.

50. Clark D, Seymour J (1999). *Reflections on palliative care*. Buckingham: Open University Press.

51. Clark D (2002). Between hope and acceptance: the medicalisation of dying. *BMJ*, **321**, 905–907.

52. Clark D (2005). *Cicely Saunders: founder of the hospice movement: selected letters 1959–1999*. Oxford: Oxford University Press.

53. Saunders (1976). Care of the dying. The problem of euthanasia. *Nurs Times*, **72**, 1003–1005.

54. Glaser B, Strauss A (1965). *Awareness of dying*. Chicago: Aldine.

55. Aries P (1974). *Western attitudes toward death: from the middle ages to the present*. Baltimore: Johns Hopkins University.

56. Kubler-Ross E (1969). *On death and dying*. New York: Macmillan.

57. Hughes JC, Robinson L, Volicer L (2005). Specialist palliative care in dementia. *BMJ*, **330**, 57–58.

58. National Health Service (NHS). *Preferred priorities for care (PPC)*. Avaiable at: http://www.endoflifecareforadults.nhs.uk/eolc/ppc.htm (accessed on 26 August 2008).

59. Henry C, Seymour J. *Advance care planning: a guide for health and social care staff*. National health Service (NHS). http://www.endoflifecareforadults.nhs.uk/eolc/files/F2023-EoLC-ACP_guide_for_staff-Aug2008.pdf (accessed on 26 August 2008).

60. Froggatt KA, Downs M, Small N (2008). Palliative care for people with dementia: principles, practice and implications, in Woods R, Clare L (eds) *Handbook of the clinical psychology of ageing*, 2nd edn. Chichester: Wiley.

61. Hughes JC, Hedley K, Harris D (2006). The practice and philosophy of palliative care in dementia, in Hughes JC (ed) *Palliative care in severe dementia*, pp. 1–11. London: Quay Books.

62. Small N, Downs M, Froggatt K (2008). Improving end-of-life care for people with dementia – the benefits of combining UK approaches to palliative care and dementia care, in Jones G, Miesen B (eds) *Care-giving in dementia: research and applications,* vol. 4. Hove, East Sussex: Brunner-Routledge.

63. Small N, Froggatt K, Downs M (2008) *Living and dying with dementia: dialogues about palliative care.* Oxford: Oxford University Press.

64. Jennings B (2004). Alzheimer's disease and quality of life, in Doka K (ed) *Living with grief: Alzheimer's disease*, pp 131–144. Washington: Hospice Foundation of America.

65. Miesen BML (1997). Awareness in dementia patients and family grieving: a practical perspective, in Miesen BML, Jones GMM (eds) *Caregiving in dementia*, vol. 2, pp. 67–79. London: Routledge.

66. Sayce L (1999). *From psychiatric patient to citizen: overcoming discrimination and stigma*. London: Palgrave Macmillan.

67. Cheston R, Jones K, Gilliard J (2003). Group psychotherapy and people with dementia. *Aging Ment Health*. **7**(6), 452–461.

68. Hockley J, Clark D (2002). *Palliative care for older people in care homes*. Maidenhead: Open University Press.

69. Hockley J, Froggatt K (2006). The development of palliative care knowledge in care homes for older people: the place of action research. *Palliative Medicine*, **20** (8), 835–843.

70. Sloane P, Hoeffer B, Mitchell C *et al.* (2004). Effect of person-centred showering and towel bath n bathing associated aggression, agitation, and discomfort in nursing home residents with dementia: A randomized, controlled trial. *JAGS*, **52**(11), 1795–1804.

71. Fossey J, Ballard C, Juszczak E *et al.* (2006). Effect of enhanced psychosocial care on antipsychotic use in nursing home residents with severe dementia: cluster randomised trial *BMJ*, **332**, 756–761.

72. Chenoweth L, King MT, Jeon Y-H *et al.* (2009). Caring for aged dementia care resident study (CADRES) of person-centred care, dementia care mapping and usual care in dementia: a cluster-randomised trial. *Lancet Neurol*, **8**(4), 317–325.

73. Cohen-Mansfield J, Creedon M A, Malone T *et al.* (2006). Dressing of cognitively impaired nursing home residents: description and analysis. *Gerontologist*, **46**, 89–96.

74. Twigg J (2009). *Clothing and dementia.* Available at: http://www.kent.ac.uk/sspssr/staff/academic/twigg/clothing-dementia.pdf (accessed on 22 March 2009).

75. Department of Health (2009). *Living well with dementia: national dementia strategy.* London: The Stationery Office.

Chapter 26

Narrative, supportive care, and dementia: a preliminary exploration

Clive Baldwin

Introduction

Narrative is, it appears, everywhere. In stating this, I am both re-stating the position that human experience is fundamentally and necessarily narrativized, that we all swim in a sea of stories, and claiming that narrative as an approach to understanding, analyzing and performing research, policy, and practice appears in disciplines as widely disparate as mathematics, psychotherapy, economics, sociology, biology, and theology (and the list goes on). The seeming ubiquity of narrative is possibly a result of the different and not always compatible definitions, performances, and operationalizations of the term. For some, narrative is a means to understand, or a window upon, human experience. For others there can be no experience that is not narrativized; that is, narrative, or rather narrativization constitutes rather than expresses experiences. For some, narrative can elucidate what it is like to be a particular Self; for others it is that very narrativization that constitutes the Self. For some, narrative is a form of data to be manipulated and analyzed to provide insight and generate new knowledge. For others narrativization is the analysis of data and is a way of knowing. Where one stands with regard to each of these positions will determine the sort of narrative work one does.

Given the ubiquity and seeming ambiguity of what is meant by narrative, it is, I think, incumbent on authors to make explicit where they stand on the questions above. While my position will become obvious in what follows, at the outset I want to make clear that, along with Bruner [1–3] and others [4] I believe that we live storied or narrativized lives both in the sense that we constitute our Selves through narrative and, along with Taylor [5], that our Selves are held within a web of narratives (interlocutions in Taylor's terminology). In understanding and pursuing this stance, which is ontological (in the sense that it is concerned with our nature as beings of this sort), I agree with Bruner (above) that there is a subsequent narrative epistemology (in the sense that narrative helps us to know things): we come to know things narratively. This way of knowing is different to the logico-scientific way of knowing, but is equally reliable, valid and important because it gives us insights into, and the resources to deal with, aspects of living that the logico-scientific method cannot. Narrative knowing, in Polkinghorne's terms is '. . . used to understand personal action and autobiography. It is the format people use to organize their understandings of each other . . .' [6].

Narrative and dementia

'People with dementia are at risk of others assuming that they do not have a narrative or if they do, of it not being understandable' [7]. The fragmentation of memory, linguistic ability and other features associated with narrativity can mean that others read this as the person with dementia no longer being able to construct or contribute to what it recognizably a narrative. I have argued

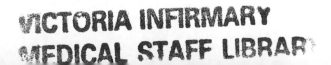

elsewhere that this 'narrative dispossession' [8] is more probably a result of a definition of narrative that relies on verbalization, extended coherence, a limited sense of narrative agency, restricted opportunities to engage in narrative activity, and narrative illiteracy on the part of those around people with dementia. Indeed, in contrast to the above quote there seems to be a small but growing literature that challenges the assumption that people with dementia do not have a narrative. On the one hand, there are the writings on the narrative activity of people living with dementia [9–11], and, on the other, an increasing autobiographical literature by people living with dementia [12–16].

Supportive care and narrative

Although there are a number of definitions of supportive care, for the purposes of this chapter I take supportive care to refer to the provision of care aimed at meeting the physical, emotional, psychological, social, and spiritual needs of those living with, or affected by, dementia, as defined by those living with or affected by dementia, from pre-diagnosis to palliation and bereavement. In other words, it is an informed and practical accompaniment on a journey, guided by those whose journey it is.

In narrative terms, supportive care can be seen as helping those affected navigate the troubled waters between different types of narrative. Frank [17] puts forward a three-fold typology of illness narratives: the restitution narrative, the chaos narrative, and the quest narrative.

The restitution narrative is probably the one that most people hold to, through the ups and downs of life. Even in serious illness it has a power to affect one's well-being. At its simplest, this narrative goes as follows: I was well, I became ill and now I am better, restored to my old self. The application of this narrative is relatively straightforward with regard to many illnesses: I have flu but will get better again. It does, however, face problems with regard to chronic and progressive conditions that have no prospect of being cured and about which restitution is inapplicable, for example, dementia. While people affected by dementia do hope for a cure, such seems unlikely, at least in the timeframe allowed for those currently affected by the condition. This does not mean, however, that the restitution narrative is irrelevant to supportive care – for there may be, even if the overall trajectory is not one of restitution, small restitutions along the way (see later). And for those who survive the person with dementia, some form of restitution is required for them to carry on.

The second type of narrative – the chaos narrative – is, for Frank, the opposite of the restitution narrative. In the chaos narrative the plot imagines life never getting better. Furthermore, the chaos narrative is far more difficult to experience, tell, and hear than the restitution narrative. Being more difficult to experience and tell, the chaos narrative might itself become fragmented, troubled, and disrupted, that is, less obviously a narrative. Being more difficult to hear, there may be fewer opportunities for telling a chaos narrative, even if one is able to, with less eliciting of these stories by those around the people directly affected, either out of avoidance or lack of narrative facility.

The final type of story Frank explores is that of the quest – seeing the onset of illness as a departure on a journey in which there is a call, tribulation transformation, and ultimately meaning. The call comes from the recognition that this is something that is a big deal, that it will not go away, and has to be faced. Following a response to this call the protagonists (the person living with dementia and/or their carers) face trials and tribulations through which they are transformed. Finally, the person returns from the experience to share that with others.

These three types of stories are not necessarily discrete, and on any journey one might find elements of each, at different times on, or about different aspects of, the journey. The art of supportive care, I will argue, is that of crafting an over-arching narrative that helps those affected navigate between these types of sub-stories. This over-arching narrative will be one that pays attention to physical, emotional, psychological, social, and spiritual needs: in other words, it will be a narrative of embodied-ness, incorporating the individual experience (emotional and psychological) within a network of narratives (social) which ultimately provides meaning (spiritual) for those involved. This is not to say that narrative supportive care can (or indeed should) provide all the answers, merely that it is a means for facilitating the journey.

And it is at this point that the observant readers of this chapter will note that in the last sentence I have removed the comma separating narrative and supportive care, bringing the two into a single concept. In this way narrative is not simply an adjunct to supportive care but a defining aspect of that care. In what follows, I outline five fundamental features of narrative supportive care.

The scope of narrative supportive care

While the reader might be forgiven for thinking that narrative is all-embracing, I think a more limited focus is appropriate for discussing supportive care. In particular, I want to address four aspects of such care which, I believe, can encompass the individual, the individual within social relations, and the individual within the organization, namely:

1 Maintaining narrative agency

2 Establishing the emergent plot

3 A sensitivity to and an appreciation of narrative webs

4 The accumulation of narrative resources.

I could, of course, expand this further to include the individual within society – and indeed I will touch upon this – but the main focus here is the performance of supportive care rather than the political context of that care. This, of course, is an artificial divide because personal narratives are also political [18,19] but extension of my argument here must await another day.

My concluding remarks will focus on the need for narrative literacy on the part of those providing supportive care.

Maintaining narrative agency

Maintaining narrative agency is probably the most straightforward aspect of narrative supportive care in that it translates relatively easily into obvious practical activities. At root, narrative agency is having the ability and opportunity to author one's own story. While the onset and progression of dementia may compromise this in some ways, there are things that practitioners can do in order to ameliorate the effects of dementia on narrativity and to create the conditions whereby narrative agency continues even when direct authorship is no longer possible. Of course, there already exist ways in which agency is projected into the future – through, for example, the legal requirement to consult individuals about decisions concerning them and advance decisions or living wills (see the Mental Capacity Act 2005) [20]). This focus on narrative agency provides a framework for the future in all its complexity, rather than simply focussing on foreseeable, specific decisions.

Elsewhere [8,19] I have indicated a number of ways in which the narrativity of people living with dementia might be enhanced. Here I repeat and extend those ways. It is my belief that the narrative agency of people living with dementia can be maintained and enhanced by:

1 Simply providing people with dementia with the opportunities to provide their narratives: making space in our busy days to talk with people having dementia, by facilitating

communication through such things as talking mats [21], and more overtly by eliciting their stories through reminiscence projects [22], and even psychotherapy [23].

2 Narrativizing other means of symbolic expression such as art, music, and dance (see for example Downs *et al.* [24] who draw attention to the communicative possibilities of sound, music, behavioural cues, and mirroring).

3 Attention to small stories that do not rely on extended communication [25], that is, the micro-scale interactions between individuals that occur throughout the day; these can indicate, if we are open to their possibilities, facets of identity, agency, and creativity on which narrative agency is based; just as Bamberg [25] sees the small interactions of adolescents as providing a way of performing, establishing, and/or maintaining their identity, the small interactions of brief conversations in the corridor, or over a cup of tea, can provide people with dementia with an opportunity to express themselves narratively – when such expressions are made meaningful within a wider life narrative.

4 Engaging with people having dementia (and others) in the co-construction of stories, [26], for example, in life history work.

The maintenance and facilitation of narrative agency can help, I believe, steer people away from being drawn into a chaos narrative. While options and abilities may become comparatively restricted, a sense of narrative agency allows some control over where the story is going. A focus on small stories can be seen as an antidote to the fragmentation of narrative and a means of establishing small restitution narratives.

Establishing the emergent plot

In 'Six characters in search of an author' [27] we find six characters who see themselves as incomplete because the writer of the play in which they were characters has died and there is no one to continue the story. They thus approach the Manager of a company of actors asking whether he will be their author so that like Sancho Panza and Don Abbondio they might have 'the fortune to find a fecundating matrix, a fantasy which could raise and nourish them: make them live for ever!' The search for a story is thus essential for a complete life.

Before narrative agency is compromised, steps can be taken to extend that agency by providing a framework for the emerging plot. Supportive care can work with individuals (and others affected) relatively early on to decide the direction in which they want the story to go and how best to effect that navigation. Such a 'plot line' could be based on the values history proposed by Rich [28]. In such histories, individuals set out the things that have been and continue to be important in their lives. This is slightly different to, and more than, the writing of and adherence to advance decisions (see the Mental Capacity Act 2005) [20]. It is more of a setting of a trajectory based on what has gone before so that the story continues to make sense. The metaphor would be a loose script and plot with and within which the actors could *ad lib* according to the dynamics of the situation, but each is charged with the responsibility of moving the plot forward. It is thus, unlike for example a living will, more about process than decision.

In Tim Burton's *Big Fish*, Edward Bloom (played by Albert Finney) lies dying. He is visited by his son Will, from whom he has been somewhat estranged over the years owing to Will's perception of his father as an insincere fraud. This perception is based on Edward's tendency to tell elaborate and bizarre tales about his life – for example, running off to the circus with Carl the Giant and escaping from Korea in the company of conjoined twins. In the final scenes of the movie, Edward is only partly conscious and is unable to continue his story so he asks Will to tell him the ending. Although lacking the narrative accomplishment of his father Will tells the story of he and his father escaping from hospital and making their way down to the river where Edward is greeted by people from his life. Will carries his father into the river and upon lowering him into the water, Edward morphs into a Big Fish and swims away. This film illustrates three important aspects of narrative: first, the importance of story in living one's life; second, the importance that the story continues in a way that emerges from the background [29]; third, the importance of the role of family or other carers in helping to maintain the narrative continuity, not only in content but in form.

In terms of supportive care, the establishment of a mutually acceptable plot that is in line with a person's previous narrative can help validate that previous narrative (that is, all is not lost) and allow for a certain narrative agency into the future. Also, drawing on the experience of others, establishing such an emerging plot may help steer the characters away from the negative features of a chaos narrative and help them find, if not a meaning, at least a way of facing the oncoming challenges (a quest narrative). For example, one carer interviewed for research into the ethical issues facing family carers of people with dementia [30], reported how such a helpful approach was taken at the day centre that his father attended. From the outset, it was acknowledged that the journey taken in living with dementia would result in the move to residential care unless the death of the individual was to occur first. This planning, in effect the establishment of an emergent plot early on in the process of living with dementia, enabled the individual and the carer to deal more easily and positively with the transitions necessarily and unavoidably involved in the journey of dementia.

Furthermore, by involving all those affected by dementia, the emerging plot need not cease upon the death of the individual but may carry on through the grieving of those around her or him. Indeed, it might extend into a restitution phase in which life, while different because of the experience, may resemble life before dementia. Some family carers may return to activities they previously enjoyed prior to 'becoming a carer'. Others may find a meaning in sharing their experiences with others through carers' support and education (the emergence of a quest narrative). In the research referred to above, a significant number of carers recounted how the experience of caring for their relative had changed them and had created a desire to help others through the difficult journey of dementia.

A sensitivity to, and an appreciation of, narrative webs

Narratives exist within a network, a web, of other stories: for example, my story about a difficult day at work is linked with the story of my line manager who provides supervision and my partner's story of having to live with a grump. The story of developing dementia is at once an individual story of illness, a couple's story of standing together and a professional story of diagnosis, prognosis, treatment, and care. Narrative webs are made up of stories of individuals, stories of others, organizational stories, meta-stories (stories that seek to provide a framework for other stories – such as the historical meta-story of dementia as one of loss of ability and self and decline until death). Such stories are not only linked but can also be incorporated into each other – we tell stories about stories – and in so doing they are moulded, transformed, distorted, fragmented, repeated, enhanced, glossed over, and so on.

An important aspect of such webs is that one can explore the web from any point. One can start, for example, from a story about attending a dementia café, which links with a story about cafés when on holiday, which links with stories about family members, which links with stories about weddings, and so on. All stories link, in some ways to other stories.

The interactions between stories can, thus, be as important as the stories themselves because stories are, in a sense, performative; that is, by recounting a story we are expecting it to have an impact, to affect others, and to affect other stories. These narrative relationships are thus imbued with not only intent (and all the emotional investment we might have placed in that) but also power.

Plummer [31] writes of a sociology of stories in which some stories establish the agendas and rhetorics, are given privilege over other stories, and act to close down the expression and even possibility of alternatives. On the other hand, some stories can open up new possibilities, empower, and give voice to other stories, can resist, recuperate, and recreate. An understanding of the nature of narrative power can help us understand the dynamics of narrative interaction and help us to focus on those stories that maintain the narrative web without pulling it out of shape. One particularly powerful narrative in the shaping of agendas and rhetorics is that of the medical model of dementia, focussing on decline and death. This meta-narrative – still dominant and politically useful in the arguments for funding for research into cause and cures – carries with it the potential to inhibit and undermine more positive stories of living with dementia that can serve individuals better in the here and now.

Another aspect of the web of narratives in which we find ourselves is the extent to which we allow others to contribute to our stories, to make a difference to our narrativized lives. Too often people with dementia are seen as receivers (of care, services, compassion, and so on) rather than active agents in a relationship, contributing as much as they receive. I would suggest that the very presence of the person with dementia is a call, to an ethical response, a response that creates us as humans. In other words, it is in responding to the Other we become human [32].

The knack, of course, is to keep the web of stories in harmony. Over-emphasis on one story might distort the web by creating damaging tension between different stories. For example, focussing on a story told through repeated psychometric testing of continuing decline in cognitive functioning can undermine other stories of retained abilities that uphold a sense of self and self-esteem. An under-emphasis on a narrative of retained ability might weaken the threads between intersections. Keeping the balance is not necessarily easy.

The accumulation of narrative resources

If narratives can be woven into a web that supports the individual and those around her or him, then the extent of one's narrative resources determines the possible patterns and diversity of those webs. The more stories one has on which to draw, the more combinations are possible, and the more links can be made. The wider the range of stories the more intricate and detailed the web.

Having a stock of stories allows us to make sense of newly emerging stories by means of comparison to those we already know. Having a range of stories helps us to identify stories that might be missed if the range were narrower (see above about identifying narrative agency). This stock of stories, in order to hold a person with dementia within a web of meaningful stories, needs to include stories of her or his past, present, and future (see above concerning the establishment of an emerging plot), stories of those around her or him (family and friends), stories of retained abilities, of meaningful interactions, of how to go about navigating the journey of dementia. In addition, on a wider scale, a stock of stories including some which challenge the negative stereotypes surrounding dementia, which celebrate aspects of life, which indicate possibilities rather than limitations, can help us resist the temptation to fit in with the current meta-narrative of dementia as one of decline, loss, and death. While death will come to us all, how we approach it can depend upon the narrative capital that we have accumulated over the years.

Concluding remarks: fostering of narrative literacy

If narrative is so important to our sense of self and the meanings we attribute to events, people, and places, it follows that if we are to enable others to tell the best story possible we must develop in ourselves the ability to recognize and work with narratives in all their diversity, strangeness, and splendour. This ability I call narrative literacy.

Narrative literacy is basically an appreciation of, and sensitivity to, the nature and process of narratives in realizing and structuring experience. It is, in this sense, the cumulative outcome of each of the four aspects of narrative discussed above. First, it is the ability to recognize and encourage narrativity in all its forms, facilitating the narrative agency of others through expression, opportunity, and co-authorship. Second, it is the ability to establish and realize a meaningful, appropriate plot that emerges from the past and presents a trajectory into the future that maintains agency, identity, character, and relationships. Third, it is an appreciation of the web-like nature of narratives, understanding how changes in one narrative might impact on others and where the points of tension between narratives exist and how. Another metaphor would be narrative quilting [33] where seemingly discrete narratives are sewn together into something that is greater than its parts. (A very visual manifestation of this would be the AIDS Memorial Quilt, consisting of over 47,000 panels, each panel marking the story of an individual and as a whole testifying to the story of the impact of AIDS [34].)

Finally, narrative literacy requires us to generate a stock of stories on which to draw – stories of individuals so that we can locate them in the wider web of the narratives of their lives (and the lives of others); stories of others so we have a broad range of stories on which to draw in our interactions with individuals; stories of ourselves that help us understand our interactions with, and the importance of, others in our lives; stories of organizations so that we can understand the context; and positive meta-stories that seek to enhance rather than diminish the narrativity of those with whom we work. These stories, accumulated through experience, reflection, contact with others, and research, can then play a role in challenging negative images and approaches to people with dementia. They can empower individuals in their journey with dementia by providing signposts, hope, inspiration, comfort, and even challenge. They can also help us resist the cultural obsession with loss and decline that seems to come to the fore with the onset and progression of dementia.

A narrative-based approach to supportive care can facilitate the intertwining of many aspects of life into a meaningful whole. It helps maintain a sense of Self, acknowledges and works with the web of relationships in which we all live, can incorporate the physical, emotional, mental, and spiritual, and can help all those involved navigate the waters between chaos and quest.

References

1. Bruner JS (1987). Life as narrative. *Soc Res*, **54**(1), 11–32.

2. Bruner J (1990). *Acts of meaning*. Cambridge, MA: Harvard University Press.

3. Bruner J (1991). The narrative construction of reality. *Crit Inq*, **18**(1), 1–21.

4. MacIntyre A (1984). *After virtue: a study in moral theory*. Notre Dame, Indiana: University of Notre Dame Press.

5. Taylor C (1989). *Sources of the self*. Cambridge: Cambridge University Press.

6. Polkinghorne DE (1988). *Narrative knowing and the human sciences*. Albany: State University of New York.

7. Small N, Downs M, Froggatt K (2008). *Living and dying with dementia*. Oxford: Oxford University Press.

8. Baldwin C (2005). The narratively dispossessed: lessons for narrative theory and methods. Paper presented at the Narrative, Memory and Aesthetics conference, University of Huddersfield, UK, April 2005.

9. Crisp J (1995). Making sense of the stories that people with Alzheimer's tell: a journey with my mother. *Nurs Inq*, **2**(3), 133–140.

10. Mills MA (1998). *Narrative identity and dementia: a study of autobiographical memories and emotions*. Aldershot, UK: Ashgate Publishing.

11. McCormack B (2002). The person of the voice: narrative identities in informed consent. *Nurs Philos*, **3**(2), 114–119.

12. Davis R (1989). *My journey into Alzheimer's disease: a story of hope*. Wheaton, IL: Tyndale House.

13. McGowin DF (1993). *Living in the labyrinth: a personal journey through the maze of Alzheimer's*. New York: Dell Publishing.

14. Bryden C (2005). *Dancing with dementia*. London: Jessica Kingsley.

15. Schneider C (2006). *Don't bury me, it ain't over yet*. Indiana: Author House.

16. Taylor R (2007). *Alzheimer's from the inside out*. Baltimore: Health Professions Press.

17. Frank AW (1997). *The wounded storyteller*. Chicago: University of Chicago Press.

18. Hearn M (2008). Mary Malone's lessons: a narrative of citizenship in federation Australia. *Gend Hist*, **16**(2), 376–396.

19. Baldwin C (2008). Narrative citizenship and dementia: the personal and the political. *J Aging Stud*, **22**(3): 222–228.

20. *The Mental Capacity Act 2005*. Norwich: The Stationery Office. Available at: http://www.opsi.gov.uk/acts/acts2005/ukpga_20050009_en_1 (accessed on 29 March 2009).

21. Murphy J, Gray CM, Cox S (2007). *Communication and dementia: how Talking Mats can help people with dementia to express themselves*. [Online]. Joseph Rowntree Foundation. Available from: URL: http://www.jrf.org.uk/sites/files/jrf/2128-talking-mats-dementia.pdf (accessed on February 2009).

22. Schweitzer P, Bruce E (2008). *Remembering yesterday, caring today: reminiscence in dementia care: a guide to good practice*. London: Jessica Kingsley.

23. Cheston R, Jones K, Gilliard J (2003). Group psychotherapy for people with dementia. *Nurs Residential Care*, **5**(4), 186–188.

24. Downs M, Small N, Froggatt K (2006). Person-centred care for people with severe dementia, in Burns A, Winblad B (eds) *Severe dementia*, pp. 193–204. London: Wiley and Sons.

25. Bamberg M (2004). Talk, small stories, and adolescent identities. *Hum Dev*, **47**(6), 366–369.

26. Keady J, Williams S (2005). Co-constructed inquiry: a new approach to the generation of shared knowledge in chronic illness. Paper presented at RCN International Research Conference. Belfast.

27. Pirandello L (1921). *Six characters in search of an author: a comedy in the making*. Trans. Storer E (1922). New York: EP Dutton.

28. Rich BA (1996). The values history: restoring narrative identity to long term care. *J Ethics Law Aging*, **2**(2), 75–84.

29. Barone T (1995). Persuasive writings, vigilant readings, and reconstructed characters: the paradox of trust in educational storysharing, in Hatch JA, Wisniewski R (eds) *Life history and narrative*, pp. 63–74. London: The Falmer Press.

30. Baldwin C (2007). Family carers, ethics and dementia: an empirical study, in Hope T, MacMillan J, Widdershoven G (eds) *Empirical ethics*, pp. 107–122. Oxford: Oxford University Press.

31. Plummer K (1995). *Telling sexual stories: power, change and social worlds*. London: Routledge.

32. Levinas E (1961). *Totality and infinity*. Pittsburgh: Duquesne University Press.

33. Moore LA, Davis B (2002). Quilting narrative: using repetition techniques to help elderly communicators. *Geriatr Nurs*, **23**(5), 262–266.

34. The NAMES Foundation (2007). The AIDS memorial quilt. [Online]. [cited on 20 February 2009]. Available from: URL: http://www.aidsquilt.org/index.htm.

Chapter 27

Persons with severe dementia and the notion of bodily autonomy*

Wim Dekkers

While persons with dementia suffer many losses in function and capacity, they do not lose their essential humanity [1; p. 223].

Introduction

Generally, dementia is a long-lasting and gradual process. While the body often remains strong for a number of years, mental capacities as well as the accumulated competencies and memories of a lifetime gradually slip away. Late stage symptoms include an inability to recognize familiar objects, surroundings, or people, increasing physical frailty, difficulties in eating and swallowing, weight loss, incontinence, and gradual loss of speech and movement control. Reflexes become abnormal and muscles grow rigid. In the end stage, people with dementia lie in bed in a foetus-like position seemingly living as a vegetative organism, being totally dependent on the care of others.

In this chapter, I shall focus on people with *severe* dementia. Before answering the question what supportive care could contribute to the well-being of these people, we must know what is meant by supportive care and what kind of human beings they are. I will concentrate on the second question, but hope to contribute to the development of a philosophical ground for a person-oriented, holistic supportive care for persons with severe dementia. I start with three preliminary remarks.

First, I do not see any problem in talking about *patients* with dementia. Except in mild cases, people with dementia are 'real' patients in the several meanings of the word. They suffer from bodily and mental problems that need medical care. Yet I am speaking of *persons* with dementia thereby using the term person in an intuitive, but philosophically relevant, meaning. Experience with severe dementia shows that even late-stage patients are in fact quite different from one another and in most cases continue to have a characteristic 'personal' interaction with their environment [2]. Julian Hughes argues that it would be odd if he thought the patients he goes to visit were not persons: what then would mark the difference between these non-person patients and person patients? And, most importantly, would we treat these two categories differently? Hughes calls his view of what it is to be a person a reflection of his daily experience: 'My clinical work involves persons: human beings with whom I interact, people with whom I have relationships' [3; p. 86]. In the same vein, my own premise is that 'person' is equivalent to 'human being'.

Second, there is a huge amount of literature dealing with the question what it means when we say someone is a person. In the Anglo-Saxon tradition the emphasis is very much on psychological criteria, i.e. rationality and consciousness. In this context, Hughes speaks about the 'Locke-Parfit

---

* This chapter is an elaboration of an earlier publication on the lived body in persons with severe dementia [26].

view of the person' (LP view) because John Locke and Derek Parfit have contributed much to the development of this view of the person [3]. This so-called LP view of the person has been criticized by many authors. Stephen Post coined the terms 'hypercognitive culture' and 'hypercognitivism' to underscore a persistent bias against deeply forgetful people that is especially pronounced in many modern philosophical accounts of the person [4]. Instead of repeating here all kinds of arguments against the LP view of the human person, I will directly focus on an alternative of which Hughes has sketched the outlines, that is, the so-called situated-embodied-agent (SEA) view of the person. The SEA view regards the human person as an embodied agent embedded in history and culture. According to the SEA view, the person is best thought of as 'a human agent, a being of this embodied kind, who acts and interacts in a cultural and historical context in which he or she is embedded' [3; p. 87]. Besides Wittgenstein, Heidegger and Taylor, it is most of all French continental thinkers, i.e. Jean-Paul Sartre, Maurice Merleau-Ponty, and Paul Ricoeur who have developed this specific view of human beings. The key element of an existential phenomenological view of human beings is their bodiliness embedded in a specific situation and historical context.

Third, it is often and easily said that people with severe dementia have lost everything that makes a being a human being. It is recognized that people with advanced dementia still have fears and longings, even if these are limited to the immediate present, but in cases of severe dementia the self (or call it the mind, the soul, or will) is often thought to be severely affected or even to be lost. The self is, so to speak, increasingly fragmented and scattered. However, with Kitwood [5] and Sabat and many other authors I shall focus on the remaining capacities of people with severe dementia and I shall view these people as human beings '. . . whose sense of self, whose dignity, dispositions, pride, and whose ability to understand the meaning of situations and to act meaningfully, remain intact to some degree' [6; p. viii]. When we talk about 'a "demented", defective, helpless, and confused patient lacking a self' [6; p. viii], we adhere to a 'defectological' view in which the afflicted person is defined principally in terms of his or her dysfunctions and of an organic mental disorder.

Many authors have struggled with the description of the nature and specific characteristics of people with severe dementia. Some presuppose a demarcation between persons and non-persons, others seem to argue that one can be more or less of a person. Hughes concludes that the SEA view holds out the possibility that the person might survive into severe dementia. At the same time he argues in line with Kitwood that we have the potential to enhance the personhood of people with severe dementia [5]. This latter possibility would imply that becoming a person and losing personhood is a gradual process. My position is that people with severe dementia cannot entirely be denied a (rudimentary) form of selfhood or personhood. They definitively are not persons in the strict sense of moral agents who are self-conscious and rational and demonstrate a minimal moral sense, but at least they can be called persons in a weaker sense [7, pp. 135–151].

Two cases

In order to view the person 'through' or 'behind' the body I will focus on bodily aspects of being severely demented by introducing the concept of bodily autonomy. Developing this concept implies a relativization of other forms of autonomy. To be clear from the outset, the principle of respect for the patient's autonomy has been of great advantage in the care of people with dementia. Nursing home residents have greatly benefited from developments that have led to explicit attention being paid to their individual preferences and rights. But this positive effect is seen in regard to only one side of the coin. The current autonomy-model reveals some serious shortcomings.

There are three reasons for this failure and all three pertain to the central focus on autonomy [8]. First, to have one's autonomy respected, an individual must have decisional capacity.

However, many people with dementia lack this capacity and thus cannot be involved in important decisions regarding their care and treatment. Second, respect for autonomy implies that great store is set on the principle of non-interference, thus bestowing individuals with a purely negative freedom. Given the (legal) possibility of saying 'no' to certain treatments, caregivers might feel that this strict obedience to the principle of respect for autonomy (understood negatively), in a way alienates them from their (more positive) nuclear responsibilities to act for the person. Otherwise people with dementia might not receive the care they are morally entitled too. Third, by articulating the values of independence and self-sufficiency so strongly, autonomy-based ethics puts a bad light on the fundamental human vulnerability, and on being dependent on care. For all these reasons, Hertogh argues [8], there is need for an alternative moral framework that is more adequate to the realities of long-term care for people with dementia. Hertogh has in mind here the ethics of care. I will move in another direction, that is, focussing on 'bodily autonomy'.

Let me start with two examples. Sabat has provided us with a nice example of so-called 'malignant social psychology' [9]. This term has been coined by Kitwood in order to describe and criticize a 'defectological' and 'dehumanizing' view of the person with dementia [5]. Sabat refers to an article in the popular press in which Jonathan Franzen describes how he, his wife and his mother took his father home for Thanksgiving dinner. His father was suffering from dementia and was staying in a nursing home. When they brought him back to the nursing home, his father said: 'better not to leave, than to have to come back'. According to Sabat, this remark was quite remarkable because it sharply contrasts with Franzen's own view of his father that 'a change in venue no more impressed my father than it does a 1-year-old'. According to Franzen, it is mostly correct that persons with dementia lose their self long before the death of the body. In light of this belief, he asserts that there was in his father a 'bodily remnant of his self discipline [. . .] when he pulled himself together for the statement he made'. According to Sabat, the idea that it was a bodily remnant of the father's self discipline that allowed him to make the insightful statement, ignores or diminishes the possibility that the father has retained the mental ability to make such an evaluative statement. Sabat considers the phrase 'bodily remnant' to imply a kind of 'reflexive, kneejerk reaction stemming from what was a "remnant" of his father's self discipline' [9; p. 294]. However, an expression such as a bodily remnant of certain mental capabilities does not necessarily refer to a reductionist interpretation as just a reflex. Besides the options of a lucid moment of Franzen's father and of a simple 'reflexive kneejerk reaction' I would like to put forward a third option, that is, the interpretation of such an expression as a meaningful behaviour.

Matthews tells about an elderly woman with dementia who recalls little of her past life and is barely aware of where she is now [10]. Nevertheless, one part of her past that she still retains is her 'ingrained sense of politeness', which is expressed in certain of her spontaneous ways of behaving. For example, she still recognizes, if not in her conscious memory, the need to keep a conversation going, the importance of not allowing an uncomfortable silence to fall. This recognition leads her to fill in with something to say even when she has lost the thread of what she was saying earlier. For those who have known her for a long time, this familiar characteristic is a part of what makes her the person she is, a surviving fragment of a once much richer identity. In persons with dementia there survives something of their adult individuality in the habits of behaviour in which it has become 'sedimented' in the course of their development to adulthood and beyond.

What struck me in these two cases is the idea of a bodily remnant and of a sedimentation of earlier personal habits and characteristics. What do we mean when we say that a character trait, individual preference, or previous experience has been sedimented in the body? Can we allot any authority to these bodily remnants? And returning to the notion of autonomy: if in the slowly deteriorating process of dementia an 'erosion of real autonomy' takes place, as Moody [11; p. 87] puts it, the question is whether and when this process of erosion stops. Should persons with severe dementia, though not autonomous in the current sense, be denied any form of autonomy? Can certain behavioural patterns be interpreted as a kind of 'bodily autonomy', as a remnant of what once was 'real' or 'rational' autonomy?

Three interpretations of 'bodily autonomy'

In contemporary medical ethics much emphasis is paid to the human being as a free, rational, and independent subject. If a human being is thought to have bodily aspects at all, these are generally not seen as having much to do with that which makes a being human. The human body has almost an exclusively instrumental value and does not seem to reveal much about the person himself. Though there are many conceptualizations of the term autonomy, it is often thought to have close ties to the concepts of decision-making capacity and competence. It seems as if 'autonomy' and the body belong to two entirely different categories. Yet, there are authors who propose one or another form of 'bodily autonomy'. Before exposing my own view of 'bodily autonomy' I shall describe two other clusters of interpretations that can be found in the literature.

Autonomy of the person over the body

The first cluster of interpretations can be summarized under the heading of 'disembodied' self or person. The body is considered more as an object among other objects in the world than as the core of the individual's own being. These interpretations take for granted the presence of a healthy body which can actually be controlled by the person. Mackenzie calls these interpretations 'maximal choice conceptions of autonomy' [12]. They include the view (1) that an agent's (bodily) autonomy is enhanced by maximizing the range of bodily options available to him or her, and (2) that any expansion of a person's bodily capacities, or of his or her instrumental control over the body, *ipso facto* enhances his or her (bodily) autonomy. This concept of bodily autonomy can refer both to voluntary movements, as deciding to go for a walk, and movements that we accomplish without voluntary decision and conscious attention.

However, a common justification for maximal choice conceptions is the equation of bodily autonomy with control over the body and the idea of ownership. Following Ricoeur [13], one can distinguish between two senses of 'belonging': (1) belonging in the sense of what one owns or possesses or has, that is, ownership, and (2) belonging in the sense of who one is, or identity. This first cluster of interpretations is based on the first sense of belonging.

Autonomy of embodied persons

The idea of ownership and control over the body has been criticized from many different angles. Mackenzie articulates the concept of bodily autonomy in terms of the phenomenological notion of an integrated bodily perspective [12]. Bodily integration rather than control over the body is constitutive of bodily autonomy, she argues. According to her, a person's body belongs to that person in the second sense of being constitutive of that person's identity, rather than in the sense of ownership. The givens of human embodiment – birth, sex, reproduction, illness, old age, decay, and death – are the condition of human selfhood. Coming to terms with these givens is part of the exercise of being an embodied person. Mackenzie's notion of bodily integration builds on the view that autonomy involves the capacity of critical reflection on one's motivational structure, and the capacity to change it in response to reflection. An integrated bodily perspective is achieved when a person is able to identify with his or her bodily perspective.

Lawton has also tried to incorporate more of a bodily element in descriptions of the self by focussing on bodily deteriorations in terminally ill patients [14]. Also her starting point is that persons do not have a body, but exist or live through their body. The understanding of embodiment as the experience of being a body and living through a body provides a helpful perspective of understanding why a patient's self is affected when various bodily capacities are lost. Expanding this way of thinking to the situation of persons with severe dementia, it is important to realize that not only the decay of bodily functions negatively influences the sense of self, but the loss of self and of cognitive capacities also negatively influences the person's bodily functions. In Lawton's view, bodily autonomy is considered a necessary (though not necessarily a sufficient) criterion for personhood.

Autonomy of the body

Similarly, in the third interpretation of 'bodily autonomy', which I want to put forward, the body is taken seriously, but now the body is considered to have more authority than in the two interpretations just mentioned. Instead of referring to control over the body, I will use the term in the sense of autonomy *of* the body, analogously to the meaning of the term 'autonomic nervous system'. Though higher brain centres can control autonomic functions, the autonomic nervous system is not directly accessible to voluntary control. This means that some body parts possess an autonomy that can only indirectly be controlled by higher brain centres.

The meaning of bodily autonomy that I want to put forward is a combination of this biomedical notion of bodily automatisms and the phenomenological idea of the lived body. Considered from this combined perspective, the human body lives its own life to a high degree being independent of higher brain functions, conscious deliberations, and intentions. It is the French philosopher Maurice Merleau-Ponty who has performed groundbreaking work in this field.

The lived body

Merleau-Ponty argues that the lived body is our only access to the outside world, the only way of being-to-the-world [15]. The lived body is the body as it is given in direct experience. It is immediately and often unconsciously felt, sensed, tasted, heard, and seen. The lived body is the expression of one's existence and is concretely lived by oneself. It is through one's lived body that one manifests oneself to the world. Whether we are consciously aware of it or not, the lived body is present as a 'true companion' in our personal existence. The lived body possesses its own knowledge of the world, which implies the existence of a 'tacit knowledge' that functions without conscious control. On a subconscious level my body provides me with a lot of information about the world.

This Merleau-Pontian idea of the lived body can be further explained by means of the metaphor of 'the body as a text' [16]. The human body can be seen as a *subject*, that is, as an interpreter (writer or reader) of texts, and as an *object*, that is, as a text to be interpreted. The body is a *subject* of experience when it functions as an interpreter in its own right, when it speaks for itself. The body interprets not only itself, but also everything in the outside world with which it is confronted via the senses. This is what Merleau-Ponty means by the notion of tacit knowledge. The content of these bodily interpretations of the world does not necessarily need to be known by the person. The human body may be considered the author of a text, but also the reader of the text that is constituted by what is happening in the outside world. The body is an *object* of experience, when one experiences one's own body. In these situations, one is more or less aware of one's own body which can then be described as a text to be interpreted. Then the person – the *I* person or another person – is the reader.

Many contemporary authors have followed Merleau-Ponty's concept of the lived body. I will mention a few of them whose theories are relevant for understanding the notions of bodily remnants and sedimentations of previous personal preferences, habits, and characteristics. According to Cspregi [17], there exists a dynamic and complex relation between the human subject and the world, a relation in which sensing and moving, space and time, reason and emotion, capabilities and opportunities are intrinsically related. 'Just like the heart in the organism, the living body is the source of an irreducible, autonomous, and creative dynamism, indispensable for the multiple relations we entertain with the world' (p. 8). Our past experiences, the painful as well as the pleasant ones, are 'inscribed in the body' (p. 113).

According to Matthews [10], a person cannot be defined in terms of consciousness alone because consciousness cannot exist on its own. Being the person, we cannot simply be equivalent to thinking I am that person. It is rather the other way around. I can think of myself as me only because I am me. Persons are beings who express their subjective thoughts, feelings and so on, in bodily form, in speech, in gesture, in behaviour, in interaction with the world.

Subjectivity exists in these physical expressions. The concept of the body-subject implies, (1) that personal life emerges from 'prepersonal' bodily existence, and (2) that our bodily existence has to be understood as the expression of our individuality. Our individuality expresses itself not just in the communication of language and consciously recalled experience, but also in our body language, our habits of behaviour, our characteristic gestures, and so on. What still remains in a person, when conscious and explicit experiences are gone, is all that originally has been conscious and reflective, but has become 'sedimented into habits' (p. 75).

Bodily remnants of autonomy in severe dementia

As far as I know, Merleau-Ponty did not deal with dementia. An important question to be solved now is whether the idea of the lived body is applicable at all when it comes to severe dementia. The person with severe dementia is extremely damaged in his or her mental and bodily existence. One can therefore argue that the specific unity of a mind and an animated body, which in a Merleau-Pontian way is thought to be essential to human beings, also gradually disappears. However, if this unity is considered an essential characteristic of human beings, by which I mean the nature of human beings as beings of this sort, it cannot (entirely) disappear. The concept of the lived body therefore makes sense here, because the Merleau-Pontian way of thinking concerns a fundamental level of being human, regardless of whether that being is young or old, healthy or diseased, fully rational or severely demented. As I explained in the introduction, my presupposition is that persons with severe dementia do not entirely lack a self or personhood.

Cognitive capabilities of persons with severe dementia gradually disappear until the moment they are no longer capable of exercising their autonomy by making explicit decisions. This does not mean, however, that their bodily knowledge, which has been developed in the course of their lives, necessarily also disappears. Tacit bodily knowledge is based on the sedimentation of life narratives. Although automatisms get gradually lost, persons with severe dementia still have routine actions stored in their body. Behavioural patterns of persons with severe dementia may be interpreted as a remainder of what once has been 'real', that is, rational autonomy. They have nothing else at their disposal than these bodily movements. Although the body in severe dementia increasingly shows dysfunctions, it still remains a lived body and a body in which previous forms of autonomy have been inscribed.

Care for persons with dementia increasingly involves the demanding ideal of emotion-oriented care. This form of care integrates several approaches such as multi-sensory stimulation, reminiscence, validation, music therapy, reality orientation, and empathic care [18]. Verbal communication is not possible with persons having severe dementia. The only way to communicate with them is through the body (see also Chapter 23). This means that one must explicitly pay attention to the bodily way in which they are 'in the world'. The methods of psychomotor and music therapy, and the practice of stimulation of the senses by means of music, light, smells and perfumes, flavours, and bodily contacts are based on these insights. By means of bodily communication, one can interpret the preferences of persons with dementia who cannot express themselves verbally any longer. Anecdotal evidence is rich with examples of the persistence of personal traits even after extensive memory loss: the enjoyment of music, food, and simple repetitive games and activities, the feel of another's hand stroking the face [19]. Pickles and Jones speak about a 'residual musicality' and a 'continuing musical self in dementia' as 'an enduring fragment of the person that the sufferer used to be' [20].

Philosophical and practical relevance

One of the elements of supportive dementia care is its multi-disciplinary character. Supportive care is also based on a holistic view of the person with dementia. In this chapter I have tried to contribute to such a holistic view by paving the way for seeing the person 'behind or through the body'. I will end with a few remarks about the philosophical and practical relevance of this chapter, which need further elaboration in the future.

On a philosophical level, the concept of bodily autonomy might be linked to what Dworkin has called 'experiential interests' as distinguished from 'critical interests' [21]. *Experiential* interests relate to the quality of our day-to-day experience, encompassing factors, i.e. pleasure, satisfaction, contentment, lack of pain, and so forth. Experiential interests are more or less identical with what Frankfurt has called 'first order desires' [22]: what we might want here and now, such as eating, drinking, sleeping, or avoiding pain. *Critical* interests relate to how we want to live our lives and could be seen as an expression of our autonomy: interests in doing or having in our life the things we consider good and in avoiding the things we consider bad, no matter what sort of experiences result from fulfilling these interests. Dworkin's critical interests are related to what Frankfurt has called 'second order desires': what we might want in the long run or in the context of our whole life, such as to be rich, healthy, or loved by fellow human beings.

There has been much debate about the role and function of experiential and critical interests in care decisions for persons with dementia. Some authors stress the role of critical interests, for example by giving priority to advance directives [21]; others focus on experiential interests and the best interest standard [23]; again others opt for a balance between the two [24]. In my view, it is not a matter of either critical or experiential interests. The idea of a continuum between the two makes much more sense. Although most behaviour of severely demented persons is probably based upon their experiential interests, critical interests might also play a role, as Jaworska argues [25]. The notions of bodily autonomy and of a sedimentation of previous individual preferences in the body might clarify that critical interests might play a role in the behaviour of persons with severe dementia.

On a practical level, the concept of bodily autonomy might function as a guide for a wise decision when one is confronted with a difficult moral dilemma in dementia care. I am thinking here of situations in which persons with severe dementia react with facial expressions, vocalizations, muscle tension and bodily defensive movements following interventions such as physical restraints and other coercive measures, the use of hypodermic or intravenous needles, the insertion of nasogastric tubes, or the use of a percutaneous endoscopic gastrostomy (PEG). In all these circumstances patient's bodily reactions must be taken seriously. Persons with severe dementia simply possess no other means to communicate. They express their wish by pushing away a spoon or by trying to pull out a feeding tube. This behaviour might be considered an expression of their bodily autonomy, a kind of negative claim against invasion and interference. That is all that is left of their 'real', rational, autonomy. The concept of bodily autonomy might support our intuitively felt hesitance to protect the security of persons with severe dementia by mechanical measures or to insert feeding tubes. The concept of bodily autonomy can be added to other arguments and considerations against too active a treatment of patients with severe dementia: the integrity of the body, respect for the patient's dignity, the social structure in which communication takes place (the wishes of family members), and societal judgements on the boundaries of acceptable treatment decisions for persons with dementia. When in a case of a serious moral dilemma in dementia care, when informed consent is not possible (by definition), when there is no advance directive, and when it is difficult to know what to do based on the idea of a substituted judgement or on best interest considerations, then notions such as bodily autonomy and wisdom of the body can be helpful in order to arrive at a wise decision.

References

1. Post SG (2006). *Respectare*: moral respect for the life of the deeply forgetful, in Hughes JC, Louw SJ, Sabat SR (eds) *Dementia: mind, meaning, and the person*, pp. 223–234. Oxford: Oxford University Press.

2. Boller F, Verny M, Hugonot-Diener L, Saxton J (2002). Clinical features and assessment of severe dementia. A review. *Eur J Neurol*, **9**, 125–136.

3. Hughes JC (2001). Views of the person with dementia. *J Med Ethics*, **27**, 86–91.

4. Post SG (1995). *The moral challenge of Alzheimer disease*. Baltimore and London: The Johns Hopkin University Press.

5. Kitwood T (1997). *Dementia reconsidered: the person comes first*. Buckingham, Philadelphia: Open University Press.

6. Sabat SR (2001). *The experience of Alzheimer's disease: life through a tangled veil*. Oxford, UK: Blackwell Publishers.

7. Engelhardt HT Jr (1996). *The foundations of bioethics*, 2nd edn. New York and Oxford: Oxford University Press.

8. Hertogh CMPH (2005). Towards a more adequate moral framework: elements of an 'ethic of care' in nursing home care for people with dementia, in Burns A (ed) *Standards in dementia care*, pp. 371–377. London and New York: Taylor & Francis.

9. Sabat SR (2006). Mind, meaning, and personhood in dementia: the effects of positioning, in Hughes JC, Louw SJ, Sabat SR (eds) *Dementia: mind, meaning, and the person*, pp. 287–302. Oxford: Oxford University Press.

10. Matthews E (2006). Dementia and the identity of the person, in Hughes JC, Louw SJ, Sabat SR (eds) *Dementia: mind, meaning, and the person*, pp. 163–177. Oxford: Oxford University Press.

11. Moody HR (1992). A critical view of ethical dilemmas in dementia, in Binstock RH, Post SG, Whitehouse PJ (eds.) *Dementia and aging: ethics, values and policy choices*, pp. 86–100. Baltimore and London: The Johns Hopkins University Press.

12. Mackenzie C (2001). On bodily autonomy, in Toombs SK (ed) *Handbook of phenomenology and medicine*, pp. 417–439. Dordrecht: Kluwer Academic Publishers.

13. Ricoeur P (1992). *Oneself as another*. Chicago and London: The University of Chicago Press.

14. Lawton J (2000). *The dying process: patients' experiences of palliative care*. London and New York: Routledge.

15. Merleau-Ponty M (1962). *Phenomenology of perception*. Trans by Smith C. London and New York: Routledge.

16. Dekkers WJM (2001). The human body, in Have HAMJ ten, Gordijn B (eds) *Bioethics in a European perspective*, pp. 115–140. Dordrecht: Kluwer Academic Publishers.

17. Csepregi G (2006). *The clever body*. Calgary: University of Calgary Press.

18. Hertogh CMPM (2004). Between autonomy and security: ethical questions in the care of elderly demented patients in nursing homes, in Jones GMM, Miesen BML (eds) *Care-giving in dementia*, pp. 375–390. New York/London: Brunner/Routledge.

19. Radden J, Fordyce JM (2006). Into the darkness: losing identity with dementia, in Hughes JC, Louw SJ, Sabat SR (eds) *Dementia: mind, meaning, and the person*. Oxford: Oxford University Press, 71–88.

20. Pickles V, Jones, RA (2006). The person still comes first: the continuing musical self in dementia. *J Consciousness Stud*, **13**(3), 73–93.

21. Dworkin R (1993). *Life's dominion*. London: Harper Collins.

22. Frankfurt HG (1971). Freedom of the will and the concept of a person. *J Philos*, **68**(1), 5–20.

23. Dresser R (1995). Dworkin on dementia: elegant theory, questionable policy. *Hastings Cent Rep*, **25**(6), 32–38.

24. Harvey M (2006). Advance directives and the severely demented. *J Med Philos*, **31**, 47–64.

25. Jaworska A (1999). Respecting the margins of agency: Alzheimer's patients and the capacity to value. *Philos Public Aff*, **28**(2), 105–138.

26. Dekkers WJM (2004). Autonomy and the lived body in cases of severe dementia, in Purtilo RB, Have HAMJ ten (eds) *Ethical foundations of palliative care for Alzheimer Disease*, pp. 115–130. Baltimore and London: The John Hopkins University Press.

Chapter 28

Advance care planning: an American view

Muriel R. Gillick

Alice Jones is an 85-year-old woman with advanced dementia living in a nursing home. She smiles when her daughters visit – just as she does when the nurse, social worker, or recreation therapist says hello to her. Her only word is 'mama'. She requires assistance with walking and toileting and is totally dependent in bathing and dressing. For the past six months, she has been fed by a nursing assistant, but increasingly she pushes away the spoon or spits out her food. A crisis was precipitated when Alice, usually a pleasant, cooperative woman, slapped the aide who tried to feed her. The nursing home staff have recommended to Mrs. Jones's daughter that she should authorize placement of a feeding tube. Her daughter is beside herself, uncertain what to do. She suspects her mother would not have wanted artificial nutrition and hydration, but she never discussed such matters and completed no advance directives. She does not think her mother would have wanted medical interventions except to promote comfort in her current condition, but on the other hand, Alice does not seem to be suffering. On the contrary, she gives every indication of enjoying simple pleasures such as holding a stuffed animal or listening to music.

Introduction

Decisions about whether to authorize potentially life-prolonging treatments for patients with dementia are amongst the most difficult choices facing families today. Typically, as in the above vignette, adult children who very much want to do the right thing for their parents feel conflicted: they are ambivalent about sustaining a dependent, regressed parent who bears little resemblance to the strong, independent figure they grew up with; they do not regard dementia as a terminal disease, analogous to advanced cancer, and thus feel obligated to authorize treatment; they would not want aggressive treatment if they themselves had dementia, but recognize that their parent seems content despite her diminished state; they do not want to inflict painful tests and treatments on an uncomprehending older person, but realize they would not hesitate to expose their children to equally unpleasant but life-prolonging medical procedures [1].

One under-utilized way to help family decision-makers is through *advance care planning*. This can be done by the patient herself before any signs of dementia have developed, or it can be carried out by the family in conjunction with the patient's physician or other members of the medical team, once dementia has been diagnosed. In the first instance, the planning process will help assure that health care decisions are in accord with the patient's values and preferences: the responsibility of the caregiver is to implement the parent's wishes rather than to determine the right course of action. In the second instance, when there is no formal advance directive, advance care planning offers the opportunity to take some of the burden off caregivers by preparing them emotionally for the kinds of decisions they are likely to be asked to make [2].

The specific form that these two kinds of advance care planning takes is shaped by cultural, legal, and institutional factors. In the *cultural* realm, African-Americans, Latinos, and Asian–Americans have been less inclined to accept advance care planning than white Americans [3]. Discussions of end-of-life care must be tailored to overcome suspicions that physicians or insurance companies are seeking to discontinue care prematurely. In the *legal* arena, each state in the United States has its own laws governing advance directives. While all states recognize the right of an individual to designate a surrogate decision-maker to act on his or her behalf in the event of incapacity, many states limit the ability of the surrogate to withhold or withdraw certain types of treatment such as artificial nutrition and hydration unless specifically authorized by the patient [4]. In terms of *institutional* factors, the type of advance care planning process most likely to be effective varies depending on whether the individual is being cared for in a state such as Oregon, with a state-wide system of advance care planning (the Physician Orders for Life-Sustaining Treatment) [5], or in a nursing home with a formalized system of levels of care such as the Veterans Administration extended care facilities [6], or in any of a number of other systems of care.

Advance care planning prior to the diagnosis of dementia

A recent survey of American adults found that Alzheimer's disease was the single most feared condition among those aged 55 and older, more feared than cancer or heart disease. Despite widespread anxiety about the possibility of developing dementia, and despite general agreement that planning was essential, 87% of those surveyed reported having made no plans for the possibility of dementia. Not only have they failed to make financial arrangements (83%), but they have also not considered where they would want to receive care (72%) [7].

Developing dementia is unfortunately not a rare occurrence as the population ages. While only 13% of those over age 65 have dementia, the rate rises to 19% of those between 75 and 84 years old and reaches 42% for those over age 85 [8]. In view of the high likelihood of developing dementia – and given that individuals who develop dementia are by definition unable to participate in decision-making (at least by the time the inevitably progressive condition moves beyond its earliest stages) – the best way to ensure that patients with dementia receive appropriate medical care is through advance care planning initiated *before* the disease develops. Interest in advance care planning rose briefly after the publicity surrounding the case of Terri Schiavo, a young woman in a persistent vegetative state whose parents sought to continue artificial nutrition over the objections of her husband: the not-for-profit organization, Aging with Dignity, reported that orders for their living will, *The Five Wishes*, reached 2000–3000/day compared to under 100/day pre-Schiavo [9]. High rates of advance directive completion are possible with a comprehensive system such as 'Respecting Choices' (used in La Crosse, Wisconsin, with an 85% response rate [10]) and 'Let Me Decide' (used successfully in 76% of elderly residents of Canadian nursing homes [11]), but engagement in planning by older patients remains far from universal. A Pew survey conducted in November, 2005, shortly after the resolution of the Schiavo case, found that only 54% of elders surveyed had a living will, though this was up from 25% in 1990 [12].

When middle aged and older adults do complete advance directives, the documents they use seldom specifically address dementia. A typical living will, for example, includes the text 'I direct my attending physician to withhold or withdraw life-sustaining medical care and treatment that is serving only to prolong the process of dying if I should be in an incurable or irreversible mental or physical condition with no reasonable medical expectation of recovery'. The words suggest the directive applies only to someone who is actively dying and refers only to treatments necessary to sustain life. A more comprehensive advance directive, the Five Wishes, asks potential patients to indicate their goals of treatment should they be close to death, in a coma and not expected to wake up, or if they have 'permanent and severe brain damage with no expectation of recovery'. The example given is 'I can open my eyes, but cannot speak or understand', which seems to refer to persistent vegetative state rather than dementia [13].

When an advance directive is completed, it seldom deals with the kinds of questions relevant to people with dementia [14]. Instructional directives, which detail the specific interventions the prospective patient finds acceptable, tend to include cardiopulmonary resuscitation, ventilators, and may list other life-sustaining treatments. The particular issues that arise in dementia, however, include the use of feeding tubes, the decision about hospitalization versus care in the home or nursing home, and, if hospitalization is acceptable, whether the patient should receive the more aggressive measures associated with an intensive care unit.

At least one validated advance directive instrument addresses both dementia and the medical interventions that many people may wish to limit in dementia. The 'Medical Directive' designed by Linda and Ezekiel Emanuel is a complex instructional directive that asks individuals, while healthy, to state which of nine medical interventions they would want in any of six clinical situations, including 'dementia and terminal illness' and 'dementia' [15]. But even this directive does not distinguish between mild and severe dementia; it implicitly fails to recognize that Alzheimer's disease is itself ultimately fatal, and it does not consider hospitalization or admission to an ICU in its list of potentially problematic interventions.

Older adults may also be prevented from engaging in advance care planning for the possibility of dementia by a limited understanding of the disease. The same poll that found adults over 55 to be frightened of dementia also revealed that 76% said they knew little about the disorder. Asking individuals to express their preference for treatment makes little sense if they do not know that dementia is a progressive, uniformly fatal disease. And it would be misguided to ask about preferences for particular interventions such as feeding tubes if the person does not recognize that the advanced stage of dementia is associated with eating difficulties but that feeding tubes neither prolong life nor maintain comfort.

One strategy both to educate older individuals about dementia and to facilitate advance care planning is a video decision aid. A pilot study found that when adults viewed a video depicting the cardinal features of advanced dementia, 89.2% said they would want comfort care in such a state, none wanted life-prolonging care, and 8.3% favoured limited care. Before viewing the video, after simply hearing a verbal description of advanced dementia, 50% asked for comfort care, 20.8% favouring life-prolongation, and 18.3% requested limited care. Subjects' knowledge of dementia, as measured by a quiz, improved after watching the video [16]. Moreover, African-Americans and Latinos, widely reported to prefer aggressive end-of-life care, also overwhelmingly favoured comfort care after seeing the video. These findings held up in a validation study comparing whites to Latinos, strongly suggesting that a previously under-recognized barrier to advance care planning is lack of health literacy, an obstacle that a suitable video can surmount [17].

At a minimum, all adults should designate a health care proxy to make medical decisions on their behalf in the event they lose capacity. Patients should be encouraged by their physicians to discuss with their proxy their preferences for care in the event of major illness. Questions about specific preferences should be tailored to the patient's clinical profile: patients with heart disease should be asked about cardiopulmonary resuscitation, patients with lung disease about ventilator treatment, and *all* patients should be asked about care in the event of dementia.

Advance care planning in early dementia

Individuals with mild dementia may still be able to participate in advance care planning, at least to a limited extent. Some of those diagnosed with Alzheimer's disease have written books [18,19]. Many live alone with minimal assistance or function quasi-independently in an assisted living facility: the prevalence of dementia in assisted living facilities has been reported to be as high as 68% [20].

Decision-making capacity is specific to the decision being made; hence, adults with mild dementia may be perfectly able to designate a surrogate decision-maker even if they are not able to hold complex discussions about preferences for care. Any patient with early dementia who has not appointed a health care proxy should be strongly advised to do so.

Some patients with mild dementia may be able to grasp the nature of advanced dementia if shown a video, which in turn allows them to select an approach to care. Preliminary data indicate that many patients with mini-mental state scores in the 20–23 range can in fact engage in this process and find it as useful and acceptable as do their cognitively intact counterparts.

Advance care planning with surrogates

Once a patient with dementia has reached a point at which he or she can no longer participate in decision-making, there is, in principle, no further role for advance care planning. Advance care planning, after all, is intended to promote autonomy in the event the patient loses capacity. To the extent there is reason to fear the health care proxy will lose capacity, an alternate surrogate should be appointed along with the primary proxy. But there is a second role for advance care planning that is often neglected: to prepare the decision-maker for problems that are likely to arise so as to avoid crisis decision-making [21]. Moreover, discussion and documentation of the *goals of care* for the person the proxy is representing has the potential to assure the patient's wishes will be respected even in a fragmented health care system. Clarifying in advance the desired approach to care can be very useful to a covering physician or if the patient is transferred from one health care facility to another.

The goals of care for a patient with dementia typically evolve as the disease progresses. Advance care planning with surrogates should therefore begin with an explanation of where the patient is along the trajectory of the disease. In addition, the proxy needs to understand the progressive nature of the disorder and to have some understanding of what the final stage entails. Decisions to consider limiting treatment are based on weighing the benefits and risks of the proposed treatment – where a burden may be patient suffering induced by the treatment, a decline in function resulting after the treatment is completed, or the possibility, provided by the treatment of an acute medical problem, to live long enough to develop more advanced stages of dementia.

Once the patient's current health status has been clarified and the typical course of the disease described, surrogates are in a position to address the overriding goal of care. In the event a new medical problem developed – whether a urinary tract infection, a gastrointestinal bleed, an acute myocardial infarction, or a malignancy – should the primary goal be prolonging life, maintaining the existing level of function, or maximizing comfort [22]?

To answer this question, the surrogate should be encouraged to draw on advance directives the patient may have completed, on conversations held with the patient before capacity was lost, and on inferences based on previously expressed values and beliefs (i.e. adherence to a religious doctrine with specific views on end-of-life care). If the surrogate is uncertain about the goals of care, the physician may find it useful to indicate what most people want in the situation facing the proxy. While data on preferences as a function of stage of disease are scant, clinical experience indicates that most individuals focus on life prolongation when dementia is mild, on function when the dementia is moderate, and on comfort when the dementia is advanced.

Some surrogates may find a more complex form of advance care planning useful. It may be insufficient merely to determine the chief goal of care: some surrogates hope that all three goals will be achieved but vary in their prioritization of the three goals. For example, surrogates who regard maintenance of function as the primary goal may see life-prolongation as secondary with comfort as a tertiary concern, or they may see comfort as more important than life-prolongation. Similarly, surrogates who regard comfort as the primary goal may see life-prolongation and function as subsidiary goals or may view comfort as the sole goal of care.

Once the goals of care have been elicited and prioritized, physicians should explain how those goals can best be translated into practice. The extremes are easiest to delineate: patients for whom life-prolongation is the primary goal of care would typically receive maximally aggressive medical treatment in the event of acute illness. Those in whom comfort is the sole goal would be treated with a hospice approach. In general, patients whose primary goal is maintenance of function would be candidates for most conventional medical treatments, excluding cardiopulmonary resuscitation, ventilatory support, admission to an intensive care unit, and major surgery. Patients with a primary but not an exclusive goal of comfort would receive simple, non-invasive but potentially life-prolonging treatments such as oral antibiotics, and potentially also blood transfusions or intravenous fluids if these were well-tolerated, but not hospital level care.

This approach to advance care planning does not determine precisely what treatment will be given in a particular situation. Rather, it establishes upper and lower boundaries of care: for the patient who develops pneumonia, for example, in whom comfort is the main but not the only goal, a ventilator is too much treatment but exclusive treatment with morphine and oxygen is too little. Care including antibiotics and intravenous fluids lies within these two extremes and might be perfectly acceptable. For the patient in whom function is the main goal, the intensive care unit is too aggressive but hospital care may well be appropriate. Determining exactly which of the available treatment options makes sense for a given patient will depend on the specific clinical circumstances and the kinds of services available, i.e. a skilled nursing facility, a visiting nurse, or physician home care. Although the details will need to be negotiated at the time an acute problem develops, having a framework in place can guide the discussion.

Reviewing and revising the advance care plan

The advance care planning process needs to be reviewed and potentially revised whenever the patient has had a significant change of status. This criterion is met if the patient develops an entirely new chronic medical problem that fundamentally changes his overall health: for example, a new diagnosis of lung cancer or a stroke; or at the point when his dementia advances. Since dementia is a gradually progressive disease with a median survival of 6.6 years, [23] physicians should engage in advance care planning when the patient moves from mild to moderate disease and again when he moves from moderate to advanced disease. While the definitions of the stages of Alzheimer's disease are imprecise [24], transitions are often signaled by a sentinel event: a person who was living alone at home, attending adult day care with a home health aide in the evening begins wandering outside his home at night, has moved into a phase where he cannot be left alone. A person in an assisted living facility who has developed incontinence may have progressed to the point where she requires nursing home care and a person who has an episode of aspiration pneumonia is likely to have moved from moderate to advanced dementia.

Revisiting advance care planning provides an opportunity to explain the new stage of the disease, to describe the problems that are most likely to occur in the near future, and to discuss preferences for care. While focussing primarily on specific technical interventions rather than the overall goals of care is generally inadvisable, educating families about the most common medical problems that can be expected in a given stage of dementia helps prepare them for decision-making.

In *early dementia*, the major concerns are related to safety. The individual who drives a car is at risk of causing an accident. The accident rate of 26.6/million vehicle miles travelled (MVMT) among persons with mild dementia is comparable to that of teenagers aged 16–19 years old (28.6 accidents/ MVMT) [25]. Hence mandatory revocation of a driver's license in this setting is problematic. Requiring special testing – usually a simulated road test in a laboratory – is also unsatisfactory as there is no compelling evidence that such tests can accurately predict risk. However, discussion with families about the anticipated increasing risk of driving over time may enable the family to come up with alternative means of transportation before any accidents occur. Other safety risks, such as injury from improperly extinguished matches or cigarettes, or from leaving the stove on, also warrant discussion.

In *moderate dementia*, health risks are associated with *behaviours* such as wandering and agitation, as well as with self-neglect. An individual with poor judgment who leaves his home and walks into oncoming traffic is at risk of an accident. Hallucinations, paranoia, and delusions are common in this stage of dementia. Alerting surrogates to anticipate these problems can pave the way for treatment. The efficacy of neuroleptic drugs to treat psychiatric symptoms has been called into question and the discovery of a risk of stroke from their use has led the Federal Drug Administration in the United States to mandate a black box warning for atypical antipsychotic medications [26]. Similar warnings have appeared in other countries (see Chapter 12 for further details). Nonetheless, these agents are often the only potentially effective pharmacologic treatments for the disturbing and disabling manifestations of dementia. Advance care planning can assure surrogates that non-pharmacologic measures will be tried first, but that when judiciously used, neuroleptics can maintain quality of life for the person with moderate dementia.

In *advanced dementia*, individuals are at high risk of feeding difficulties, aspiration pneumonia, and pressure ulcers. A clear understanding of the natural history of the final stage of dementia is useful in promoting a palliative approach to what is essentially a terminal illness. As illustrated in the vignette introducing this chapter, families are often particularly distressed when patients develop difficulty eating. They worry when their parent is receiving less than the recommended number of calories per day that she will suffer. The advance care planning process can anticipate feeding difficulties, explaining that the ability to perform activities of daily living is lost in a predictable sequence, with loss of independence in mobility, toileting, and feeding characteristic of the most advanced stage of dementia [27]. Surrogate decision-makers need to understand that patients who reject food or who have trouble swallowing do not appear to experience discomfort: extrapolation from the experience of dying cancer patients with swallowing problems suggests that at the very end of life, hunger is rarely experienced [28].

Moreover, an observational study of patients with advanced dementia in Dutch nursing homes who stopped eating and drinking and who were not given artificial nutrition and hydration found that discomfort was associated with other symptoms such as dyspnoea rather than with the absence of food and drink alone [29]. Finally, caregivers should understand that tube feeding has not been shown to prolong life in patients with advanced dementia, strongly suggesting that feeding difficulties are a marker of advanced disease and that providing artificial nutrition will not alter the natural history of the disease [30]. Hand feeding is the recommended approach to patients with advanced dementia and feeding problems [31].

Once surrogates realize that the patient has progressed to a new phase of dementia, the advance care planning process encourages reconsideration of the goals of care. While many, if not most, families favour life-prolonging care in early dementia, they often modify their primary goal to maintaining function and independence in moderate dementia. When an individual develops advanced dementia, surrogates should be encouraged to consider comfort as the main goal of care. A hospice approach to treatment is appropriate at this juncture, providing support to families, management of symptoms to patients, and avoiding burdensome procedures and hospitalizations [32].

Conclusion

Systematic advance care planning – beginning when an older adult is cognitively intact, addressed again when the earliest symptoms of dementia appear, and then revisited with the surrogate at each stage of the illness – can avoid both under-treatment and over-treatment of the individual with dementia. It allows physicians to respect the patient's wishes and provides support to caregivers over the many years that the disease unfolds.

References

1. Mitchell SL (2007). A 93-year-old man with advanced dementia and eating problems. *JAMA*, **298**(21), 2527–2536.

2. Perkins HS (2007). Controlling death: the false promise of advance directives. *Ann Intern Med*, **147**(1), 51–57.

3. Crawley LM (2005). Racial, cultural, and ethnic factors influencing end-of-life care. *J Palliat Med*, **8**(S1), S58–S69.

4. Sabatino C. *Health care power of attorney and combined advance directive legislation*. Available at: www.aba.net. (accessed on 18 February 2009).

5. Tolle SW, Tilden VP (2002). Changing end-of-life planning: the Oregon experience. *J Palliat Med*, **5**(2), 311–317.

6. Volicer L, Rheaume Y, Fabiszekwski K, Brady R (1986). Hospice approach to the treatment of patients with advanced dementia of the Alzheimer type. *JAMA*, **256**(16), 2210–2213.

7. MetLife Foundation Alzheimer's Survey. *What America Thinks, 2006*. Available at: http://www.metlife.com/WPSAssets/20538296421147208330V1FAlzheimersSurvey.pdf (accessed on 28 August 2008).

8. Alzheimer's Association. *Alzheimer's disease facts and figures 2007*. Available at: www.alz.org/national/documents/Report_2007FactsandFigures.pdf (accessed on 29 August 2008).

9. Grady D (2005). The best way to keep control is to leave instructions. *NY Times*, March 29.

10. Hammes BJ, Rooney BL (2004). Communication, trust, and making choices: advance care planning four years on. *J Palliat Med*, **7**(2), 335–340.

11. Molloy WM, Guyatt GH, Russo R *et al.* (2000). Systematic implementation of an advance directive system in nursing homes: a randomized controlled trial. *JAMA*, **283**(11), 1437–1444.

12. The Pew National Center for the People and the Press. *Strong public support for right to die*. Available at: http://people-press.org/report/266/strong-public-support-for-right-to-die (accessed on 27 August 2008).

13. Aging with Dignity. *Five wishes*. Available at: http:///www.agingwithdignity.org/5wishes.html. (accessed on 29 August 2008).

14. Gillick M (2006). The use of advance care planning to guide decisions about artificial nutrition and hydration. *Nutr Clin Pract*, **21**(2), 126–133.

15. EPEC. *The medical directive*. Available at: www.medicaldirective.org (accessed on 25 August 2008).

16. Volandes AE, Lehmann LS, Cook EF, Shaykevich S, Abbo ED, Gillick MR (2007). Using video images of dementia in advance care planning. *Arch Intern Med*, **167**(8), 828–833.

17. Volandes AE, Ariza M, Abbo ED, Paasche-Orlow M (2008). Overcoming educational barriers to advance care planning in Latinos using video images. *J Palliat Med*, **11**(5)**,** 700–706.

18. McGowin D (1993). *Living in the labyrinth: a personal journey through the maze of Alzheimer's.* New York: Delacorte Press.

19. DeBaggio T (2003). *Losing my mind: an intimate look at life with Alzheimer's.* New York: The Free Press.

20. Rosenblatt A, Samur QM, Steele CD *et al.* (2004). The Maryland assisted living study: prevalence, recognition, and treatment of dementia and other psychiatric disorders in the assisted living population of central Maryland. *J Amer Geriatr Soc*, **52**(10)**,** 1618–1625.

21. Gillick MR (1995). A broader role for advance medical planning. *Ann Intern Med*, **123**(8), 621–624.

22. Gillick MR (2001). Choosing appropriate medical care for the elderly. *J Am Med Dir Assoc*, **2**(6), 305–309.

23. Wolfson C, Wolfson DB Asgharian M *et al.* (2001). A reevaluation of the duration of survival after the onset of dementia. *N Engl J Med*, **344**(15), 1111–1116.

24. Scalan SG, Resiberg B (1992). Functional assessment staging (FAST) in Alzheimer's disease: reliability, validity, and ordinality. *Intr Psychogeriatr*, **4**(Suppl 1), 55–69.

25. Dubinsky RM, Stein AC, Lyons K (2000). Practice parameter: risk of driving and Alzheimer's disease (an evidence-based review) *Neurology* **54**(12), 2205–2211.

26. Meeks TW and Jeste DV (2008). Antipsychotics in dementia: beyond 'black-box' warnings *Curr Psychiatr*, **7**(6), 51–65.

27. Chen J-H, Chan D-C, Kiely DK, Morris JN, Mitchell SL (2007). Terminal trajectories of functional decline in the long-term care setting. *J Gerontol A Biol Sci Med Sci*, **62**(5)**,** 531–536.

28. McCann RM, Hall WJ, Groth-Juncker A (1994). Comfort care for terminally ill patients: the appropriate use of nutrition and hydration. *JAMA*, **272**(16), 1263–1266.

29. Pasman HR, Onwuteaka-Philipsen BD, Kriegsman DM, Ooms ME, Ribbe MW, van der Waal G (2005). Discomfort in nursing home patients with severe dementia in whom artificial nutrition and hydration are forgone. *Arch Intern Med*, **165**(15)**,** 1729–1733.

30. Mitchell SL, Kiely DK, Lipsitz LA (1997). The risk factors and impact on survival of feeding tube placement in nursing home residents with severe cognitive impairment. *Arch Intern Med*, **157**(3), 327–332.

31. Gillick MR (2000). Rethinking the use of feeding tubes in patients with advanced dementia. *N Engl J Med*, **342**(3)**,** 206–210.

32. Luchins DJ, Hanrahan P (1993). What is appropriate care for end-state dementia? *J Amer Geriatr Soc*, **41**(1)**,** 25–30.

Chapter 29

Advance care planning and palliative care in dementia: a view from the Netherlands

Cees Hertogh

Introduction

As in the countries around us, the number of elderly people with dementia in the Netherlands is rising sharply. In recent years this fact has caused government, care organizations, and non-governmental organizations (NGOs), i.e. the Alzheimer's Society, to focus increasingly and more actively on how the care for this vulnerable group of elderly can be improved. Pleas are made for early diagnosis and timely intervention; and much of the effort is aimed at taking care of people in their own environment as long as possible by means of support for informal carers, the development of day care and informal meeting centres for people with dementia, and active case management. This leads to an emphasis on mild to moderate dementia, which sometimes creates the impression that dementia is a stationary condition, or that it can be stabilized. Nothing could be farther from the truth, of course. The disease is accompanied by a progressive loss of all learned skills and the majority of patients are admitted into a nursing home in the final stage of their illness. In the Netherlands, 70% of all people with dementia will be admitted into this care facility at some point in the course of the disease.

   In a way, nursing home admission can therefore be considered one of the final complications of the disease. That is the subject of this chapter. It will address in particular the care model for people with dementia as it has been developed in the Dutch nursing homes. This model is unique in the sense that the Netherlands, unlike most other countries, has a medical specialty that concentrates specifically on this patient population. We will address this specialty first. Subsequently, several factors will be discussed that have influenced the development and further elaboration of the medical care policy for nursing home patients with dementia. Against this background we will then explain how this care is given shape by Dutch nursing home medicine/elderly medicine.

Nursing homes and nursing home medicine

In a population of approximately 17,000,000, the Netherlands has some 345 nursing homes with a total capacity of about 66,000 beds. Half of those beds are in so-called dementia special care units; the other beds are earmarked for geriatric rehabilitation and long-term care for somatic patients, the majority of whom are frail elderly with chronic conditions. Nursing home care is financed through the so-called Exceptional Medical Expenses Act or AWBZ, an income-related care insurance to which every person in the Netherlands contributes. What is special about this insurance is that it not only entitles one to nursing care, but also to medical (and paramedical) treatment.

For that reason nursing homes, as early as the 1960s, started hiring physicians whose principal site of practice was in the nursing home, in a ratio of 1 physician for every 100 residents.

These physicians were in a unique position to gain experience with the medical care for a group of patients in advanced and final stages of chronic diseases. To this end they developed a multi-dimensional model of medical and multi-disciplinary care provision. The formal recognition in 1989 of this field by the authorities and the KNMG (Royal Dutch Medical Association) as 'nursing home medicine' marked an important milestone in the professionalization of this specialty. Since then, all physicians who want to practice this specialty must first complete an additional 2-year post-academic specialty training course, which was recently extended to 3 years. However, it was clear right from the start that the name 'nursing home medicine' did not do justice to the geriatric content of the field. This focus on the elderly has only sharpened in the past decades, while the field of the 'nursing home physician' has expanded considerably in that same period, also outside the walls of the nursing home. Nursing home physicians are now also active in hospitals, where they are involved in the so-called sub-acute or post-acute care of frail elderly who require specific medical aftercare and rehabilitation after the hospital treatment is completed. In addition the nursing home physician is involved in the care and support of frail elderly people who still live at home, for example as consultants to the general practitioners (GPs), or as physician in a home care team. For all of these reasons it was recently decided to change the name of the field from 'nursing home medicine' to 'elderly medicine' (in Dutch: ouderengeneeskunde).

A summary of the main characteristics of the specialty is provided in Box 29.1 [1,2].

These characteristics indicate the aspects by which the profession distinguishes itself from related fields such as GP medicine, rehabilitation medicine, and (hospital-based) clinical geriatrics (which focusses mainly on short-term clinical interventions). In particular, the *proactive approach* and the *triadic care-giving relationship* must be mentioned [1]. Elderly medicine is proactive, because interventions are not (merely) incident-driven, but preventive and anticipatory, i.e. focussing also on expected future developments in the health of the elderly patient. Active monitoring of the elderly person with chronic conditions and multi-morbidity, among other things by means of regular multi-disciplinary evaluations, is therefore an essential element in elderly medicine. Another elaboration of the proactive approach is advance care planning: a process of periodical consultation between physician, patient, and the patient's relatives about goals and boundaries of future care, taking into consideration the patient's preferences, and the prognosis for his condition(s). This also indicates to some degree how the care-giving relationship differs from the traditional doctor-patient relationship. For an essential element of clinical practice in elderly medicine is the relationship with and active involvement of the care system. After all, requests for help are frequently not made by the elderly patient himself, but rather his relative(s) or (in)formal carers sound the alarm or notice that something is wrong. Conversely, in

Box 29.1 Definition of 'elderly medicine'

Problem-oriented and pro-active medical care for frail elderly with chronic conditions and multi-morbidity

In a triadic care giving relationship

By means of both patient-oriented and care-oriented interventions

Aimed at the highest attainable level of functional autonomy and the best possible quality of life her interventions the elderly medicine physician often uses the care system surrounding the elderly person, whether it be informal caregivers such as relatives and loved ones, or a formal system such as the carers in the nursing home or home care staff. In a way, both physician and patient are dependent on the quality and strength of this care system, and part of the physician's responsibility is to assess whether the medical and nursing care required by the elderly patient can be provided safely within this system, or whether additional care, or perhaps admission into a hospital or nursing home, is indicated.

Finally, a third distinguishing characteristic of elderly medicine is that the physician in this field is frequently confronted with ethical decisions when determining the goals and limits of medical care. For, all her medical decisions are decisions in the context of a declining life course. It always involves finding the correct balance between 'overtreatment' and 'undertreatment', i.e. between medical interventions unilaterally focussed on prolonging life and too much therapeutic restraint with the risk of providing insufficient medical care. This is especially true in the case of patients with dementia in nursing homes.

Motives for adopting a palliative care approach in dementia

There are various reasons why physicians in nursing home care of people with dementia explicitly opted for a palliative care model in the 1990s. These can be categorized into medical and care-related reasons on the one hand, and societal reasons on the other.

Medical considerations

In recent decades, research in Dutch nursing homes has resulted in a more profound understanding of the course of dementia after admission to the nursing home. Starting from an average duration of illness of 7 years, a patient with dementia in the Netherlands, on average, lives at home for 5 years and spends his last 2 years in a nursing home. There can be large variations in the duration of stay: some patients die shortly after admission; very occasionally a patient is still alive 10 years later. The duration of stay depends partly on the age on admission, gender, type of dementia, and degree of need for care or assistance. In the Netherlands, Koopmans and Van Dijk both conducted research into the predictive value of various patient characteristics on admission with their results largely in agreement [3,4]. Van Dijk found that the mortality risk for men was twice as high as the risk for women, and that for every year added to his age on admission, the patient's mortality risk increased by 3%. Both studies confirmed the clinical experience that comorbidity results in a considerable increase in the mortality risk, the major conditions being: atrial fibrillation, malignancies, chronic heart failure, diabetes mellitus, and parkinsonism. Vascular dementia was accompanied in Koopmans' study by a two times higher mortality risk than Alzheimer's disease. The most frequent causes of death were dehydration, pneumonia, and cardiovascular disease, together accounting for more than three-quarters of all deaths. One remarkable finding in Koopmans' study was that only one in seven patients with dementia survived to end-stage dementia, that is to stage 7d or higher on the Functional Assessment Staging (FAST) scale of Reisberg et al. [5] This is the stage where the patient is fully dependent and mute. Communication is no longer possible and patients display the characteristics of what was once known as the Kluver-Bucy syndrome. In these cases, swallowing disorders often herald the beginning of the end of life and such patients usually die of the combined consequences of dehydration, cachexia, and (aspiration) pneumonia.

In a very high proportion of patients with dementia, there are also changes in eating behaviour in the final stage, ranging from excessive eating (hyperphagia) to reduced eating and drinking as a consequence of apraxia, dysphagia, anorexia, or sometimes the deliberate refusal of food.

Other more or less direct consequences of dementia are the occurrence of functional neurological disorders, such as (oppositional) paratonia (German: 'Gegenhalten'), hypertonia, myoclonus, and epileptic seizures.

All of these findings combined – and there may be more from research conducted elsewhere – justify the notion that dementia is not only an incurable, but also a deadly disease process that is accompanied for most patients by a considerably reduced life expectancy. In addition to a less favourable prognosis for comorbid conditions, a number of inevitable complications occur in the course of the illness trajectory that may herald the end of life. Ryan argued as early as 1992 that when a severely demented patient dies as a result of pneumonia, the underlying dementia rather than the pneumonia should be considered 'the old man's best friend' [6].

For the treating physician, a thorough understanding of the course and the complications of dementia is essential. He needs to weigh continuously each treatment decision in the context of a progressive disease with the risk of repetition and new complications. Not being familiar with the course of the illness trajectory may cause overly aggressive medical intervention and ultimately even unnecessarily taxing hospitalization of patients with severe dementia, as described by, among others, Mitchell and colleagues [7].

Care-orientated considerations

Care-related motives for a palliative approach are to a high degree connected with how the relatives or loved ones of patients are supported and informed about the consequences of dementia. Not only do doctors (GPs and medical specialists) regularly lack an understanding of the terminal nature of this condition, the patient's relatives are usually also unfamiliar with what the final stage of the disease entails. This is not altogether surprising, considering the lack of balance in terms of public information on dementia. In addition, for family members the decision to institutionalize a dear one brings with it several adaptive challenges and is often accompanied by feelings of guilt. They not only have to cope with the loss of proximity of their loved one, they also have to accommodate themselves to a new role in handing over their former caregiver responsibility to the nursing home staff, while at the same time the progression of the dementia confronts them with difficult moral decisions with regard to the last stage of the disease. At the moment of nursing home admission family caregivers often experience a lack of information, not only with regard to the specific decisions to be made, but also with regard to the natural course of the disease, which makes it difficult for them to anticipate the future. And with limited knowledge regarding the disease trajectory one should not be surprised that health care proxies often insist on aggressive medical treatment or hospital admission in case of acute illness of their demented relative. In addition, there are often negative reports in the media on the quality of care in nursing homes. In some cases this is definitely justified, especially in the current climate of understaffing and sparse budgets. But these reports also regularly demonstrate the huge lack of knowledge on the nature of the disease and its natural progression.

For example, in 1997 there was a huge outcry in the Netherlands about the supposed policy of nursing homes allowing patients with dementia to die from dehydration 'deliberately' by administering insufficient fluids and forgoing artificial rehydration. The immediate cause of this turmoil was a complaint made by the family of a nursing home resident who accused the nursing home staff of deliberately allowing the patient to dehydrate. The incident roused a lot of emotion among the general public and even resulted in a discussion in the Dutch parliament. It led the Minister of Health to commission a research study into the decision-making process, the clinical course, and quality of dying of patients with severe dementia as a result of dehydration. This study showed that the particular case that caused the commotion was indeed based on an atypical incident and it confirmed once again that forgoing artificial rehydration in the end stage of dementia is generally not associated with discomfort or suffering in the dying patient [8,9]. Despite these findings, however, the issue still reappears in the media at regular intervals. One lesson that should be learned from this is the importance of emotional support of relatives of nursing home patients with dementia, of providing sound information about the expected course of the disease, and of shared decision-making.

Societal factors

Above we addressed the way in which the care for people of dementia in the nursing home is influenced by popular notions and societal prejudices. Careful information and solid communication could perhaps remedy this situation. However, a society that closes its eyes, more or less deliberately, to the tragedy of an autumn of life with dementia and that – borrowing an expression from Stephen Post [10] – is characterized by a hypercognitive orientation, will always have problems with a disease that undermines its core values as ruthlessly as dementia. For dementia is inevitably accompanied by a loss of self-determination and autonomy. Those who suffer from it lose control of their own inner selves and their lives, and they end up completely dependent on the care of others. Many people in our society, especially the elderly, fear this prospect and are looking for means to be spared this eclipse of their personality. One way of influencing a possible future with dementia is by means of an advance directive.

Under the Dutch Medical Treatment Act, that came into effect in 1995, written advance treatment directives or living wills are considered to be the optimal instrument for patients to retain control in health care situations and medical treatments after they have become incompetent, because such a directive comes closest to regular informed consent. In case of incompetence, a living will representing the patient's competent beliefs should govern the outcome of current treatment issues and the physician is more or less obliged to comply with its content. This applies in particular to negative living wills, i.e. a non-treatment advance directive. However, one problem with this type of advance directive is that it is often formulated fairly robustly, namely as a 'treatment refusal', prohibiting all medical treatment, except the alleviation of pain, breathlessness and other discomforts. However, following such a directive to the letter may result in the patient manoeuvring himself into a situation in which he forgoes appropriate care. For example, what would respecting a treatment refusal mean in the case of a hip fracture, or a bleeding gastric ulcer? So a negative advance directive does not suffice to develop the care for people with dementia in their final years of life in an appropriate and ethically sound way. After all, forgoing medical treatment does not automatically result in a good death. Extensive consultation with relatives and proxies is also indicated here, in order jointly to determine how the patient's wishes are best honoured.

Apart from the negative advance directive, the Netherlands also knows a so-called positive advance directive, which describes what treatments or actions the author of the advance directive would wish for under certain conditions. The most prominent example of a positive living will is the euthanasia declaration in case of dementia. The societal debate on this subject reached a new stage with the adoption in 2002 of the Euthanasia Act, because this law states that a living will can replace an oral request for euthanasia in case of incompetence.

However, nursing home physicians/specialists in elderly medicine were being confronted with the request for active life-termination of incompetent patients with dementia and a euthanasia directive long before that time. After a commission of the Royal Dutch Medical Association (in which nursing home physicians/specialists in elderly medicine were not invited to participate!) opened the door for honouring such written requests in the early 1990s, the then Dutch Association of Nursing Home Physicians (NVVA) felt the need to formulate its own opinion on the subject. This resulted in the establishment of the Committee on Medical Decision-Making in Dementia, which presented its report in 1997 [11]. In this report, the professional community emphatically opted for a palliative care model that tries to accommodate both the norms of the patient (respect for autonomy and advance directive) and the medical-professional standards of good care (beneficence and non-maleficence).

Palliative care in advanced dementia

The palliative care concept was originally developed in the field of oncology and is often closely associated with terminal care, that is, with end-of-life care. This is erroneous because the WHO definition of palliative care covers a much broader domain of application, and it involves much more than pain management and symptom relief. According to this 1990 definition, palliative care entails 'integral multi-disciplinary care for patients with incurable diseases, aimed at reaching and maintaining optimal quality of life for both patients and their relatives'. Essential to this definition is also that palliative care 'neither intends to hasten nor postpone death' [12].

This clearly indicates that palliative care must also be available for patients who, although they have an incurable disease, are not yet in the terminal stages of their illness. The essence of this type of care is the orientation on well-being and perceived quality of life. Prolonging life may be a side effect of palliative care, but never a primary objective. For example, in the context of palliative care, incurably ill oncology patients are treated for heart failure or infections with medicines that, in addition to alleviating complaints, also have a life-prolonging effect. The degree to which this is acceptable naturally depends not only on the patient's wishes and the prognosis for the primary illness, but also on the expected effect on well-being of the intended treatment.

In a similar vein, palliative treatment is indicated in dementia. In this case also, the irreversibility and the ultimately deadly course of the disease are evident, which is why the decision-making regarding medical action should always take into account the course of the disease. For, as was indicated earlier, each successful treatment of a comorbid illness (ascending urinary tract infection, hyperglycaemia, lower respiratory tract infection) also means continuing life with the progressing dementia. This fact implies that as the disease progresses, it must be continually assessed whether – and to what degree – a life-prolonging side effect of medical intervention that is aimed primarily at well-being is acceptable.

Another important characteristic of palliative care is the care for loved ones and relatives. This care aims to involve them as much as possible in the organization of the patient's care and to help them cope with the consequences of the disease. Therefore, palliative care also presumes a triadic care-giving relationship, as outlined above, as a characteristic of elderly medicine. Thus, there is an obvious correspondence between the description of the field of 'elderly medicine' at the beginning of this chapter and the view of palliative care formulated here. This is by no means a coincidence. Both turn away from purely disease-orientated medical action and opt instead for a broad approach, in which not only the patient and his problems, his possibilities and limitations, but also his values and relationships are central.

With this definition underlying it, the Dutch care model for palliative care in dementia consists of three elements:

1 An individual care plan, in which the goals and boundaries of medical care are recorded, as determined in consultation with the patient's family

2 Periodic consultation with relatives/loved ones of the patient, during which the care plan is evaluated and, if necessary, adjusted based on the course of the disease

3   A further differentiation within the covering framework of the palliative care approach between two policies: a (wider) palliative treatment policy and a (more restricted) symptomatic policy [11,13].

This distinction between a palliative and a symptomatic policy calls for some clarification. Roughly two basic intentions can be distinguished in the domain of clinical interventions: (1) interventions aimed at prolonging life expectancy and (2) interventions aimed at improving the well-being or quality of life of the patient. In elderly medicine both intentions often coincide or overlap, but in view of a palliative care approach in dementia, a further articulation and differentiation between both intentions in the individual treatment policy acquires specific importance precisely because palliative care is far from identical to terminal care. Therefore, given the variations in duration of survival following nursing home admission, there is no reason to withhold life-prolonging medical treatment automatically from nursing home patients with dementia, with the exception of artificial ventilation and cardio-pulmonary resuscitation, interventions that are clearly contraindicated in late dementia. Thus, in line with the WHO definition, a palliative treatment policy is defined as:

> A medical policy aimed primarily at safeguarding optimal wellbeing and an acceptable quality of life of the patient with dementia. This goal is achieved by: optimal treatment of intercurrent ailments, comorbidity, and complications of the dementia, in which prolonging life as a side effect of medical treatment is acceptable in view of the patient's quality of life [13].

The main intention of this policy is therefore aimed at the well-being of the patient, but the means to be used to this end are not *a priori* limited by their possible life-prolonging effects. This is exactly the difference with a symptomatic policy: symptomatic care entails *a medical policy in which a life-prolonging side effect is emphatically unwanted.* Such a policy implies only alleviating symptoms and signs of discomfort and so limits the choice of therapeutic options to reach this goal. The decision in favour of one of the two treatment policies is made in consultation with the family, based on the assessment of the course of the dementia, the patient's condition and life expectancy, as well as his (precedent) wishes and preferences.

Since most patients at the time of admission to the nursing home are no longer capable of overseeing their whole situation, their participation in the decision-making regarding medical intervention can only be limited. This does not alter the fact that in the context of a triadic relationship, shared or supported decision-making should be pursued whenever possible, even if only on elements of the care plan. A decision to limit medical treatment to symptomatic relief will, however, almost always be situated at a stage of the disease in which only proxy decision-making with relatives is possible.

Place of antibiotic therapy and artificial rehydration

Physicians in Dutch nursing homes are generally reserved when it comes to prescribing antibiotics and implementing artificial rehydration. Tube feeding is relatively rare because eating behaviour disorders in the advanced stages of dementia are generally considered an unavoidable and irreversible complication of the primary illness. Artificial rehydration is only applied as a temporary, supporting treatment, for example in the case of a respiratory or urinary tract infection with a favourable prognosis. Whether or not antibiotics are prescribed in the treatment of respiratory tract infections in actual practice depends mainly on the agreed policy. Although recent epidemiological research suggests that antibiotic treatment (mostly oral) in case of pneumonia decreases discomfort even when death is imminent, this generally is not sufficient reason in clinical practice to prescribe these medicines [14]. On the contrary, the decision not to provide

Box 29.2 Comparison of palliative and symptomatic treatment policies (ANR = artificial nutrition and rehydration)

Palliative treatment policy	Symptomatic treatment policy
Focus on comfort, not on prolonging life	Focus on comfort, not on prolonging life
Life-prolonging 'side effects' are acceptable or even co-intended	Life-prolonging 'side effects' are considered unacceptable
Includes administration of antibiotics, temporary ANR	Excludes antibiotics and temporary ANR
Excludes (permanent) tube feeding, cardio-pulmonary resuscitation, artificial ventilation	Excludes these and also antibiotics and temporary ANR
Examples	**Examples**
Administration of antibiotics in treatment of pneumonia, supported, if necessary, by artificial rehydration	Oxygen and morphine to relieve symptoms; palliative sedation in case of refractory symptoms
Optimal treatment and monitoring for comorbid diseases (e.g. diabetes, chronic heart failure)	Critical assessment and (if acceptable from a symptom-relief perspective) discontinuation of chronic life-sustaining medication for comorbid diseases

antibiotic therapy is in line with a so-called symptomatic policy. To the loved ones of the patient, this decision marks a major transition in the care policy, not just in terms of content, but also emotionally, because this brings death within their field of vision as an imminent reality. Direct symptom alleviation by means of analgesics and/or sedatives then makes more sense than the prescription of antibiotics, which in this situation would be at the very least counter-intuitive. Box 29.2 shows the different accents of a palliative treatment policy and a symptomatic treatment policy related to various treatment possibilities.

The role of advance directives

The above has shown that advance directives are always a reason for consultation about the care policy, if possible with the patient himself, but at the very least, with his representative. Although the law suggests differently, at least as far as the negative advance directive is concerned, these directives can never be interpreted as instructions for the caregiver. From an ethical perspective, advance directives are best viewed as an instrument for advance care planning. In the case of an incompetent dementia patient, the discussion will take place between the treating physician and the patient's representative. The goal of this discussion is to find out the patient's intentions and to determine the best way the care policy can be made to correspond with those intentions. In most cases, it will prove possible to align the tenor of a negative advance directive with the principles and objectives of palliative care as described above.

It is no different for positive advance directives, and the euthanasia directive, in particular. Although the enactment of the Euthanasia Law in 2002 allowed physicians to act upon such directives, cases of euthanasia in incompetent dementia patients with an advance directive for euthanasia have been virtually absent so far. The fundamental reason for this absence is that the practice of euthanasia is essentially rooted in joint decision-making and mutual assessment of the patient's condition by both doctor and patient. Every physician who has ever had to deal with euthanasia will agree that this ultimate form of relief of suffering is only possible in the context of a relationship of trust and mutual understanding. An advance directive for euthanasia can never replace this. Even in the face of obvious suffering, ending a demented patient's life out of respect for the directive is morally inconceivable without the reciprocity that is essential to this act of mercy. In addition, most proxies of dementia patients with advance euthanasia directives indicate explicitly that they don't want the directive to be executed, not even when the patient's situation clearly corresponds with the circumstances intended in the directive.

Thus, if advance directives for euthanasia have a place in end-of-life practice, their role is restricted to the earlier stages of certain subtypes of dementia, in which case they might help to create a window of opportunity for reciprocity and shared decision-making.

In the situation of advanced dementia the possible role of an advance directive for euthanasia is equivalent to that accorded to an advance non-treatment directive.

Conclusion

The strength of the Dutch care model for nursing home patients with dementia is shown in, among other things, the very low rate of hospital admissions of people with dementia in the Netherlands compared to other countries, such as the United States. Also, aggressive medical treatments such as tube feeding are extremely rare here and antibiotics are more frequently withheld than in most other countries [15]. In addition, it has been demonstrated, against popular belief and prejudice, that careful symptomatic treatment of dehydration does not result in discomfort. Thus, there is some reason to conclude – cautiously – that a palliative care approach based on the elements discussed above can be successful.

Recent qualitative research by Helton *et al.* supports this conclusion [16]. According to these authors, this success is because Dutch nursing homes are staffed with specially trained physicians, who take on an active role in advance care planning, not only through regular and intensive discussions with proxies, but also by being open and frank about the course of the dementia process and by putting more emphasis on keeping the patient comfortable than on the possibilities of medical technology.

However, there is also criticism to answer. A crucial question is whether this active approach to decision- and policy-making truly represents an adequate ethic. This is a morally complex matter, but in essence the answer to this question depends on how one values the role of the physician in the decision-making process. The Dutch model tends towards an ethic of communication in which the physician is both a moderate autonomist and a moderate welfarist. According to this ethic the role of the physician is not restricted to informing the family on the diverse treatment options at stake, but is, indeed, to recommend a course of action instead of abandoning the decision to them. This attitude reflects yet another dimension of the triadic caregiving relationship that is so essential to elderly medicine. Others, however, hold the opinion that through this active engagement in advance care planning and decision-making, Dutch physicians in elderly medicine fall victim to the ancient vice of medical paternalism, because – as Helton *et al.* [16] suggest – they are alleged to be too directive in their communication. But perhaps this criticism is also a reflection of different cultural values: there is, indeed, more than an ocean between the US and the Netherlands [15].

Finally, although there is much room for practice improvement through further research, palliative care begins with the recognition that the curative power of medicine is limited and that modesty should be one of the basic virtues of the doctor. This maxim is already found in the ancient Hippocratic writings. Crucial to good medical care, in dementia as in all other diseases, is that physicians learn to recognize the limits of their art, or in the words of Hippocrates: that they learn to recognize the moment in the course of the disease where the patient is overwhelmed by his disease and any further medical treatment is futile. However, what Hippocrates failed to include in his maxims, is that recognizing the limits of the art can never be an excuse for abandoning the patient. Indeed, the limits of the art are also a stimulus for its continuation under new conditions and with other, but surely not inferior, goals.

References

1. Hertogh CMPM (1999). *Functionele geriatrie*. Maarsen: Elzevier/De Tijdstroom. (*Functional geriatrics*, in Dutch).

2. Hertogh CMPM (2006). Medical care for chronically ill elderly people: nursing home medicine as functional geriatrics, in Jones GGM, Miesen BML (eds). *Caregiving in dementia: research and applications*, vol 4, pp. 219–239. New York/London: Routledge.

3. Koopmans RTCM (1994). *Het leven, ziek zijn en sterven van dementerende verpleeghuispatiënten. Een onderzoek naar morbiditeit, functionele status en mortaliteit*. Thesis, Nijmegen, Radboud University Nijmegen. (*Life, illness and death of demented nursing home patients: studies in morbidity, disability and mortality*, in Dutch).

4. Dijk PTM van. (1994). *Prognosis of patients with dementia after admission to a Dutch nursing home*. Thesis, Rotterdam, Erasmus University Rotterdam.

5. Koopmans RTCM, Ekkerkink JLP, van der Weel C (2003). Survival to late dementia in Dutch nursing home patients. *J Am Geriatr Soc*, **51**, 184–187.

6. Ryan DH (1992). Death in dementia: a study of causes of death in dementia patients and their spouses. *Int J Geriatr Psychiatr*, **7**, 465–472.

7. Mitchell SL, Kiely DK, Hamel MB (2004). Dying with advanced dementia in the nursing home. *Arch Int Med*, **164**, 321–36.

8. The Anne Mei (2005). *In de wachtkamer van de dood*. Amsterdam: Thoeris. (*In the waiting room for death*, in Dutch).

9. Pasman HR, Onwuteaka-Philipsen BD, Kriegsman DM, Ooms ME, Ribbe MW, van der Wal G (2005). Discomfort in nursing home patients with severe dementia in whom artificial nutrition and hydration is foregone. *Arch Intern Med*, **165**, 1729–1735.

10. Post SG (2000). *The moral challenge of Alzheimer disease: ethical issues from diagnosis to dying*, 2nd edn. Baltimore: Johns Hopkins University Press.

11. Dutch Association of Nursing Home Physicians (NVVA) (1997). *Medische zorg met beleid*. Utrecht: NVVA. (*Policy statement on end-of-life-care in demented patients in nursing homes*, in Dutch).

12. World Health Organization (WHO) (1990). Cancer pain relief and palliative care. *WHO Tech Rep Ser*, 804.

13. Hertogh CMPM (2005). End-of-life care and medical decision making in patients with dementia, in Burns A (ed) *Standards in dementia care – european dementia consensus network (EDCON)*, pp. 339–354. London/New York: Taylor & Francis.

14. Steen JT van der, Pasman HR, Ribbe MW, van der Wal, G, Onwuteaka-Philipsen BD (2009). Discomfort in dementia patients dying from pneumonia and its relief by antibiotics. *Scand J Infect Dis*, **41**(2), 143–151.

15. Steen JT van der, Kruse RL, Ooms ME *et al.* (2004). Treatment of nursing home residents with dementia and lower respiratory tract infection in the United States and the Netherlands: an ocean apart. *J Am Geriatric Soc*, **52**, 691–699.

16. Helton MR, van der Steen JT, Daaleman TP, Gamble GR, Ribbe MW (2006). A cross-cultural study of physician treatment decisions for demented nursing home patients who develop pneumonia. *Ann Fam Med*, **4**, 221–227.

Chapter 30

Living and dying at home with dementia

Adrian Treloar and Monica Crugel

Dementia: a terminal illness

It is now well recognized that dementia is a terminal illness that is both associated with early death and also causes death in its own right. Despite this, it is relatively rare for those who die with dementias to be certified as dying from dementia. This is despite patients with dementia having a life expectancy of about 4.5 years [1]. The progressive loss of mental ability leads to inabilities in terms of self-care, mobility, and nutrition, but also triggers further physical losses owing to the poor nutrition and poor levels of physical activity. But beyond this, the increasing disability leads to an increase in infections, vascular events, falls, and so forth. This is, in part, caused by physical frailty, but is also caused by the inability of the patient to describe emergent symptoms which would normally lead to a more rapid accessing of treatments for infections and other remedial conditions. An increasing inability to communicate leads to a reduced frequency of treatment, which is provided later as a result of the illness itself.

Of course, physical conditions such as infections, or major operations, also trigger delirium. Accumulating evidence suggests that delirium does not often fully resolve in those who have a pre-existing dementia [2]. Hence, for the person with dementia, the prognosis is often significantly worsened than it would be in someone without dementia [3]. For those who do not die during the course of an illness such as pneumonia, dementia progresses and, in the end causes death by a variety of means. These include the loss of the ability to swallow, epileptic fits, and the effects of the severe frailty seen in advanced dementia.

It has been suggested that the illness trajectory for dementia is slower than that of other conditions [4]. In fact, whereas the mean life expectancy of dementia is around 4.5 years [1], survival from many cancers is substantially longer. But it may well be that illness progression is, somehow, more predictable in cancer than in dementia. So predicting death in dementia may be more difficult than in cancer. This, in turn, may make it harder to identify the time to have discussions about the end of life with patients or carers.

Supportive, palliative, and end-of-life care is poorly understood

However, we should be careful not to base a discussion of dying with dementia purely around the question of life expectancy. Dying is only a part of the issue here. Distress is common in dementia and as one moves towards the end of life, supportive care and reducing distress become a central part of the endeavour. The question of life expectancy focusses upon a single outcome, whereas an alternative approach is to focus on needs, key among which may be the relief of distress. Indeed, the definition of end-of-life care (see Box 30.1), talks more of symptom relief than it does of life expectancy. It also clearly fits the care of people with advanced dementia. The only issue that does not easily emerge from the definition is that a lot of the distress in dementia is caused by both mental and physical pain. Yet, it is important to provide good symptom relief for both in dementia.

> **Box 30.1 End-of-life care**
>
> Helps all those with advanced, progressive, incurable illness to live as well as possible until they die. It enables the supportive and palliative care needs of both patient and family to be identified and met throughout the last phase of life and into bereavement. It includes management of pain and other symptoms and provision of psychological, social, spiritual and practical support [5].

Dementia is now recognized as a condition for which palliative care is poorly available [5,6]. But it is not often understood that dementia is a condition in which palliative care needs occur. Very few patients die in hospices with dementia [6], and it has been sensibly argued that long-stay dementia wards are, in fact, units that could deliver palliative care [7]. Care at home is perhaps even less frequently obtained [8], and we are aware of very few services that support this work. Barbara Pointon has already pointed out in Chapter 4 of this volume how unsupported people can sometimes feel when living with dementia at home.

So there is a real need to develop methods and understanding of how people with dementia can be supported at home until they die. Whilst the expertise of palliative care is clearly relevant, much of the expertise to make this possible will also come from dementia services themselves.

Priorities of care and advance care planning

Advance care planning (discussed more fully in the preceding two chapters) is a patient-centred and patient-driven dialogue with care professionals that can enable effective care to take place. The importance of advance care planning has already been mentioned in Chapter 13 in connection with hospital admissions. The aim is to enable patients and their carers to set out their hopes concerning the future management of the disease and their lives, and to avoid particular pitfalls that they think might appear. A number of tools have been developed to assist this and the Preferred Priorities of Care guidance aims to support timely discussion about future care [9]. Many patients will express a desire to complete (more general) advance statements and (more specific) advance decisions to refuse treatment. Advance refusals have been found to provide helpful guidance and advice once capacity has been lost, but they may also be hazardous [10]. For example, a blanket refusal to receive antibiotics in severe dementia may not recognize the fact that many infections will not be terminal events, but will only cause distress, which would be alleviated by oral antibiotics. In such circumstances, it would be critical to consider the reasons why an advance refusal might be invalid, so as to prevent unintended harm coming to the patient. The *Mental Capacity Act 2005* [11], which relates to England and Wales, offers the following useful criteria to judge when an advance refusal would be invalid:

1 If the patient withdraws the decision at a time when he or she had the capacity to do so

2 If the patient, under a lasting power of attorney created after the advance decision was made, conferred authority on the donee(s) of the power of attorney to give or refuse consent to the treatment to which the advance decision relates

3 If the patient does anything else clearly inconsistent with the advance decision remaining his or her fixed decision (Section 25(2)).

Further, an advance decision is not applicable if:

1 The person has the capacity to give or refuse consent to the treatment

2 The treatment is not the treatment specified in the advance decision

3 Any circumstances specified in the advance decision are absent

4 There are reasonable grounds for believing that circumstances exist which the person did not anticipate at the time of the advance decision and which would have affected his or her decision had he or she anticipated them (Sections 25(3–4)).

The various ways in which decisions are made in different contexts for those who cannot make decisions will be a matter for individual legislatures. Perhaps the hardest task will be to work out how and when someone ought to move to hospital for acute care and when they might be best managed at home.

We have found that most carers of people with advanced dementia at home decide that they will keep their loved ones there unless there is an absolutely compelling reason to admit them to hospital. Such reasons might be acute breathlessness or a fractured hip; but frequently chest infections will either be untreated, or treated at home with oral antibiotics. The distress of hospital admission is greater than carers often feel is warranted by the gain. Hospital acquired infections are also an argument in themselves against hospital admission.

In drawing up an advance care plan to do with the prospect of a hospital admission, it is sensible to have specific medical scenarios in mind, which would lead to questions in a process that is more likely thereby to be truly helpful. Thus, sensible questions to stimulate thought might be:

1 Would hospital admission be appropriate to treat an inter-current illness such as a chest infection?

2 Would hospital admission be appropriate to treat a (simple) fracture?

3 Would hospital admission be indicated for dehydration, particularly if associated with apparent distress?

4 Would cardiopulmonary resuscitation, ventilation, or intensive care medicine be appropriate?

5 Would aggressive treatment such as cancer chemotherapy, where there are severe potential side effects, be appropriate?

6 Would complex surgical procedures be appropriate?

7 Would treatment be deemed appropriate to alleviate distress in the face of imminent death?

Having had such discussions, as in the case of people dying with other conditions at home, it is hoped that the distress of a trip to an emergency department at about the time of death is avoided and death can occur with family, friends, and in the comfort of one's home.

Assessment of needs in advanced dementia

As well as the assessment of cognition in dementia, a whole raft of needs must be considered for anyone with advanced dementia living at home. There ought to be a full and detailed assessment. Areas to be considered might fall under the following headings:

1 *Medical*: a full assessment of physical health; decisions will be required on the need to treat conditions such as heart failure, lung disease, and the like, which (untreated) may worsen the abilities of the patient and increase their distress; an assessment of the presence of physical pain (see Chapter 14).

2 *Psychiatric*: assessment of the relevance of anti-dementia drugs; consideration given to the presence of psychosis or depression; assessment and treatment of mental distress.

3 *Physical care*: assessment of the need for personal care, help with mobility, continence, washing, dressing, and so forth; assessment of feeding and the need for nutritional support.

4 *Emotional and spiritual needs*: assessment of the need for emotional support; the possibility of meaningful activities and occupation; spiritual care and support.

5 *Financial support*: assessment of need for benefits, social care, and health funding.

6 *Carer support*: assessment of the needs of unpaid cares, such as husbands, wives, sons, daughters, and so on.

7 *Needs arising from poor care*: assessment of symptoms that arise from poor care, poor understanding, and fear, which can arise as a result of the cognitive difficulties of advanced dementia.

Assessment should be carried out by a suitably qualified person who can access the appropriate services as and when required.

Promoting living well with dementia

Perhaps, the greatest aim of all is to promote living well with dementia. Given that dementia is a terminal illness, it will be absolutely the case that care will both anticipate and accept natural death. However, an essential part of palliative care is to cherish life and to that end rehabilitation and re-enablement are crucial [12]. This will be no less the case in dementia, and ought to be striven for where support could increase the quality of life and function of a person dying with dementia. The only reason for not pursuing such a course would be if the effort entailed were burdensome to the point where the benefit of the intervention would be outweighed. But normally, good care and support will merely make living easier and relieve burdens on both patient and carer.

Understanding of the illness

To care for people with dementia requires carers, both formal and informal, to have a suitable understanding of the condition. As dementia moves towards the end of life, communication becomes even more difficult, but important (as discussed in Chapter 23). The challenges of care change with time. With increasing physical frailty and physical dependency the challenges change, for instance, from dealing with depressive and emotional symptoms, through wandering and 'challenging behaviour', towards physical dependency. However, it has been our experience with patients having severe dementia looked after at home that behaviours that challenge continue to affect many patients with advanced dementia right up to the days and weeks before death. As a result, both good nursing and an understanding approach by all carers are essential. Ongoing training in appropriate skills to help carers and families modify the environment for patients with dementia to maintain functioning and reduce behavioural disturbance has been shown to be effective [13]. Individualized person-centred occupational therapy interventions have also been shown to improve quality of life and carer burden [14]. There are other possible ways in which a more appropriate approach might be inculcated: Dementia Care Mapping and person-centred care, for instance, have already been discussed in Chapters 13 and 25.

Understanding distress

As the illness progresses there will, naturally, be a transition from a more actively therapeutic approach towards a more palliative one. In this context, it becomes more and more important both to recognize distress and to understand it. Jordan and Lloyd-Williams have already discussed distress and pain in dementia in Chapter 14. To emphasize a point from their discussion, pain may be the physically noxious type, or it may be mental pain. In palliative care the concept of 'total pain' was coined by Dame Cicely Saunders, who defined it as the suffering that encompasses all of a person's physical, psychological, social, spiritual, and practical struggles [15].

This broad characterization means that the causes of pain or distress must be considered in an equally broad fashion. The reflex use of antipsychotic medicine, for instance, would be inappropriate in the absence of a proper, holistic assessment (see Chapter 12). We have found that treating distress is a central part of supportive and palliative care for people with dementia. The treatments are directed by informed guesses as to the cause or causes of the distress and should normally include the best possible nursing care, best possible communication, and responses that lower anxiety. But the treatments will also include anti-depressants, as well as analgesics, titrated according to response and, in the right circumstances, anti-psychotics, too. While recognizing very clearly the harm they do, the All Party Parliamentary Group on dementia in the UK concluded that the use of anti-psychotics can be justified because they are effective in reducing severe distress in people with dementia, which squares with our experience and that of many in the field [16], albeit other approaches to agitation might be more appropriate in certain circumstances (see Chapter 17). It would be utterly wrong to leave severe suffering untreated for fear of the risk of side effects. In line with the *Mental Capacity Act 2005* [11], Section 6, sedative drugs could be justified if the prevention of harm means that the use of such drugs is a proportionate response and there are no less restrictive measures to relieve the sort of harm we are considering, namely mental suffering.

Resistance in the face of care

Resistance will be a common feature in response to even the best care of people with dementia. Often enough, resistance can be reduced by a gentle approach, withdrawing, and offering care later. Other aspects of best practice have been outlined earlier in this book. If procedures (like dressing ulcers) are painful then analgesia half an hour beforehand may help. If food is refused, offering it again half an hour later may work well. Similarly, if washing and dressing is refused, trying again a little later may work, provided the care package and carers are able to be there and support this approach. But in the end, washing, dressing, warm clothes, and comfort must be provided and so, in those who really do resist, clear, compassionate, and firm nursing are needed to achieve basic care. Quite poorly paid carers have considerable skills at enabling such care to be provided with the minimum of resistance and distress. The best carers, perhaps those with the most compassion, end up with the patient accepting happily what they have resisted so resolutely.

In the legal framework governing England and Wales, basic care cannot be refused; so warmth and comfort, washing and dressing, and so forth, might have to be imposed if those who lack capacity resist it and cannot be more easily persuaded to accept it. Similarly, restraint would be deemed appropriate if the patient would suffer harm as a result of resisting care, as long as the level of restraint is proportionate to the harm to be avoided.

Covert medication

Concealing medication is a tactic often used in nursing and residential homes and also considered by many carers to be ethically right and necessary [17]. Such methods can enable effective care to be given to those who lack capacity in the least restrictive and least distressing manner. But processes, guidance, and policy on this ought to be followed [18]. The worst outcome is faced if these measures are pursued secretly. However, part of the process of deciding upon the use of covert medication is to assess the need for medication and the modes of administration. Many medicines, such as statins, low dose aspirin, and anti-hypertensives may be discontinued in advanced dementia without detriment to the patient. Others may be switched to more easily taken forms, such as orodispersible tablets, low volume drop formulations, and antibiotics that require few doses. A five-day course of ampicilin, for example, may be hugely more challenging and distressing for patients with dementia than four doses of Azithromycin in a small volume. If efficacy is equivalent, and treatment indicated, the extra cost can be easily justified.

Providing comfort and care at home

The provision of care and comfort at home must embrace all of the facets of supportive care seen in other illnesses, as well as meeting some specific challenges that exist in dementia. Perhaps, the two greatest of these are the inability to express oneself as a result of cognitive impairment and severe distress both for patients and for carers. In Greenwich, we have set out to support people at home with advanced dementia and have now successfully provided care, in total, for over 50 people, the majority of whom have died at home. Some of the key features of that care are outlined below.

Social support

Carers who look after their loved ones at home require good quality support. It has been noted in the general palliative care literature that the attributes of family caregivers play an important role since they will largely have to bear responsibility for the provision of care to their dying relatives [19]. They must, therefore, be able to do the task. To provide good quality care at home for those dying with cancer requires carers who are mentally robust. We, too, have found this, even where the main carers were in their 90s and physically frail. It does not appear to work well when the main carer has a degree of dementia or some other mental illness. Social support (see also Chapter 18 above) will potentially need to include:

1 Help with washing, dressing, toileting, and feeding

2 Help with cleaning, bed-making, shopping, and other daily tasks

3 Respite care

4 Carer breaks

5 Carers or volunteers to sit with the patient while the carer goes out.

Good training of carers, who are thereby helped to understand the challenges of advanced dementia, is also very important. A key aspect of social support, however, is financial support, which will come from different sources in different countries. The distribution of scarce resources and the financial support available to individuals dealing with dementia is crucial as far as the quality of care goes, even if it is not the whole story.

Physical support

Physical support includes the appropriate use of medication (see Chapter 12); but, especially as dementia worsens, and crucially if the intention is for the person to remain at home, the right appliances can make an enormous difference to the ease with which care can be given and with which it is accepted [20]. The increasing availability of hospital beds within the community, as well as waterproof mattresses and various other aids, has revolutionized care for advanced disability at home. The days when an incontinent patient had to be nursed and mobilized from a low sprung mattress, which became soggy with urine despite the best waterproof covers, are now things of the past. Home functional assessments and advice on assistive devices are useful [21]. Skills training for carers can decrease risk of falls and improve functional ability, social participation, and quality of life. Structured interventions are more useful than non-specific counselling [22]. We have found that recognizing the need for appliances is crucial. For physical frailty people

Box 30.2 Equipment to support dementia care at home

Commode

Special waterproof and pressure relieving mattresses

Hospital bed with adjustable height

Mattress elevator for sitting up in bed

Shower bath aids

Zimmer frame

Wheelchair

Continence pads

Continence sheets

Other continence aids

Chair

Cushion

Toilet raiser

Adjustable electric chair

Electric hoist

Shower wet room

Shower stool

often recognize the need for appliances, but those with dementia are not always recognized as needing special beds and hoists and so forth until the carers are exhausted as a result of their struggle. One carer told us that when it became too hard to mobilize their father from the bed, they raised the bed by placing it on a wardrobe, which had been laid flat. When the professional involved saw this, the carers were told it was unsafe and the bed had to be put back on the floor; but no help was given to provide a bed that would rise up, thus enabling their father to be helped to mobilize. Such errors are made by professionals in all disciplines and all such errors are unacceptable.

Key equipment required to support dementia at home are shown in Box 30.2. In terms of adaptations to the home, we always recommend, earlier on in dementia, that a wet room be fitted in preference to a shower, as access and care can be hugely simplified later on as a result.

Dietary support

Come what may, if patients are not fed, they will become frail and lose weight. Tube feeding will rarely be indicated in dementia, and in the UK such measures are rarely undertaken (see discussions in Chapters 13, 27, and 28). But oral feeding using well produced and presented food, cut up into small pieces and given while hot with adequate carer support to enable feeding to continue, is important. Repeated opportunities to eat are also essential [20,23]. Nutritional therapy given to elderly patients with comorbidities can improve their functional abilities [24]. As dysphagia progresses, swallowing difficulties may well indicate thickened fluids; our carers have recommended thick soups, spoon-fed for those with very advanced dementia. Proprietary dietary supplements may also be very useful, although the flavours can sometimes be unappealing. Some of our carers recommend just liquidizing foods such as meat and vegetables so that they can be eaten more easily. If this is done, we recommend that they are liquidized as individual foods and not just mixed together in one big slush!

As has been found in hospitals, the availability of carers at meal times can mitigate some of the problems associated with hunger and weight loss. Perhaps of greatest importance, and easiest to achieve at home, is the option of repeatedly offering food to the person outside of institutional meal times so that they eat as and when they wish.

Advance discussion of the process of dying

Illness contingency planning is an important means to help patients to stay home until they die. But when death occurs, the patient will normally be with someone who has not previously seen a death, let alone in a loved one. It is, therefore, important to discuss the process of dying with the key carers so that they feel more confident in managing this.

Most people will die over a period of days following a downturn in their ability to eat and drink, having gradually become weaker. Cheyne-Stokes (or periodic) respiration, where the breathing can alternate between being rapid and shallow and being absent, may be seen and should be discussed in advance. Few carers struggle to identify the moment of death, but it is important to warn people that 'agonal' gasps may be taken for up to half an hour after death. It is also a good idea to recommend that, if the death is expected and the patient peaceful, they merely sit with the patient and comfort them in their last moments. Ringing the GP or ambulance at that stage may merely mean that a professional arrives and changes the plan, moving the patient to hospital at the point of death.

After death, carers should be pre-informed about how death is certified and how to contact undertakers for removal of the body. Some patients die more rapidly – cardiac arrests do occur in people with dementia as in any other illness. In these circumstance, if the discussion has been had about death and dying, and the conclusion has been reached that hospital is inappropriate, then the management should remain palliative and at home.

Support for dying (allowing to die but not promoting it)

The fundamental basis of palliative and supportive care is to cherish life while accepting natural death. This fits well with the care of people with dementia at home. It is right both to accept the increasing disability and to limit care to that which is less burdensome and likely to bring benefit. For if good quality care, with sensible feeding, carer support, and use of medicines does lead to a longer period of comfort with the family, or to a shorter period of better quality of life with reduced distress, then this constitutes excellent and effective supportive care. And this is quite the opposite of actions where death is aimed at as the primary intent.

Lessons for institutional care

Much of what has been described in this chapter applies not only to home care but also to nursing and residential care. Home care is not appropriate for all. But for some it provides a better opportunity for good care and quality of life than does nursing or residential care. For some patients, there will be a period of behaviour that challenges that might require a secure setting with extra staff. We have cared for several people at home after discharge from specialist dementia nursing care. Here were people who had indeed been through a period when they could not have been managed at home, but then they settled enabling them to return home. For others, it was merely that the quality of care in a nursing care home was so low that carers could not bear to see their loved ones in these institutions. It is important not to promote home dementia care as the right option for all; it is merely the right option for some, where those close to the person are able to provide care, safety, and support at home.

Nonetheless, we do think that almost everything described in this chapter would also apply to the best care in institutional settings. The key difference is that the main carer or next of kin is further from control and influence. Therefore, it is terribly important to engage carers of those in institutional care so that their concerns and fears can be heard and poor care rectified as soon as it is noted. This, indeed, was part of the message of Chapter 19, where the objective of care in the institution, as at home, is to maintain the person's identity through the intimacy of personal knowledge and contact.

Conclusions

Supporting patients with dementia is a key and central part of the patient journey. In the UK, the skills to enable that support to be given at home are currently poorly grasped and limited to a few committed individuals. With better understanding and knowledge among professionals, the option to choose home-based care may be increased. A broad range of support is needed: excellent care overall, including social care, aids and appliances, good nutritional strategies, as well as ongoing medical care, psychiatric care, and the alleviation of distress, whether caused by mental or physical pain. Ongoing support and encouragement from professionals dedicated to supporting advanced dementia care at home seems essential.

References

1. Xie J, Brayne C, Matthews FE, The Medical Research Council Cognitive Function and Ageing Study Collaborators. (2008). Survival times in people with dementia: analysis from population based cohort study with 14 year follow-up. *BMJ*, **336**, 258–262.
2. Treloar A (1998). Delirium: prevalence, prognosis and management. *Rev Clin Gerontol*, **8**, 241–249.
3. Morrison RS, Siu AL (2000). Survival in end-stage dementia following acute illness. *JAMA*, **284**(1), 47–52.
4. Murray SA, Kendall M, Boyd K, Sheikh A (2005). Illness trajectories and palliative care. *BMJ*, **330**(7498), 1007–1011.
5. National Council for Palliative Care (NCPC) (2006). *Exploring palliative care for people with dementia*. London: NCPC.
6. National Audit Office (2007). *Improving services and support for people with dementia*. London: National Audit Office.
7. Hughes JC, Robinson L, Volicer L (2005). Specialist palliative care in dementia. *BMJ*, **330**(7482), 57–58.
8. Treloar A, Newport J, Venn-Treloar J. Specialist palliative care in dementia. *BMJ*, **330**(7492), 672.
9. NHS End of Life Care Publications. Preferred Priorities for Care (PPC). Available at: http://www.endoflifecareforadults.nhs.uk/eolc/ppc.htm (accessed on 29 March 2009).
10. Department of Health, End of Life Care Programme (2007). *Advance care planning: a guide for health and social care staff*. London: Department of Health. Available at: http://www.endoflifecareforadults.nhs.uk/eolc/eolcpub.htm (accessed on 29 March 2009).
11. *The Mental Capacity Act 2005*. Norwich: The Stationery Office. Available at: http://www.opsi.gov.uk/acts/acts2005/ukpga_20050009_en_1 (accessed on 29 March 2009).
12. The National Council for Palliative Care (2006). *Fulfilling lives: rehabilitation in palliative care*. London: NCPC. Available at: http://www.ncpc.org.uk/publications/pubs_list.html (accessed on 11 March 2009).

13. Gitlin LN, Hauck WW, Dennis MP, Winter L (2005). Maintenance of effects of the home environmental skill-building program for family caregivers and individuals with Alzheimer's disease and related disorders. *J Gerontol A Biol Sci Med Sci*, **60**(3), 368–374.

14. Dooley NR, Hinojosa J (2004). Improving quality of life for persons with Alzheimer's disease and their family caregivers: brief occupational therapy intervention. *Am J Occup Ther*, **58**(5), 561–569.

15. Richmond C (2005). Dame Cicely Saunders. *BMJ*, **331**(7510), 238.

16. All-Party Parliamentary Group on Dementia (2008). *Always a last resort: inquiry into the prescription of antipsychotic drugs to people with dementia living in care homes.* London. Available at: http://www.alzheimers.org.uk/downloads/ALZ_Society_APPG.pdf (accessed on 29 March 2009).

17. Craig GM (1994). On withholding nutrition and hydration in the terminally ill: has palliative medicine gone too far? *J Med Ethics*, **20**(3), 139–145.

18. Treloar A, Philpot M, Beats B (2001). Concealing medication in patients' food. *Lancet*, **357**, 62–64.

19. Fakhoury W, McCarthy M, Addington-Hall J (1996). Determinants of informal caregivers' satisfaction with services for dying cancer patients. *Soc Sci Med*, **42**(5), 721–731.

20. Treloar A, Crugel M, Adamis D (2009). Palliative care of dementia at home is feasible and rewarding – results from the 'Hope for Home' study. *J Demen Care – Spec Issue Palliat Care.* Available at: http://wwwcareinfoorg/dementiacare/

21. Steultjens EMJ, Dekker J, Bouter LM, Jellema S, Bakker EB, van den Ende CHM (2004). Occupational therapy for community dwelling elderly people: a systematic review. *Age Ageing*, **33**(5), 453–460.

22. Nobili A, Riva E, Tettamanti M *et al.* (2004). The effect of a structured intervention on caregivers of patients with dementia and problem behaviors: a randomized controlled pilot study. *Alzheimer Dis Assoc Disord*, **18**(2), 75–82.

23. Weddle D, Wellman NS, Shoaf LR (1996). Position of the American Dietetic Association: nutrition, aging, and the continuum of care. *J Am Diet Assoc*, **96**(10), 1048–1052.

24. Cederholm T (2002). Treatment of protein-energy malnutrition in chronic disorders in the elderly. *Minerva Gastroenterol Dietol*, **48**(3), 247–263.

Chapter 31

Namaste care and dying in institutional settings

Joyce Simard and Ladislav Volicer

Introduction

Namaste Care is a programme designed to improve the quality of life for residents living in institutional settings [1]. Great strides have been made in helping people with early and moderate dementia live with quality to their lives. However, with the exception of Namaste Care, programmes and services for people who are in the advanced or terminal stage of a dementing illness and living in an institutional setting have been slow to emerge. Although nursing facilities have experienced a significant growth in the number of residents with advanced dementia, this population has seemingly lost their voice both literally and figuratively to communicate pain and discomfort and to express feelings. Pain is under-treated in nursing home residents (see Chapter 14), and this under-treatment is most common in residents within the terminal stages of dementia [2]. The process of dying with a dementing illness may take months. During this last stage of life, residents often rely on staff to take care of their most basic needs. Even the most caring staff is often at a loss as to how to address the resident's psychosocial needs. The Namaste Care Programme helps staff in an institutional setting to provide quality services that are holistic and meet the physical and emotional needs of their residents. It helps to make the last days and months of life comfortable by surrounding residents with people who care for and about them as individuals, giving them a 'voice'.

When first diagnosed, the person with dementia is offered support from a variety of organizations (see Chapter 18) and medications (see Chapter 12). Although these medications do not stop the disease, they can slow the progression for many patients and should be counted as part of good quality supportive care [3]. Many other medications and some vaccines that show promise of even more effective treatments are in the 'pipeline'. People with early stage dementia are invited to support groups, they speak and write about their experience of living with memory loss [4] and have opportunities to access community services designed to keep them as independent as possible for as long as possible. In the United States people with early dementia are a very vocal advocacy group. They visit state and federal legislators demanding more money for research and additional services to support them living at home. The person with early stage dementia has a voice, sometimes a very loud voice!

When the middle stage of the disease is reached the person with dementia may be admitted to a long-term care facility with a specialized dementia unit. Good dementia care is expected by families. Many resources are available now to help design dementia-specific programmes in both nursing facilities and assisted living communities. The Alzheimer's Association has published guidelines for quality care in residential settings [5] and many books and educational courses are available for health care staff. Families have been educated to know what to expect from a good dementia programme. Many families participate in support groups and advocacy groups demanding that the government increase money for research and improved community services. The family becomes the voice for the person with dementia.

With the life expectancy rising and improved medical care available, people with dementia are living longer and transitioning to the advanced stage of their disease. It is in this stage that the 'voice' of the person with dementia and of their families begins to fade. Families are exhausted by the emotional toll that results from years of watching their loved one gradually fade away. This heart-wrenching experience has been described as 'a long good-bye' and a 'never ending funeral' [6]. They feel hopeless when advised that nothing can be done to help their loved one: that the burdens of medical interventions outweigh their benefits [7].

Medical interventions in advanced dementia

Some medical interventions that may be routinely used in cognitively intact individuals may not be appropriate in residents with advanced dementia. These interventions, which have been discussed in earlier chapters of this book, include cardiopulmonary resuscitation (CPR), transfer to an acute care setting, use of tube feeding, and treatment of generalized infections with antibiotics. CPR after cardiac arrest in a nursing home results in less than 2% of the residents surviving until they return to their facility. Even this potential benefit may not be desirable in residents with severe dementia because CPR is a stressful experience for those who survive. They may experience CPR-related injuries such as broken ribs, and may be deemed to require mechanical ventilation. The intensive care unit environment is not conducive to appropriate care for demented patients who are confused and often develop delirium. In addition, patients who are discharged alive from the hospital after CPR are much more impaired than they were before the cardiac arrest [8].

Transfer to an emergency room or hospital exposes them to serious risks. Even cognitively intact hospitalized elderly individuals develop depressed psychophysiological functioning that includes confusion, falling, not eating, and incontinence [9]. As discussed by Sampson in Chapter 13, hospitalization for treatment of infections and other conditions may not represent optimal management. Immediate survival after an episode of pneumonia is similar in residents receiving treatment in a long-term care facility and in a hospital [10], and longer term outcomes are actually better in residents treated in a nursing home [11]. Similarly, a larger proportion of hospitalized residents had worsening of their functional status or died at 2 months after the episode of pneumonia [12].

Residents with advanced dementia are unable to feed themselves and often develop swallowing difficulties that provoke choking on food and liquids. They may also start refusing food by not opening their mouths when they are fed. As Gillick has indicated in Chapter 28, there is little evidence to support the use of tube feeding in severe dementia. Tube feeding does not prevent aspiration pneumonia and might increase its incidence because it does not prevent aspiration of nasopharyngeal secretions and of regurgitated gastric contents [13]. Tube feeding also does not prevent occurrence of other infections. Nasogastric tubes may cause infections of sinuses and the middle ear. Gastrostomy tubes may cause cellulitis, abscesses, and even necrotizing fasciitis and myositis. Contaminated feeding solutions may cause gastrointestinal symptoms and bacturiuria. Tube feeding does not prevent malnutrition, and it does not increase the survival rate in residents with progressive degenerative dementia. Insertion of a tube may actually cause death from arrhythmia during insertion of a nasogastric tube and from perioperative mortality in percutaneous endoscopic gastrostomy tube placement. The occurrence of pressure ulcers is not decreased by tube feeding; rather, it may be increased because of the use of restraints and increased production of urine and stool. There is also no evidence that tube feeding promotes healing of pressure ulcers or improves functional status of residents with severe dementia [14]. In addition to the lack of benefits, tube feeding increases discomfort of the residents by both the tube presence and by the use of restraints that are often necessary to prevent tube removal. Tube feeding also deprives the patient of the taste of food and contact with the caregivers during the feeding process.

Antibiotic therapy is quite effective in the treatment of an isolated episode of pneumonia or other systemic infections. In most patients, it is possible to limit antibiotic therapy to oral preparations that are equally, if not more, effective as parenteral therapy [15]. It is preferable to limit the use of intravenous therapy in residents with severe dementia who do not understand the need for intravenous cannulae, try to remove them, and often have to be restrained or given psychotropic drugs to allow treatment to continue. In patients who have poor oral intake, intramuscular administration of cephalosporins can be used for treatment of infections. However, the effectiveness of antibiotic therapy is limited by the recurrent nature of infections in advanced dementia. Antibiotic therapy does not prolong survival in cognitively impaired residents who are unable to ambulate even with assistance and who are mute [16,17]. Antibiotics are also not necessary for maintenance of comfort in demented residents who can be maintained equally well with analgesics and anti-pyretics, and oxygen if necessary [18,19]. In addition, antibiotic use is not without adverse effects. Residents may develop gastrointestinal upset, diarrhoea, allergic reactions, hyperkalaemia, and agranulocytosis. Diagnostic procedures such as blood-drawing and sputum suctioning, which are necessary for rational use of antibiotics, cause discomfort and confusion in residents with dementia who do not understand the need for them.

Under such circumstances, families are often counselled that aggressive medical interventions may not be appropriate for their loved ones. As a consequence, they often feel hopeless that nothing can be done to improve the quality of life for their family members. Namaste Care was developed to provide hope for the families that something still can be done to improve the quality of life of residents with advanced dementia. In this way, it can be seen as a necessary component of continuing supportive care.

Namaste care overview

The Namaste Care Programme gives 'voice' to residents who can no longer speak and helps to ensure that the last stage of life is peaceful and comfortable in the presence of others. Residents have different values, wants, needs, and desires. Namaste Care recognizes that each person is a unique individual and honours them for who they were and who they are. 'Namaste' is a Hindu term meaning 'to honour the spirit within'. Namaste staff, called Namaste Carers, recognizes that in spite of the resident's inability to communicate with appropriate words they 'speak' with sounds, facial expressions, and movements. They continue to have a 'voice'. Namaste Carers take time to get to know each resident; the residents are never viewed as being in a vegetative state or as the shell of their former self.

Richard Taylor, a retired psychologist who was diagnosed with probable Alzheimer's disease (AD) and has become a strong voice for people in the early stage of the disease, has helped us understand how people with advanced dementia might be feeling.

> Please consider and reconsider these concerns of mine: everyone living with Alzheimer's disease is and will be until the moment of their death, a whole and complete human being. Every day of my life I will be, in my own mind Richard. I am neither half-full nor half-empty. I am Richard. I am not fading away. Will you always treat me as Richard? Or will there come a time when I am seen as Richard's shell? I want and need to give and receive love. Even when I can't remember your name, will you please love me? [4].

No person in Namaste Care is ever viewed or treated as if they were a shell. People are honoured until they take their last breath, and then, they continue to be honoured until they physically leave the facility.

Namaste Care uses a person-directed [20] approach to care ensuring that residents are honoured as individuals. For example, one resident was quite the 'social butterfly' and always wore hats and gloves when she went out with her friends before she was diagnosed with probable AD. Almost to the day she died, her caregivers made sure she had make-up on and wore colourful hats and her white gloves. When she was welcomed to the Namaste Care Room, she made a grand entrance. Even though she could no longer speak, her beautiful smile widened and her eyes twinkled as the Namaste Carer welcomed her with a flourish, complimenting her stylish clothing. In spite of the profound impact of AD, this woman somehow was aware that she was still a 'social butterfly'.

Namaste Care is a 7-day-a-week 'enhanced' nursing programme. Activities of daily living (ADLs) are offered as 'meaningful activities'. Several nurses have remarked that when they went to nursing school, they were taught to give massages and take time to listen to their patients. They got to know them as individuals, not as 'the patient in room 200'. Now with the amount of paper-work required in institutional settings and the chronic staffing shortages that seem to be so prevalent, they rarely have an opportunity to provide, or model for staff, nursing care the way they were taught. Namaste Care activities return nursing to the basics of individualized care, slowed down with the emphasis on a loving touch approach. On the opening day of a Namaste Care Programme a Director of Nursing (DON) was showing the Namaste Carer how 'loving touch' can produce minor miracles. One resident was so agitated; she would not allow staff to clean her hands properly without a battle. Her hands were tightly clenched and in a desperate need of washing. The DON had taken a basin of warm water and lovingly coaxed the resident to open her hand by speaking softly to her and gently helping her swirl her hand in the warm soapy water. The resident not only opened her hand but gave the DON a beautiful smile. With tears in her eyes, the DON remarked that this was how she was taught to provide nursing care and the reason why she became a nurse in the first place.

Namaste care room

The Namaste Care Programme is usually staffed by a licensed (or qualified according to state or country regulations) nursing assistant. Often the programme begins with existing staff so the budget is not adversely affected. The programme needs a space that is free of distractions so that the peaceful feeling of the milieu is maintained. Some programmes are fortunate enough to have a room dedicated to the programme; in other instances where space is limited, the dining room or a day room that has other uses is the only option available. When a room has been dedicated for Namaste Care, it has all of the items and furnishing needed and opening the programme in the morning just requires staff to gather fresh linens, snacks, and beverages. In this instance, it is also possible to have comfortable recliners, real plants, and items like serenity fountains and nursing supplies out in the open, as the room is locked when a staff person is not present. If the room also has other uses, it is important to take the resident out of the room and change the atmosphere by lowering the lights, playing soothing music, infusing the room with the scent of lavender and gathering all the supplies needed so that the Namaste Carer never leaves residents unattended. Changing the 'feel' of the room is an important aspect of the programme. Even in the advanced stage of dementia, residents' behaviour usually becomes calm when they are taken into a room that they can sense is peaceful.

Morning programme

Person-directed care is the approach used throughout the programme. Residents are taken to the Namaste Care room by their assigned nursing assistant where the Namaste Carer greets each resident by name and touches them. Greetings are personalized so that one resident may be welcomed by using their first name 'Good morning Hilda', or a special name they like, for instance 'Grandma I am so glad to see you', and given a hug. Other residents are welcomed more formally by using their professional title, 'Good morning Doctor Smith' or 'Welcome Mrs. Conner' and offered a handshake. Occasionally, residents do not want to be touched. When that is the case, staff simply greets them verbally, makes eye-contact and respects their wishes not to be touched.

Each resident in a wheelchair is transferred to a recliner and made comfortable with pillows. Quilts or soft blankets are tucked around them so that they feel secure. If residents are wearing uncomfortable shoes, they are removed and soft slipper socks are placed on their feet. The resident may be offered a lollypop as long as they have no problems with swallowing and are not in danger of biting the lollypop and chocking. It's amazing that in spite of significant memory loss and inability to speak, eyes twinkle when they are given this treat. When appropriate, residents are offered life-like stuffed animals. Women prefer cats, small dogs and rabbits, whereas the men like large dogs. The stuffed animals the programme uses are as real looking as possible so that they do not look like a child's toy. Residents will pet them and have conversations with these new 'friends'. One non-verbal resident began to 'talk' to a small life-like puppy that breathes when petted. She also began to answer questions from staff after not responding to them verbally for several months. Sometimes residents refuse to give their pets up when they are taken from the room for lunch and dinner. Dolls are used if they resemble a real baby, with soft skin. All efforts are made to use 'adult' items like handbags and books, but if the residents find comfort and pleasure in holding a 'baby' or 'pet', those items are made available to them.

When the Namaste Carer is confident that the residents they are working with are comfortable, another resident is greeted. The carer is constantly assessing residents for pain and discomfort. If a resident does not seem comfortable at any time during the Namaste Care Programme, nurses are asked to assess the resident for pain or other causes of discomfort. Occasionally, the residents will look uncomfortable in the lounge chair no matter how they are placed in the chair. A rehabilitation or occupational therapist may be asked to recommend a more comfortable chair or try a different positioning. Namaste Care recognizes that quality of life is not possible if a person is uncomfortable; therefore, continual assessment for pain and discomfort is a priority for the Namaste Carer.

When the majority of the residents are in the room, the Namaste Carer begins to provide ADLs recognizing that the process is more important than the task. They slow down the process of providing care, make eye-contact, and speak to the resident as care is given. Whenever possible and safe, gloves are not used. Loving touch is more effective without a rubber or latex barrier. Each resident has a container with brush, comb, lip balm, nail clipper, and other personal items like perfume or aftershave lotion they had used in the past to make providing ADLs efficient and personalized. Each day residents' faces are gently washed and moisturized as skin becomes dry with ageing. If men need to be shaved, it is accomplished the 'old fashioned' way, with a warm moist towel softening the skin, shaving cream, a safety razor, and aftershave lotion. Hair is brushed or combed with gentle movements and lip balm is applied to help eliminate cracked lips. The Namaste Carer moves from one resident to another pausing to greet new residents and monitor everyone in the room. During this time, many of the residents are blissfully sleeping, exhausted by the morning routine of waking up, being groomed, changed, and fed breakfast. When they do open their eyes they seem to be aware that they are not alone and look around the room.

Maintaining weight and hydrating residents in the advanced stage of dementia is usually a time consuming task for staff as they have many residents to care for and residents with advanced dementia tend to take only small sips of beverages. Residents usually need to be fed or assisted during meals. In most nursing facilities, the number of residents who need to be fed has risen dramatically in the past few years, whereas the number of staff assigned to care for them has not. Part of the Namaste Care Programme involves offering beverages and snacks to help increase hydration and prevent weight loss. Beverages are offered throughout the day. One programme has suggested that the increase of liquids has resulted in fewer infections for residents in Namaste Care. If the resident is losing weight, drinks with high calorie content are offered, for others, the carer gives them a fruit juice they prefer. In the afternoon, ice cream and high calorie puddings are served. Slices of oranges are available for residents to suck. The smell of an orange usually stimulates the appetite and most orange slices disappear quickly! Quality of life for many residents includes access to treats that are sweet and beverages that they enjoyed in the past.

Throughout the morning, soft music is playing, lights are low, and the scent of lavender permeates the room. The staff speaks with quiet voices when they enter the room. The Namaste Care room is always open to others so that the staff feels comfortable taking residents in after the programme has started or taking them out for a bath or shower at any time. Families are always invited in to visit with their loved one. The mood in the room is quiet and tranquil until just before lunch. Then lights are brightened, music is changed to more lively tunes such as love ballads of the forties or songs from musicals they may remember. Nursing assistants enter the room to transfer residents from their lounge chairs to wheel chairs and take them to the dining room. The Namaste Carer says good-bye to each resident and thanks them for coming to be with her. She also invites them back after lunch. This is another example of 'honouring the spirit within'. Most residents do not understand the words, but they may understand the respectful tone of the Namaste Carer's voice. When the room where Namaste Care takes place is also used for dining, staff change the appearance of the room by placing tablecloths on tables, and change the scent in the room to something more stimulating, for instance, lemon or a food related scent like baking bread or coffee.

Afternoon programme

After lunch, nursing assistants take residents to their rooms so that they can be groomed and toileted or changed. Some residents need to go to bed because they are at risk of skin problems; most are taken back to the Namaste Care room. Residents are usually tired after lunch and will sleep. They spend many long hours in bed isolated from others after dinner and all night so, from a psychosocial aspect, returning to the Namaste Care room where they are comfortable yet with others is in keeping with the goal of maintaining quality of life.

In the afternoon there are fewer residents in the programme, so the Namaste Carer can offer more time-consuming activities like soaking and moisturizing their feet and legs or providing nail care. A nature video may be playing with the sounds of a rain forest or the carer may read poetry or a special spiritual or religious passage that is meaningful to the resident. At about 3 pm, the Namaste Carer changes the mood of the room to stimulate residents in preparation for dinner. Lights are turned up and the music is livelier. Range of motion exercises are done to the beat of the music and fun items are introduced to wake up residents and hopefully produce smiles. Items like chattering false teeth, blowing bubbles, funny looking puppets produce happy expressions. Some creative Namaste Carers have crazy wigs or may put on a clown nose or strange glasses, to get a laugh from residents.

Often families visit in the afternoon. Prior to the Namaste Care Programme, the staff reports that families visited less and visits were shorter as their loved one stopped recognizing them and were unable to communicate. Perhaps as Richard Taylor feared, they began to see a 'shell' rather than a person. Namaste Care now encourages and teaches families and visitors how to interact with the residents in ways that continue to be meaningful, like brushing their hair or feeding them treats. Family visits began to lengthen and relationships with other families developed. Prior to the Namaste Care Programme, family visits usually took place in the isolation of a resident's room, or in a corner of the day room. Now family members interact with other families who may be experiencing some of the same feelings and informal support groups begin to develop. In one programme, the Namaste Carer has what she calls 'The Men's Club'. Several husbands visit at the same time in the afternoon. Without their wives living at home with them, they seemed like 'lost souls'. She now has comfortable seating for the men and serves them snacks because they look like they are not eating properly. They 'help' her move chairs so she lets them know they are important to her. These men are now looking and sounding less depressed and have begun to become friends with each other.

The Namaste Care room usually closes at 4 pm. Each resident is bid farewell and thanked for joining the group. Some Namaste Carers are required to complete paperwork, but this is minimal and can be completed quickly. The object of this programme is to be present for the resident and not be saddled with other tasks. Family and staff satisfaction is high in the Namaste Care Programmes. Administrators and Directors of Nursing report fewer family calls with complaints and many facilities have seen an increase in referrals from this unique programme. Comparison of data collected as the Minimum Data Set before and after enrollment in the Namaste Care Programme showed that residents who are withdrawn or have reduced social interaction have improved interest in the environment. Their participation in the programme decreased some indicators of delirium, and decreased the need for administration of anti-anxiety medications [21].

Dying with Namaste Care

The final component of Namaste Care is the dying experience and after-death care. When residents enter the terminal stage and are actively dying they may be moved to a Namaste Care private room. This provides the family private space to be with their loved one during the last days and hours of life. When a private room is not available, the privacy curtain can enclose the dying person with as much seclusion as is possible or the roommate can be engaged in another area of the institution. One creative facility places a silk rose on the door to let all staff know that there is someone in the room who is dying so they enter the room respectfully. The dietary department is notified so that food and beverages can be offered to families. Families are asked if they would like staff to inform clergy, other faith leaders, or friends of the situation. If no family is available the facility tries to make sure the person is not alone during the dying process.

The room might be personalized by the Namaste Carer who may suggest music the resident seemed to enjoy and items they found comfort in holding while they were in the Namaste Care room. Nursing assessments are provided on a regular basis to monitor for pain and discomfort. A peaceful, pain-free passing is the goal for staff during this time. Nurses also help families to understand what is happening during the dying process and may give them lotion and mouth swabs to help keep arms, legs, and lips moisturized and make the family feel needed. Every effort is made to have someone with the family at the moment of death. When the family is ready to leave the room, they are asked if they would like to stay until their loved one leaves the institution. If they stay, families become part of the Namaste Care after death ritual. The body is prepared, and the funeral home staff arrives. A quilt or flag, if the resident was a veteran, is placed on the body and family and staff accompany the deceased to the hearse. This farewell helps to bring closure to the staff who have been part of an extended family for the resident and provides comfort to the family.

Until the resident leaves the institution Namaste Care 'honours the spirit within'. The programme's goal of individualized person-directed care extends to the last moments of life and gives 'voice' to the resident with advanced or terminal dementia. It helps families feel that until the moment of death, something can always be done to help their loved ones maintain some quality to their lives. Namaste Care helps to extend the notion of supportive care from the time of diagnosis until and beyond the time of death. The Namaste Care Programme ensures that no resident in its care will ever be viewed as the 'shell' of who they were. The 'social butterfly', the person who can still smile when offered a lollypop, and the resident who appears at peace when tucked into a comfortable lounge chair answer the question 'Is it possible to live with quality to your life even with a dementing illness?' with a resounding 'Yes'.

References

1. Simard J (2007). *The end-of-life Namaste care programme for people with dementia*. Baltimore, London, Winnipeg, Sydney: Health Professions Press.

2. Husebo BS, Strand LI, Moe-Nilssen R, Borgehusebo S, Aarsland D, Ljunggren AE (2008). Who suffers most? Dementia and pain in nursing home patients: a cross-sectional study. *J Am Med Dir Assoc*, **9**, 427–433.

3. Raina P, Santaguida P, Ismaila A *et al.* (2008). Effectiveness of cholinesterase inhibitors and memantine for treating dementia: evidence review for a clinical practice guideline. *Ann Intern Med*, **148**, 379–397.

4. Taylor R (2007). Personal correspondence with JS.

5. Tilly J, Reed P. *Dementia Care Practice Recommendations for Assisted Living Residences and Nursing Homes – Phases 1 and 2*. http://www.alz.org/national/documents/brochure_DCPRphases1n2.pdf (accessed on 1 August 2008).

6. Combs LM (2008). *The long goodbye and beyond*. Winston-Salem, NC: Combs Music.

7. Volicer L (2008). End-of-life care for people with dementia in long-term care settings. *Alzheimer's Care Today*, **9**, 84–102.

8. Applebaum GE, King JE, Finucane TE (1990). The outcome of CPR initiated in nursing homes. *JAGS*, **38**, 197–200.

9. Gillick MR, Serrell NA, Gillick LS (1982). Adverse consequences of hospitalization in the elderly. *Soc Sci Med*, **16**, 1033–1038.

10. Naughton BJ, Mylotte JM, Tayara A (2001). Outcome of nursing home-acquired pneumonia: derivation and application of a practical model to predict 30 day mortality. *JAGS*, **48**, 1292–1299.

11. Thompson RS, Hall NK, Szpiech M (1999). Hospitalization and mortality rates for nursing home-acquired pneumonia. *J Family Pract*, **48**, 291–293.

12. Fried TR, Gillick MR, Lipsitz LA (1997). Short-term functional outcomes of long-term care residents with pneumonia treated with and without hospital transfer. *JAGS*, **45**, 302–306.

13. Finucane TE, Christmas C, Travis K (1999). Tube feeding in patients with advanced dementia: a review of the evidence. *JAMA*, **282**, 1365–1370.

14. Gillick MR (2000). Sounding board – rethinking the role of tube feeding in patients with advanced dementia. *N Engl J Med*, **342**, 206–210.

15. Hirata-Dulas CA, Stein DJ, Guay DR, Gruninger RP, Peterson PK (1991). A randomized study of ciprofloxacin versus ceftriaxone in the treatment of nursing home-acquired lower respiratory tract infections. *JAGS*, **39**, 1040–1041.

16. Fabiszewski KJ, Volicer B, Volicer L (1990). Effect of antibiotic treatment on outcome of fevers in institutionalized Alzheimer patients. *JAMA*, **263**, 3168–3172.

17. Luchins DJ, Hanrahan P, Murphy K (1997). Criteria for enrolling dementia patients in hospice. *J Am Geriatr Soc*, **45**, 1054–1059.

18. Hurley AC, Volicer B, Mahoney MA, Volicer L (1993). Palliative fever management in Alzheimer patients: quality plus fiscal responsibility. *Adv Nurs Sci*, **16**, 21–32.

19. Van der Steen JT, Ooms ME, Van der Wal G, Ribbe MW (2002). Pneumonia: the demented patient's best friend? Discomfort after starting or withholding antibiotic treatment. *J Am Geriatr Soc*, **50**, 1681–1688.

20. Kitwood T (1998). Toward a theory of dementia care: ethics and interaction. *J Clin Ethics*, **9**, 23–34.

21. Simard J, Volicer L (2009). Effects of Namaste care on residents who do not benefit from usual activities. *Am J Alzheimers Dis Other Demen*. Published on 30 March 2009 at: doi:10.1177/1533317509333258

Chapter 32

The principles and practice of supportive care in dementia

Julian C. Hughes, Mari Lloyd-Williams, and Greg A. Sachs

Introduction

The notion of supportive care in dementia is broad and deep. In Chapter 1, we characterized supportive care at a conceptual level, which gives the notion its depth: a full mixture of biomedical dementia care, with good quality, person-centred, psychosocial, and spiritual care under the umbrella of holistic palliative care throughout the course of the person's experience of dementia, from diagnosis until death and, for families and close carers, beyond. In Chapter 11, we highlighted the issues (Box 11.1, on page 100) and ingredients (Box 11.2, on page 103) of supportive care. We introduced the 'Sheffield model' of comprehensive supportive care [1,2], which makes a distinction between an explanatory model, spanning disease-directed, patient-directed, and family-directed therapies, and the logistical step, which considers how care is delivered to the patient and the family.

Whilst in Chapter 1 we outlined how comprehensive supportive care was closely aligned with and encompassed many aspects of palliative care, we argued that it is more than simply palliative care. In subsequent chapters, we saw how there was remarkable consistency regarding the elements of supportive care for people with dementia – across perspectives (patient, caregiver, health care professionals); care settings (hospital, community, clinic, and long-term care); nations; and disease aetiologies (developmental disorders, Huntington's disease, HIV, and Alzheimer's disease). In some ways, the specific physical complications of Huntington's disease (HD), which can be addressed by a team involving neurology, occupational, and physical therapy, or the complex medication regimen that can help prevent opportunistic infections and HIV-associated dementia, illustrate how supportive care can involve aggressive physical and biological treatments, more often associated with disease-directed approaches than with palliative care. Rather than being isolated examples related to the unusual features of HD and HIV, the *appropriate application* of aggressive biomedical treatments (at the right stage of disease and consistent with the goals of care of specific patients and families) is a component of supportive care for patients with dementia of all aetiologies. We shall briefly explore this below in the context of treatments arising in patients with typical late-onset dementias such as Alzheimer's disease (AD) and vascular dementia (VaD).

Curative intents

Even without the availability of highly effective treatments for AD and VaD, aggressive attention to both the consequences of dementia and comorbid conditions can be an important component of supportive care. First, patients with dementia are at increased risk for many of the other geriatric syndromes, such as falls and delirium [3,4]. While the increased risk directly attributable to cognitive impairment may not be modifiable, attention to other contributing factors can lower the risk of both falls and delirium in selected patients using clinically proven strategies [5,6]. Depression is another condition that appears in significant numbers of patients with dementia. While we do not have strategies to prevent depression in patients with dementia, it is a treatable condition, so screening for depression in patients with dementia is part of high quality care [6]. Second, while data may have to be extrapolated from other populations, such as from studies of primary and secondary prevention of stroke in patients without cognitive impairment, efforts to reduce the risk of common medical conditions and their complications can play an important role in supportive care. Treatment of hypertension, diabetes, and hyperlipidemia, smoking cessation, and daily aspirin can lower the risk of stroke and may avert events that would accelerate cognitive decline in patients with either AD, VaD, or mixed dementias [7]. Especially early in the course of dementia, it would be inappropriate to forgo such treatments because one is adhering either to a nihilistic approach in the face of a progressive dementia or to a palliative care approach that focusses solely on symptom management. Decreasing the risk of falls, delirium, and stroke may diminish morbidity and suffering, so these efforts clearly are warranted, at least as long as the treatment benefits outweigh their burdens.

As the dementia progresses, however, goals of care shift, treatments become more burdensome because of cognitive impairment, and remaining life expectancy shrinks. These forces combine to shift care towards the more palliative approach and to remove much aggressive treatment of comorbid conditions from the care plan of most patients with dementia [8]. Some kinds of care, such as routine cancer screening or treatment of osteoporosis may simply no longer make sense in light of life expectancy and time horizons needed for such care [9,10]. The art of supportive care, and a distinguishing feature from palliative and hospice care, lies in being able to provide the required biomedical treatments early on and in managing the transition away from them as the disease progresses. This transition places a premium on advance care planning, communication with families, and guiding and supporting decision-making.

In the remainder of this final chapter, we shall flesh out the explanatory model of supportive care in specific ways, and then, say something further about logistics.

Explanatory models

Models are representations of reality and, as such, are simplifying. In terms of explaining supportive care in dementia, we need to think about (at least) three layers of understanding. The *first layer* (as depicted in Box 32.1) is influenced by the biomedical model, is more obviously applicable to conditions such as cancer, but is nonetheless relevant to dementia.

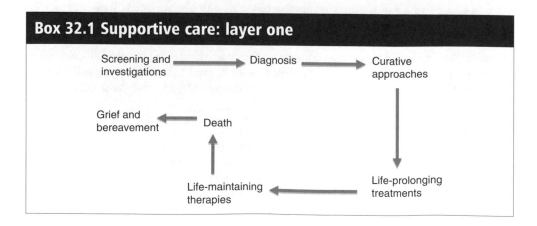

Box 32.1 Supportive care: layer one

We have already seen that there are a number of ways in which curative intent is an appropriate stance in dementia care. In the future, it may be that new ways to reduce amyloid plaque burden or the phosphorylation of tau (see Chapter 2), or to encourage neuroprotection, might emerge [11]. Meanwhile, life-prolonging treatments in dementia form part of what Hertogh called (in Chapter 29) a 'palliative treatment policy', according to which the aim would primarily be comfort, but life prolongation would be a concomitant. 'Life-maintaining' is all about the quality of life and not about prolonging life: Hertogh's 'symptomatic treatment policy' (see page 278), which would include attention to good communication (see Chapter 23) and many of the other psychosocial approaches covered in various chapters of this book. This would involve the sort of compassionate and holistic approach epitomized by Namaste care as described in the previous chapter. This level of understanding of supportive care for dementia, however, does not capture the required complexity. In Box 32.1, for example, grief and bereavement come after death, but as Frank records (in Chapter 22) in dementia these emotions and reactions are experienced in a very particular anticipatory way.

The *second layer* of understanding of supportive care in dementia focusses on the more holistic approach of palliative care, where due attention is given to the biological, psychological, social, and spiritual aspects of care. Here, the importance of the individual context comes to the fore, but there will be differing patterns. Biological concerns will be important at the time of diagnosis and in considering particular treatments throughout the course of the disease, not least in the terminal phase. The person's individual psychology will always be important, but – as many of the chapters in this book attest – is all too often overlooked, either because medical solutions seem easier, or because the person's psychology (manifestations of his or her self) seem too readily to slip from view (see Chapter 24). The social standing of persons cannot be ignored: if there are times when the person with dementia takes centre stage, the supporting cast is usually the family; and there are other moments in the drama when the family (or friends or close carers) become the main focus of supportive concern. Finally, the spiritual elements of care need to be emphasized too (see Chapter 21). There may be an existential crisis at the time of diagnosis, even if it is not seen in these terms. The process of advance care planning, much discussed in previous chapters, is an opportunity not solely to discuss future treatments, but also to order one's life and to decide on priorities. Later in the disease, it may be that religious observances provide comfort to patients and their families; but even in the absence of religious beliefs, the meaning of a person's life and death becomes increasingly salient.

The relative importance of these different facets of care will vary with time (as depicted in Figure 32.1) and between people.

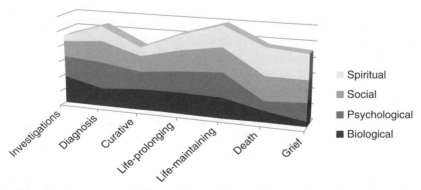

Fig. 32.1 Changing importance of different facets of supportive care through one person's experience of dementia

The *third layer* of understanding of supportive care forces us to view not only the process in time, where the simplifying assumption is that different stages of the disease (as if 'dementia' is a single entity) are passed through in some sort of ordered fashion (with different forms of 'management' neatly applicable), not only the various facets of holistic, palliative care, which will need to vary between individuals and change over time for individuals, but also the embedding context of supportive care in any given situation. This sort of surround brings in culture, social constraints, law, ethics, politics, and so on. This is the level of understanding that makes the model real because it situates supportive care in particular contexts in the world. (The importance of contexts was, of course, highlighted by Shaji's account of dementia care in developing countries in Chapter 10.) Thus, we are led to consider the logistics of supportive care.

Logistical steps

As we said in Chapter 11, and as emphasized by our comments about the embedding surround, the exact details of supportive care will be different in different places, within and between countries. We have already highlighted the issues and ingredients of supportive care in dementia. In addition, we have mentioned possible examples of how to provide supportive care. We shall touch on these again now, but with the disclaimer that we are not suggesting any particular model of care. There will be various ways to provide supportive care, in large part dictated by the local social and political health care economy. Key features of any model, however, should be continuity of care, timely access to services of all sorts, and advance care planning.

Ahmedzai suggests that teams or networks of care might be 'virtual' [1]. In other words, they need not exist as single entities located at a particular place. In theory, the leadership of such a supportive care network might be passed on as the disease and the needs of the individual change. In practice, this might lead to the same loss of continuity that accompanied the split between curative and palliative services in the older cancer care model. So it might be better for there to be a single key worker appointed at the time of diagnosis who would follow people throughout the course of the disease, but who would often simply co-ordinate care rather than deliver it.

Of course, the notions of 'key worker', 'care manager', or 'care co-ordinator' have been around for some years, yet there have still been deficiencies in dementia care. Optimistically, perhaps, we would suggest that the problem has been framing the role. The key worker or care coordinator, if for instance, this is a community psychiatric nurse (CPN), comes from a particular background (see Chapter 16 in this volume). For a CPN to be called upon to deal with the complexities of some aspects of social care can seem like an inappropriate use of resources. That is, the notion that someone in a specialized role should be able to offer assistance, even if only by making a further referral, in all the circumstances that might arise throughout the course of a person's dementia does not seem practicable, unless case loads are to be minimal. In the framework of supportive care, the key worker would not necessarily be a specialist worker, although they would need to acquire knowledge and understanding in order to help people find the support they required. Furthermore, in the US, which is still dominated by a fee-for-service, private practice mode of financing and care delivery, a major barrier has been the inability to pay for the services of a care manager or care coordinator. Outside of managed care or demonstration projects, a private care manager has been accessible only to those with substantial financial resources.

Recently a national 'Dementia Strategy' has been launched in the UK, which puts forward the possibility of 'Dementia Advisers': people who would be able to provide a point of contact and continuity of care for people with dementia and their carers [12]. Recall that Wallace (Chapter 3) and Pointon (Chapter 4) both commended the idea from their perspectives as a person with dementia and a former carer. A Dementia Adviser would not necessarily be providing hands-on clinical or social care, but would be working closely with other services. Perhaps, a Dementia Adviser would be equivalent to a 'key worker' or 'care co-ordinator', but unburdened by specialized responsibilities and, therefore, able to encourage seamless working between professionals. Depending on how the role develops, perhaps a Dementia Adviser would provide the key point of reference necessary for supportive care to be meaningful throughout the course of the illness. The options would seem to be:

1 A single dementia care adviser (or care co-ordinator), perhaps accessible mainly via telephone or email, who provides no (or very little) specialized 'hands-on' care, but provides continuity and advice concerning all avenues of care

2 A single dementia care adviser (or care co-ordinator) who provides specialized care, but who also provides continuity and advice concerning other avenues of care

3 Dementia care advisers (or care co-ordinators) who provide specialized care, who also provide advice concerning other avenues of care, but who pass care on to another dementia care adviser when the social or clinical situation changes.

The first of these options is likely to be efficient, but depending on caseloads may or may not seem particularly personal and may lack the specialist skills to engage, for instance, in the sort of care planning that can then be pursued throughout the course of the illness. The second option would allow potentially supportive relationships to be formed, encouraging good care planning with continuity of care, but would lack efficiency because caseloads would have to be small. The third option allows personal, supportive relationships, bigger caseloads, but less continuity of care.

While the US currently does not have an analogous 'Dementia Strategy', there are some who hope that the growing support for the model known as the 'Patient Centered Medical Home' (PCMH) will offer both a framework and enhanced financial reimbursement to facilitate care. Thus:

> In the advanced medical home model, patients will have a personal physician working with a team of health care professionals in a practice. For most patients the personal physician would most appropriately be a primary care physician, but it could be a specialist or subspecialist for patients requiring on-going care for certain conditions, . . . In most cases, primary care physicians, with their office care team, are ideally suited to provide principal care and be a patient's care coordinator . . . Rather than being a 'gatekeeper' who restricts patient access to services, a personal physician leverages the key attributes of the advanced medical home to coordinate and facilitate the care of patients . . . Personal physicians advocate for and provide guidance to patients and their families as they negotiate the complex health care system [13; p. 5].

Similarly, in the UK (as discussed in Chapter 15) and elsewhere, the role of the general practitioner (GP) must be regarded as central to any effective implementation of supportive care. Many GPs would not have the knowledge or experience necessary to provide specialist diagnostic skills, nor understanding of the range of therapeutic options, nor associated expertise in terminal care. A general practice could arrange itself so that different practitioners specialize, in which case one GP might wish to take on a pivotal role as the 'dementia specialist', co-ordinating and advising on care. But this would require a significant change, at least in the UK, if such a system were to become the norm. In discussing general practice, Evans and Robinson (Chapter 15) mentioned the collaborative care model, pioneered in the US, with its core components: 'a care manager (or key worker) to provide information and co-ordinate care, the use of care pathways (evidence-based protocols) for common areas of dementia management, and timely access to specialist advice' (see page 142). Meanwhile, the PCMH also raises the possibility of either primary care practices or groups of practices being organized in ways that facilitate access to dementia specialty care.

Alternatively, the 'home' (which is virtual) for frail older adults, especially those with dementia, might need to be based upon several practices with the expertise and resources to provide supportive dementia care.

These are not the only options for supportive care. The Dutch system, described by Hertogh (Chapter 29), which has seen 'nursing home medicine' change to 'elderly medicine', presents the possibility of a specialized service for frail older people reaching out into the community, but with feet firmly in both institutional long-term and acute hospital settings. Although much of the emphasis in our discussion in this chapter has been on the medical input and oversight of services, it would seem much more likely that day-to-day care coordination would be undertaken by a nurse, perhaps by a specialized nurse such as the Admiral nurses now available in the UK (see Chapter 16), or it might be the sort of care coordination provided by the nurse researchers in the PEACE programme (described in Chapter 5). Furthermore, much of the care that people with dementia require is social and there is no reason why social workers (see Chapter 18) or suitably trained workers from the voluntary sector might not act as dementia care advisers or coordinators.

What seems inevitable, however, is that, in order to achieve the logistical step of supportive care, at some level a specialist service must emerge dedicated to the care of people with dementia. Such a service might be based in social services, in primary care, in nursing home care, or in hospital practice, and it could be run by a variety of practitioners. But it would have to be inter-disciplinary; it would have to have the ingredients outlined in Chapter 11 in order to deal with the multitude of issues that emerge in dementia care; it would have to have immediate access to and liaison with specialists in a variety of medical and social care settings; it would have to facilitate and encourage advance care planning and its implementation; it would have to be available to people with dementia and their carers from the time of diagnosis until after death.

Conclusion

Supportive care in dementia might be achieved in small steps: it might simply involve the introduction of a nurse to liaise with and offer training to a group of nursing homes on the care of people with dementia. Such a project in the UK in Croydon has already demonstrated important gains in terms of its palliative and supportive approach [14]. It is certainly the case that carers of people with dementia appreciate supportive care, as shown by these quotes from participants in the PEACE programme (see Chapter 5):

> The team approach [was done especially well]. They were attentive to my needs – always available to answer questions.
>
> [The doctor] helped me make the decision to keep her home. I knew he was just a phone call away. That gives you a lot of courage.
>
> The staff was very supportive. [The doctor] was away and the covering doctor was very supportive – gave me options which I really appreciated.
>
> Not just the last two weeks, but the personal touches. I never saw anything I didn't like.

As in so many aspects of care, it is the 'personal touches' that count for so much. These quotes also indicate the importance of advice and support with decision-making. Even when there is a 'covering doctor', there is a sense of partnership. So, much of this comes down to the right (supportive) approach.

Yet a fully-fledged move to supportive care for the person with dementia would represent a much bigger step. For what is at stake is our whole attitude to people with dementia and even to ageing. Supportive care represents a broad view; it is a broad view of the person with dementia [15], who must be seen in all of his or her biological, psychological, social, and spiritual complexity, where care is aimed broadly, holistically, impeccably, and with enthusiasm, but also with clinical judgement. As such, supportive care involves ethical decisions, but these are based on our standing as mutually engaged, interdependent human beings. Supportive care for the person with dementia is an imperative for our age.

References

1. Ahmedzai SH (2005). The nature of palliation and its contribution to supportive care, in Ahmedzai SH, Muers MF (eds). *Supportive care in respiratory disease*, pp. 3–33. Oxford: Oxford University Press.

2. Ahmedzai S, Walsh D (2000). Palliative medicine and modern cancer care. *Semin Oncol*, **27**, 1–6.

3. van Doorn C, Gruber-Baldini AL, Zimmerman S *et al.* (2003). Dementia as a risk factor for falls and fall injuries among nursing home residents. *J Am Geriatr Soc*, **51**, 1213–1218.

4. Inouye SK (2006). Delirium in older persons. *N Engl J Med*, **354**, 1157–1165.

5. Tinetti ME, Baker DI, McAvay G *et al.* (1994). A multifactorial intervention to reduce the risk of falling among elderly people living in the community. *N Engl J Med*, **331**, 821–827.

6. Feil DG, MacLean C, Sultzer D (2007). Quality indicators for the care of dementia in vulnerable elders. *J Am Geriatr Soc*, **55**, S293–S301.

7. Erkinjuntti T, Román G, Gauthier S *et al.* (2004). Emerging therapies for vascular dementia and vascular cognitive impairment. *Stroke*, **35**, 1010–1017.

8. Brauner DJ, Muir JC, Sachs GA (2000). Treating nondementia illness in patients with dementia. *JAMA*, **283**, 3230–3235.

9. Holmes HM, Cox Hayley D, Alexander GC *et al.* (2006). Reconsidering medication appropriateness late in life. *Arch Int Med*, **166**, 605–609.

10. Walter LC, Covinsky KE (2001). Cancer screening in elderly patients: a framework for individualized decision making. *JAMA*, **285**, 2750–2756.

11. Sano M (2009). The future of dementia treatment, in Weiner MF, Lipton AM (eds). *Textbook of Alzheimer disease and other dementias*, pp. 435–442. London and Washington, DC: American Psychiatric Publishing.

12. Department of Health (2009). *Living well with dementia: a national dementia strategy*. London: Department of Health.

13. Barr M, Ginsburg J (2006). The advanced medical home: a patient-centered, physician-guided model of health care: a policy monograph of the American college of physicians. American College of Physicians. Available at: http://www.acponline.org/advocacy/where_we_stand/policy/adv_med.pdf (accessed on 31 March 2009).

14. Pace V (2008). A partnership approach within a local area: the Croydon Project. *Creative partnerships: improving quality of life at the end of life for people with dementia. A compendium*, pp. 22–24. London: The National Council for Palliative Care.

15. Hughes JC (2001). Views of the person with dementia. *J Med Ethics*, **27**, 86–91.

Index